# Molecular Research of Alzheimer's Disease

# Molecular Research of Alzheimer's Disease

Editor

**Lorenzo Falsetti**

MDPI • Basel • Beijing • Wuhan • Barcelona • Belgrade • Manchester • Tokyo • Cluj • Tianjin

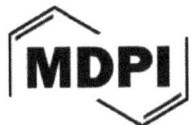

*Editor*
Lorenzo Falsetti
Azienda Ospedaliera
Universitaria Ospedali Riuniti
Ancona, Italy

*Editorial Office*
MDPI
St. Alban-Anlage 66
4052 Basel, Switzerland

This is a reprint of articles from the Special Issue published online in the open access journal *Biomedicines* (ISSN 2227-9059) (available at: https://www.mdpi.com/journal/biomedicines/special_issues/Alzheimer_Molecular).

For citation purposes, cite each article independently as indicated on the article page online and as indicated below:

LastName, A.A.; LastName, B.B.; LastName, C.C. Article Title. *Journal Name* **Year**, *Volume Number*, Page Range.

ISBN 978-3-0365-8438-6 (Hbk)
ISBN 978-3-0365-8439-3 (PDF)

© 2023 by the authors. Articles in this book are Open Access and distributed under the Creative Commons Attribution (CC BY) license, which allows users to download, copy and build upon published articles, as long as the author and publisher are properly credited, which ensures maximum dissemination and a wider impact of our publications.
The book as a whole is distributed by MDPI under the terms and conditions of the Creative Commons license CC BY-NC-ND.

# Contents

**About the Editor** . . . . . . . . . . . . . . . . . . . . . . . . . . . . . . . . . . . . . . . . . . . . . . . . . . vii

**Preface** . . . . . . . . . . . . . . . . . . . . . . . . . . . . . . . . . . . . . . . . . . . . . . . . . . . . . . . . ix

**Lorenzo Falsetti**
Molecular Research on Alzheimer's Disease
Reprinted from: *Biomedicines* 2023, 11, 1883, doi:10.3390/biomedicines11071883 . . . . . . . . . . 1

**Filippa Lo Cascio, Paola Marzullo, Rakez Kayed and Antonio Palumbo Piccionello**
Curcumin as Scaffold for Drug Discovery against Neurodegenerative Diseases
Reprinted from: *Biomedicines* 2021, 9, 173, doi:10.3390/biomedicines9020173 . . . . . . . . . . . . 5

**Liqing Song, Evan A. Wells and Anne Skaja Robinson**
Critical Molecular and Cellular Contributors to Tau Pathology
Reprinted from: *Biomedicines* 2021, 9, 190, doi:10.3390/biomedicines9020190 . . . . . . . . . . . . 29

**Grazia Ilaria Caruso, Simona Federica Spampinato, Giuseppe Costantino, Sara Merlo and Maria Angela Sortino**
SIRT1-Dependent Upregulation of BDNF in Human Microglia Challenged with Aβ: An Early but Transient Response Rescued by Melatonin
Reprinted from: *Biomedicines* 2021, 9, 466, doi:10.3390/biomedicines9050466 . . . . . . . . . . . . 55

**Gabriela Dumitrita Stanciu, Razvan Nicolae Rusu, Veronica Bild, Leontina Elena Filipiuc, Bogdan-Ionel Tamba and Daniela Carmen Ababei**
Systemic Actions of SGLT2 Inhibition on Chronic mTOR Activation as a Shared Pathogenic Mechanism between Alzheimer's Disease and Diabetes
Reprinted from: *Biomedicines* 2021, 9, 576, doi:10.3390/biomedicines9050576 . . . . . . . . . . . . 71

**Lihong Cheng, Hiroyuki Osada, Tianyan Xing, Minoru Yoshida, Lan Xiang and Jianhua Qi**
The Insulin Receptor: A Potential Target of Amarogentin Isolated from *Gentiana rigescens* Franch That Induces Neurogenesis in PC12 Cells
Reprinted from: *Biomedicines* 2021, 9, 581, doi:10.3390/biomedicines9050581 . . . . . . . . . . . . 91

**Shao-Xun Yuan, Hai-Tao Li, Yu Gu and Xiao Sun**
Brain-Specific Gene Expression and Quantitative Traits Association Analysis for Mild Cognitive Impairment
Reprinted from: *Biomedicines* 2021, 9, 658, doi:10.3390/biomedicines9060658 . . . . . . . . . . . . 107

**Víctor Antonio Blanco-Palmero, Marcos Rubio-Fernández, Desireé Antequera, Alberto Villarejo-Galende, José Antonio Molina, Isidro Ferrer, et al.**
Increased YKL-40 but Not C-Reactive Protein Levels in Patients with Alzheimer's Disease
Reprinted from: *Biomedicines* 2021, 9, 1094, doi:10.3390/biomedicines9091094 . . . . . . . . . . . 121

**Shang-Der Chen, Jenq-Lin Yang, Yi-Heng Hsieh, Tsu-Kung Lin, Yi-Chun Lin, A-Ching Chao and Ding-I Yang**
Potential Roles of Sestrin2 in Alzheimer's Disease: Antioxidation, Autophagy Promotion, and Beyond
Reprinted from: *Biomedicines* 2021, 9, 1308, doi:10.3390/biomedicines9101308 . . . . . . . . . . . 135

**Ioanna Tsantzali, Fotini Boufidou, Eleni Sideri, Antonis Mavromatos, Myrto G. Papaioannou, Aikaterini Foska, et al.**
From Cerebrospinal Fluid Neurochemistry to Clinical Diagnosis of Alzheimer's Disease in the Era of Anti-Amyloid Treatments. Report of Four Patients
Reprinted from: *Biomedicines* 2021, 9, 1376, doi:10.3390/biomedicines9101376 . . . . . . . . . . . 157

**Lorenzo Falsetti, Giovanna Viticchi, Vincenzo Zaccone, Emanuele Guerrieri, Gianluca Moroncini, Simona Luzzi and Mauro Silvestrini**
Shared Molecular Mechanisms among Alzheimer's Disease, Neurovascular Unit Dysfunction and Vascular Risk Factors: A Narrative Review
Reprinted from: *Biomedicines* **2022**, *10*, 439, doi:10.3390/biomedicines10020439 . . . . . . . . . . . **171**

**Ioanna Tsantzali, Aikaterini Foska, Eleni Sideri, Evdokia Routsi, Effrosyni Tsomaka, Dimitrios K. Kitsos, et al.**
Plasma Phospho-Tau-181 as a Diagnostic Aid in Alzheimer's Disease
Reprinted from: *Biomedicines* **2022**, *10*, 1879, doi:10.3390/biomedicines10081879 . . . . . . . . . . **187**

# About the Editor

**Lorenzo Falsetti**

Dr. Lorenzo Falsetti is an Internal Medicine specialist and a researcher working in the Clinical and Molecular Sciences Department of the Marche Polytechnic University. Among his scientific interests, he is actively involved in research in Emergency Medicine, Internal Medicine, ultrasonography, and Neurology, with a particular interest in neurodegenerative disorders. In this last field, he is interested in studying the role of classical vascular risk factors, blood–brain barrier breakdown, neurovascular unit dysfunction and carotid atherosclerosis in the determination of Alzheimer's disease onset and progression.

# Preface

The current Special Issue is directed to all the neurologists and other specialists involved in Alzheimer's Disease research and care. The papers aim to review old and new molecular pathways in Alzheimer's Disease that can be used as potential alternative targets to improve both diagnosis and treatment of this neurodegenerative disorder. In fact, although the effectiveness of anti-amyloid therapy is still controversial, it has been shown to improve the quality of life and reduce AD progression in mild or moderate forms of the disease. However, potential adverse effects include urinary tract infections, nervous system disorders, intracranial hemorrhage, and amyloid-related imaging abnormalities. These treatments seem to reduce the burden of brain amyloid, which is the final waste product of complex molecular pathways that lead to AD neurodegeneration.

This Special Issue first discusses the current and future molecular methods suggested to improve AD diagnosis. Patients who cannot be selected for specific treatments or studies due to mixed or atypical presentations should undergo cerebrospinal fluid (CSF) biomarker interpretation to differentiate AD from other forms of dementia, such as vascular forms. By integrating clinical, neuropsychological, and radiological data with the AT(N) biochemical profiling system (amyloid, tau pathology, and neural loss), researchers and physicians can refine AD diagnosis for both research and clinical purposes, even in atypical clinical presentations. Current molecular research also proposes novel serum plasma markers, such as plasma phospho-tau-181, which will be adopted to refine AD diagnosis and to predict its progression, without the need for an invasive lumbar puncture for CSF biomarker determination. However, this novel marker of disease deserves extensive validation, and the optimal method of determination should be standardized to determine its exact sensitivity or specificity values.

The second topic covered deals with the complex molecular pathways associated with AD pathophysiology. Identifying innovative molecular targets could lead to more effective treatments to reduce both the incidence and the progression of this neurodegenerative disease. An increased deterioration of cognitive function has been observed in patients showing a status of comorbidity, considering vascular risk factors, such as diabetes, hypertension, dyslipidemia, and cigarette smoking, which are associated with neuroinflammation, neurovascular unit dysfunction, and blood–brain barrier breakdown. Evidence suggests that AD and its associated comorbidities share molecular pathways leading to a faster cognitive decline. One of the most intriguing molecular overlaps between neurodegenerative and systemic diseases is symbolized by diabetes mellitus. Insulin resistance translates into a chronic signaling activation of the mechanistic target of rapamycin (mTOR), leading to blood–brain barrier dysfunction, tau hyperphosphorylation, and amyloid plaque formation. Thus, the insulin receptor could represent a potential target to improve neurogenesis. Several other genes involved in oxidative stress and mitochondrial dysfunction have been associated with mild cognitive impairment and AD, representing targets of interest for future investigations.

Another typical aspect of AD is characterized by neuroinflammation, especially in its later stages. Microglia seem to play a pivotal role in the neuroinflammatory component observed in AD neuropathology. Of note, melatonin and other similar molecules act on neuroinflammatory pathways and seem able to upregulate SIRT1-mediated brain-derived neurotrophic factor with regard to prolonged microglial exposure to Aβ42. This could translate into a reduced expression of inflammatory markers, such as IL-1β and (TNF)-α, with a subsequent downregulation of the proinflammatory pathway, which is mediated by NF-κB. Other molecules, such as curcumin, have been shown to be effective in reducing inflammation, oxidative stress, and the aggregation of amyloidogenic proteins.

Despite actual knowledge, more insights into the molecular mechanisms leading to the amyloid cascade are still needed to improve diagnostic methods and to explore novel therapeutic agents acting on different molecular targets of the neuropathogenetic cascade of Alzheimer's disease.

**Lorenzo Falsetti**
*Editor*

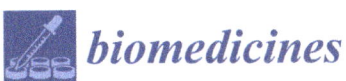 

*Editorial*

# Molecular Research on Alzheimer's Disease

Lorenzo Falsetti

Internal and Subintensive Medicine Department, Azienda Ospedaliero-Universitaria delle Marche, 60131 Ancona, Italy; lorenzo.falsetti@ospedaliriuniti.marche.it

Alzheimer's disease (AD) is the most common form of dementia worldwide. Despite its prevalence and incidence, there are few and limited specific treatments for this disabling and progressive disorder. Anti-amyloid therapy effectiveness is still controversial, but it seems to improve quality of life and reduce AD progression in mild or moderate forms, at the cost of potentially serious adverse effects, especially urinary tract infection, nervous system disorders, intracranial hemorrhage, and amyloid-related imaging abnormalities. However, this treatment seems able to reduce the burden of brain amyloid, which represents the final waste product of complex molecular pathways, leading to AD neurodegeneration. The first topic discussed in this Special Issue is related to current and future molecular methods suggested to improve AD diagnosis. Often, patients cannot be selected for specific treatments, studies, or enrolled in clinical trials due to mixed or atypical presentations: in these settings, AD diagnosis should be enriched with cerebrospinal fluid (CSF) biomarker interpretation, which still represent the cornerstone for differential diagnosis in the setting of neurodegenerative diseases, allowing one to differentiate AD from other forms of dementia, such as vascular forms [1]. Moreover, integrating clinical, neuropsychological, and radiological data with the AT(N) biochemical profiling system (amyloid, tau pathology, and neural loss) allows the researcher and the physician to refine AD diagnosis for both research and clinical purposes, allowing one correctly frame the patient, even in atypical clinical presentations. Current molecular research is also proposing novel serum plasma markers, such as plasma phospho-tau-181, that, in the near future, will be adopted to refine AD diagnosis and to predict its progression, without the need for an invasive lumbar puncture for CSF biomarker determination [2]. Still, this novel marker of disease deserves extensive validation: especially, the optimal method of determination should be standardized to determine its exact sensitivity or specificity values. The second topic covered in this issue of Biomedicines, "Molecular Research of Alzheimer's Disease", deals with the description of the complex molecular pathways associated with AD pathophysiology. Identifying innovative molecular targets could lead to more effective treatments to reduce both the incidence and the progression of this neurodegenerative disease. Most AD cases are not inherited and become clinically evident in elderly, multicomorbid subjects. In this setting, the pathophysiology of AD neurodegeneration seems complex and seems to be associated with the disruption of several molecular pathways, compromising the function of neuronal, glial, and neurovascular units. An increased deterioration of cognitive function has been observed in patients showing a status of comorbidity, considering—among a patient's associated disorders—vascular risk factors, such as diabetes, hypertension, dyslipidemia, and cigarette smoking, which are associated with neuroinflammation, neurovascular unit dysfunction, and blood–brain barrier breakdown [3]. Evidence suggests that AD and its associated comorbidities share molecular pathways, leading to a faster cognitive decline: one of the most intriguing molecular overlaps between neurodegenerative and systemic diseases is symbolized by diabetes mellitus. Alterations in the insulin signaling pathway and glucose resistance in AD subjects' brains are common and typical, and AD is commonly referred as to type 3 diabetes mellitus. Insulin resistance translates into a chronic signaling activation of the mechanistic target of rapamycin (mTOR), leading to blood–brain barrier dysfunction, tau hyperphosphorylation, and amyloid plaque formation. Thus,

**Citation:** Falsetti, L. Molecular Research on Alzheimer's Disease. *Biomedicines* **2023**, *11*, 1883. https://doi.org/10.3390/biomedicines11071883

Received: 20 June 2023
Accepted: 25 June 2023
Published: 3 July 2023

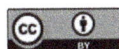

**Copyright:** © 2023 by the author. Licensee MDPI, Basel, Switzerland. This article is an open access article distributed under the terms and conditions of the Creative Commons Attribution (CC BY) license (https://creativecommons.org/licenses/by/4.0/).

the insulin receptor could represent a potential target to improve neurogenesis. Some molecules, such as amarogentin, seem able to interact with this receptor, representing potential candidates for future clinical studies [4]. Other classes of newer drugs, such as SGLT-2 inhibitors [5] and sestrins [6], could be considered to reduce mTOR activity, acting after the insulin receptor cascade and slowing neurodegeneration. Sestrins seem able to also act in other commonly disrupted pathways in AD, such as, for example, by improving antioxidation and adjusting autophagy. Several other genes involved in oxidative stress and mitochondrial dysfunction have been associated with mild cognitive impairment and AD [7], representing targets of interest for future investigations. Another typical aspect of AD is characterized by neuroinflammation, especially in AD's later stages [8]. As in most tau-dependent neurodegenerative diseases, the interplay between astrocytes, microglia, and neurons often shift from an early, neuroprotective, tau-clearing phenotype with an exacerbated autophagy-lysosomal pathway to a "loss of function" phenotype, leading to neuronal excitotoxicity, often associated with a neuroinflammatory phenotype, which is related to increased tau pathology, oxidative stress, and increased amyloid deposition [9]. Microglia seem to play a pivotal role in the neuroinflammatory component observed in AD neuropathology. Of note, melatonin and other similar molecules act on neuroinflammatory pathways and seem able to upregulate SIRT1-mediated brain-derived neurotrophic factor with regards to prolonged microglial exposure to A$\beta$42. This could translate into a reduced expression of inflammatory markers, such as IL-1$\beta$ and (TNF)-$\alpha$, with a subsequent downregulation of the proinflammatory pathway, which is mediated by NF-$\kappa$B [10]. Other molecules, such as curcumin, have been shown to be effective in reducing inflammation, oxidative stress, and the aggregation of amyloidogenic proteins [11]. Albeit interesting, most of the published papers in this issue show evidence at a preclinical stage, and further clinical studies are required to validate and to extend the interesting results collected in this issue of Biomedicines. Despite actual knowledge, more insights into the molecular mechanisms, leading to the amyloid cascade, are still needed to improve diagnostic methods and to to explore novel therapeutic agents acting on different molecular targets of the neurodegenerative cascade of Alzheimer's disease.

**Conflicts of Interest:** The authors declare no conflict of interest.

## References

1. Tsantzali, I.; Boufidou, F.; Sideri, E.; Mavromatos, A.; Papaioannou, M.G.; Foska, A.; Tollos, I.; Paraskevas, S.G.; Bonakis, A.; Voumvourakis, K.I.; et al. From Cerebrospinal Fluid Neurochemistry to Clinical Diagnosis of Alzheimer's Disease in the Era of Anti-Amyloid Treatments. Report of Four Patients. *Biomedicines* **2021**, *9*, 1376. [CrossRef] [PubMed]
2. Tsantzali, I.; Foska, A.; Sideri, E.; Routsi, E.; Tsomaka, E.; Kitsos, D.K.; Zompola, C.; Bonakis, A.; Giannopoulos, S.; Voumvourakis, K.I.; et al. Plasma Phospho-Tau-181 as a Diagnostic Aid in Alzheimer's Disease. *Biomedicines* **2022**, *10*, 1879. [CrossRef] [PubMed]
3. Falsetti, L.; Viticchi, G.; Zaccone, V.; Guerrieri, E.; Moroncini, G.; Luzzi, S.; Silvestrini, M. Shared Molecular Mechanisms among Alzheimer's Disease, Neurovascular Unit Dysfunction and Vascular Risk Factors: A Narrative Review. *Biomedicines* **2022**, *10*, 439. [CrossRef] [PubMed]
4. Cheng, L.; Osada, H.; Xing, T.; Yoshida, M.; Xiang, L.; Qi, J. The Insulin Receptor: A Potential Target of Amarogentin Isolated from Gentiana rigescens Franch That Induces Neurogenesis in PC12 Cells. *Biomedicines* **2021**, *9*, 581. [CrossRef] [PubMed]
5. Stanciu, G.D.; Rusu, R.N.; Bild, V.; Filipiuc, L.E.; Tamba, B.-I.; Ababei, D.C. Systemic Actions of SGLT2 Inhibition on Chronic mTOR Activation as a Shared Pathogenic Mechanism between Alzheimer's Disease and Diabetes. *Biomedicines* **2021**, *9*, 576. [CrossRef] [PubMed]
6. Chen, S.-D.; Yang, J.-L.; Hsieh, Y.-H.; Lin, T.-K.; Lin, Y.-C.; Chao, A.-C.; Yang, D.-I. Potential Roles of Sestrin2 in Alzheimer's Disease: Antioxidation, Autophagy Promotion, and Beyond. *Biomedicines* **2021**, *9*, 1308. [CrossRef] [PubMed]
7. Yuan, S.-X.; Li, H.-T.; Gu, Y.; Sun, X. Brain-Specific Gene Expression and Quantitative Traits Association Analysis for Mild Cognitive Impairment. *Biomedicines* **2021**, *9*, 658. [CrossRef] [PubMed]
8. Blanco-Palmero, V.A.; Rubio-Fernández, M.; Antequera, D.; Villarejo-Galende, A.; Molina, J.A.; Ferrer, I.; Bartolome, F.; Carro, E. Increased YKL-40 but Not C-Reactive Protein Levels in Patients with Alzheimer's Disease. *Biomedicines* **2021**, *9*, 1094. [CrossRef] [PubMed]
9. Song, L.; Wells, E.A.; Robinson, A.S. Critical Molecular and Cellular Contributors to Tau Pathology. *Biomedicines* **2021**, *9*, 190. [CrossRef] [PubMed]

10. Caruso, G.I.; Spampinato, S.F.; Costantino, G.; Merlo, S.; Sortino, M.A. SIRT1-Dependent Upregulation of BDNF in Human Microglia Challenged with Aβ: An Early but Transient Response Rescued by Melatonin. *Biomedicines* **2021**, *9*, 466. [CrossRef] [PubMed]
11. Lo Cascio, F.; Marzullo, P.; Kayed, R.; Palumbo Piccionello, A. Curcumin as Scaffold for Drug Discovery against Neurodegenerative Diseases. *Biomedicines* **2021**, *9*, 173. [CrossRef] [PubMed]

**Disclaimer/Publisher's Note:** The statements, opinions and data contained in all publications are solely those of the individual author(s) and contributor(s) and not of MDPI and/or the editor(s). MDPI and/or the editor(s) disclaim responsibility for any injury to people or property resulting from any ideas, methods, instructions or products referred to in the content.

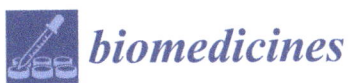 

*Review*

# Curcumin as Scaffold for Drug Discovery against Neurodegenerative Diseases

Filippa Lo Cascio [1,2], Paola Marzullo [3], Rakez Kayed [1,2] and Antonio Palumbo Piccionello [3,*]

1. Mitchell Center for Neurodegenerative Diseases, University of Texas Medical Branch, Galveston, TX 77555, USA; filocasc@utmb.edu (F.L.C.); rakayed@utmb.edu (R.K.)
2. Departments of Neurology, Neuroscience and Cell Biology, University of Texas Medical Branch, Galveston, TX 77555, USA
3. Department of Biological, Chemical and Pharmaceutical Sciences and Technologies-STEBICEF, University of Palermo, 90128 Palermo, Italy; paola.marzullo@unipa.it
* Correspondence: antonio.palumbopiccionello@unipa.it; Tel.: +39-09123897544

**Abstract:** Neurodegenerative diseases (NDs) are one of major public health problems and their impact is continuously growing. Curcumin has been proposed for the treatment of several of these pathologies, such as Alzheimer's disease (AD) and Parkinson's disease (PD) due to the ability of this molecule to reduce inflammation and aggregation of involved proteins. Nevertheless, the poor metabolic stability and bioavailability of curcumin reduce the possibilities of its practical use. For these reasons, many curcumin derivatives were synthetized in order to overcome some limitations. In this review will be highlighted recent results on modification of curcumin scaffold in the search of new effective therapeutic agents against NDs, with particular emphasis on AD.

**Keywords:** curcumin; Alzheimer's disease; amyloid; tau

## 1. Introduction

For last two centuries, natural occurring products have attracted the attention of many researchers due to their health benefits in the prevention and treatment of several diseases [1]. In 1815 Vogel isolated a yellow pigment, called curcumin, from the rhizome of Curcuma Longa, an East Indian plant [2]. Curcumin is the most abundant polyphenol and the most biologically active molecule found in the turmeric root; other minor components, known as curcuminoids, are demethoxycurcumin, bisdemethoxycurcumin, and cyclocurcumin [3]. Curcumin is one of the main elements of the Southeast Asian diet and it has been widely used for centuries as a traditional Indian and Asian medicine. After its first extraction, several studies showed that this polyphenolic molecule exhibits a broad spectrum of biological activities. Curcumin offers several health benefits, including anticancer [4], hypoglycemic activities [5], as well as the ability to be used as an analgesic, antiseptic or antimalarial [6]. In addition, curcumin has been shown to have anti-inflammatory [7], antioxidant [8,9], and antiamyloidogenic properties, which are relevant for the treatment of Alzheimer's disease (AD), and related diseases [10,11].

Worldwide, 50 million people have dementia. Unfortunately, this number is expected to increase exponentially, affecting 152 million people by 2050 [12]. AD is the most prevalent progressive neurodegenerative disease associated with age and the most common form of dementia [13], contributing to 60–70% of cases. AD is characterized clinically by progressive loss of memory, language problems, social withdrawal, deterioration of executive functions and eventually death [14,15]. Histopathologically, as Alzheimer's disease progresses, the brain shrinks dramatically and is characterized by cortex damage, and progressive degeneration of limbic and cortical brain structures, mainly in the temporal lobe [15]. This atrophy also affects the cortical association areas and the hippocampus, which is critical for the formation of new memories [16]. As a result of this pattern of

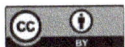

cortical thinning, it is also possible to observe an enlargement of ventricles and a functional alteration of Wernicke's and Broca's areas [17]. A common characteristic of age-related neurodegenerative diseases, including AD, is the pathological accumulation of unfolded and aggregation-prone proteins in the brain, which are considered the major cause of synaptic loss and progressive neuronal death observed in these disorders [18]. The two major systems involved in proteostasis maintenance are the autophagy-lysosomal system and the ubiquitin proteasome system [19]. However, these two systems have been found to be impaired in many neurodegenerative diseases, including AD. Therefore, the failure of these systems in maintaining proteostasis may also contribute to the pathological aggregation of proteins as well as formation of insoluble and fibrillar amyloid inclusions [20].

The major neuropathological features of AD are synaptic and neuronal degeneration and the presence of amyloid plaques and neurofibrillary tangles (NFTs).

Neuritic plaques are polymorphous aggregates made up of the amyloid Aβ peptide (Aβ) aggregates. The ≈4 kDa Aβ fragment originates from the transmembrane amyloid precursor protein (APP) by concerted proteolytic cleavage of β- and γ-secretase [21]. Monomeric Aβ1-40 (Aβ40) and Aβ1-42 (Aβ42) species can aggregate to form Aβ oligomers that can further aggregate and assembly into amyloid fibrils [22]. A growing body of evidence suggest that the oligomeric/prefibrillar Aβ peptide is the neurotoxic species that trigger the amyloid cascade, leading to the damage and eventual death of neurons associated with AD [23–25]. On the other hand, NFTs are intracellular inclusions of hyperphosphorylated tau, a microtubule associated protein. In its native state tau is a monomeric protein [26]. Tau is a natively unfolded protein involved in microtubule stabilization and axonal transport. However, under pathological conditions, tau can undergo abnormal post-translational modifications, including phosphorylation or acetylation [27,28]. As result of these modifications, tau detaches from the microtubules causing their disassembly, cytoskeletal instability, and axonal transport perturbation [29,30]. Unbound tau can self-aggregate forming soluble tau oligomers that assemble into paired helical filaments (PHFs) [31–33]. The PHFs mature into fibrils that constitute the intracellular NFTs, observed in the brain of AD patients [27]. Increasing evidence suggests that synaptic dysfunction and neuronal loss precede the formation of NFTs [34–39], indicating that the smaller and prefibrillar aggregates, tau oligomers, may be responsible for the toxic effects during the early stage of AD and other tauopathies [40,41]. Therefore, tau oligomers are considered to be highly toxic and to seed tau misfolding, thus propagating the pathology seen across different neurodegenerative diseases [38,42].

Despite the many efforts made to develop new treatments and therapeutic approaches to prevent the onset of the disease and to reverse the disease process, to date, there are no effective therapeutics. Nowadays, the therapeutic strategies available are only symptomatic treatments that counterbalance neurotransmitter disturbance, thus ameliorating a few of the clinical symptoms associated with the disease. The established treatments available are acetylcholinesterase inhibitors (e.g., Donepezil or Tacrine), antagonists of glutamate NMDA receptor (e.g., Memantine), agonist of nicotinic or muscarinic receptors, antioxidants and anti-inflammatory agents [43,44].

Growing evidence demonstrates a protective effect of curcumin against Aβ plaque formation; however, the mechanism of action is not yet fully clarified. Some studies have classified curcumin as an inhibitor of Aβ aggregation, others as disaggregating and destabilizing of amyloid fibrils [45]. In addition, curcumin has been shown to hamper Aβ oligomerization but not its fibrillization [46]. Recently, curcumin has been shown to attenuate amyloid-β aggregate-associated neurotoxicity by promoting the formation of "off-pathway" nontoxic soluble oligomers and prefibrillar proteins [47].

Curcumin has also been shown to exert a neuroprotective role by inhibiting tau aggregation. Indeed, curcumin has been shown to inhibit tau oligomerization, disintegrate preformed tau oligomers, inhibit β-sheet formation, and disaggregate tau filaments [48,49]. In addition, in vitro studies have shown that curcumin prevents the aggregation of other amyloidogenic protein, including α-synuclein (α-syn), which is a presynaptic protein involved in PD. PD is a debilitating neurodegenerative disorder characterized by the gradual loss of dopaminergic neurons in the substantia nigra pars compacta and clinically characterized as movement disorder. α-syn accumulates abnormally and aggregates in the cytosol as Lewy bodies and in the neuronal processes as Lewy neurites [50]. Several studies have showed that curcumin inhibits α–syn aggregation and reduces α-syn-induced cytotoxicity [51,52].

The neuroprotective effect of curcumin is certainly due to its ability to modulate the aggregation pathways and toxicity of amyloidogenic proteins and mitigate inflammation and oxidative stress, known to be key factors in the progression of neurodegenerative disorders [53,54].

This review attempts to explore the protective role of curcumin and its related compounds in the treatment of neurodegenerative disorders as a potential modulator of pathogenic pathways associated with AD and related diseases.

## 2. Physicochemical Characteristics of Curcumin

Due to the relevant biological and health benefits of curcumin, several chemists proposed a potential structure of curcumin. In 1913 Lampe et al. synthesized curcumin for the first time [55]. A general procedure for the synthesis of curcumin with a higher yield was later reported by Pabon [56]. In this reaction scheme 2,4-diketones, such as acetyl acetone, reacts with conveniently substituted aromatic aldehydes, particularly vanillin aldehyde, to synthesize curcumin. To prevent a Knoevenagel condensation due to the high acidity of the α-methylene group, the reaction is carried out in the presence of boron oxide as a complexing agent for the dienolate group. In this way, the condensation reaction involves terminal alkyl groups of di-ketone and primary or secondary amines, usually $n$-butylamine, are used to deprotonate these groups. Alkyl borates act as drying agents to remove the water formed by condensation reaction between boron complex and aromatic aldehyde. In the final step, boron complex gives the final product in acidic conditions. The reaction is refluxed, using aprotic solvent such as ethyl acetate (Scheme 1).

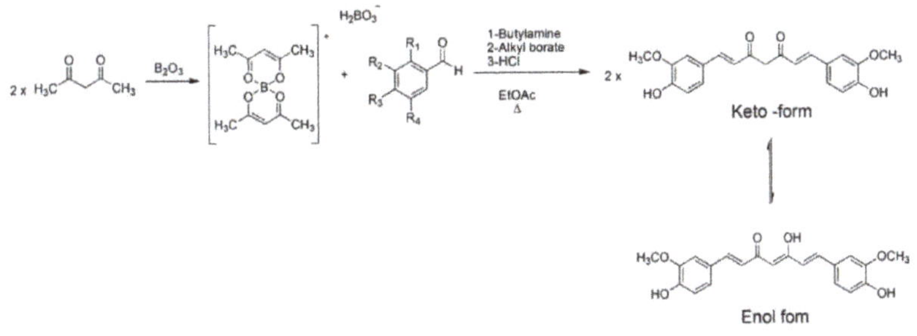

**Scheme 1.** Synthesis of curcumin with Pabon's method.

Several research groups follow the general method proposed by Pabon with slight modifications. For example, boron oxide has been replaced with boric acid with a lower yield [57,58]. An alternative procedure, reported by Rao et al., replaced boron oxide with borontrifluoride to obtain curcuminoid difluoroboronites that can be then hydrolyzed using aqueous methanol at pH 5.8 to get curcuminoid compounds [59]. To synthesize polyhydroxy curcuminoids, it is necessary to protect the hydroxyls groups on the starting benzaldehyde. These groups were protected as ethers and deprotected using aluminum chloride [60]. Curcumin is a low molecular mass polyphenolic compound (368.38 g/moL) with a melting point of 183 °C [61]. The IUPAC name of curcumin is 1,7-bis(4-hydroxy-3-methoxy-phenyl)-1,6-heptadiene-3,5-dione and is also known as diferuloyl methane. Curcumin is a hydrophobic molecule with a log $p$ value of 3.29. It is insoluble in water and soluble in polar organic solvent, like methanol, ethanol, dimethylsulfoxide, dimethylformamide, or ethyl acetate. It is partially soluble in hexane or cyclohexane [62].

Curcumin is a symmetrical molecule composed of two aromatic rings substituted with o-methoxy phenolic groups and a β-diketone moiety as a central linker. The heptadienone linkage exhibits keto-enol tautomerism (Scheme 1) that influences physicochemical and antioxidant properties of curcumin [63,64]. Curcumin is present in its bis-keto form in acidic and neutral pH conditions (pH 3–7) due to the presence of an acid proton linked to a highly activated carbon between the two aromatic rings. Conversely, under basic conditions (pH > 8), the enol form predominately and curcumin acts as an electron donor. Indeed, the antioxidant activity of curcumin is attributed to its enolic form [65]. X-ray crystallography studies confirmed that the enol form has a lower energy as compared to the diketone tautomer and it is the exclusive form in solution [66]. Moreover, keto-enol tautomer can exist as syn and anti isomers with the syn-enol form being more stable. In the syn form the two methoxy groups are on the same side with respect to keto-enol and hydroxy groups. Thus, it is possible to identify a polar surface with either a phenolic or enol group and a nonpolar area with methoxy groups [67].

Curcumin, as well as other polyphenolic compounds, displays a strong absorption in the visible region with a maximum absorption around 410–430 nm and another band with maximum absorption at 265 nm. In the presence of nonpolar solvents, including hexane or cyclohexane, a blue-shift of the absorption spectrum is observed. Conversely, in polar solvents, such as methanol or DMSO, the peak is shifted towards the lower frequencies [65]. These observations can be justified by the shift of the keto-enol tautomerism towards the enol form in a polar solvent or towards the bis-keto form in nonpolar solvent. The enol form exhibits a larger electronic delocalization and, therefore, a red-shifted absorption peak is observed [68].

## 3. Curcumin Bioavailability: Metabolic Reactions and New Formulations

Despite the relevant biological activities of curcumin, several studies have revealed a low oral bioavailability due to its poor solubility in water, low permeability and absorption, fast metabolism, and excretion in vivo. Oral administration of curcumin in rats (500 mg/kg) showed 1% of bioavailability in rat plasma [69]. In addition, several clinical studies have revealed extremely low serum levels following oral administration [70,71]. However, curcumin bioavailability improves once it is injected intravenously in rats [72].

The gastrointestinal tract represents the first physical barrier that limits the oral absorption due to the presence of the mucus layer and the tight junction proteins [48]. In addition, following oral administration, curcumin is rapidly metabolized by both conjugation and reduction pathways in the body, resulting in the formation of several pharmacologically inactive metabolites. Indeed, O-glucoronide or O-sulphate have been the principal curcuminoid metabolites found in the plasma following oral administration in rats. Furthermore, bioreduction products such as dihydrocurcumin or tetrahydrocurcumin and their conjugates formed by alcohol dehydrogenase were identified by HPLC and mass spectrometry analyses [73]. The α,β-unsatured β-diketo moiety of curcumin can be susceptible to degradation by hydrolysis at room temperature in neutral or alkaline conditions (pH $\geq$ 7). Several degradation products, including ferulic acid, ferulic aldehyde, vanillin, vanillic acid, and feruloylmethane, are also found in the serum; however, the amount of conjugated metabolites is more than the amount of reduction products. Probably in biofluids the β-keto function is not free but bound to proteins and, therefore, is not hydrolysable [62,74]. Curcumin is also photoreactive and undergoes photodegradation when exposed to sunlight, forming similar products to those found following hydrolytic degradation [75,76].

Several preclinical studies have suggested curcumin as a potential therapeutic approach for AD and related diseases; however, no clinical trials have been successful. The failure of these studies may be due to curcumin low brain bioavailability after oral administration and fast metabolism [77,78]. Consequently, alternative formulations and new drug delivery systems, including liposomes and nano-based approaches, have been developed to increase curcumin brain delivery. Most of the new delivery systems proposed are characterized by the presence of a central hydrophobic pocket in which curcumin binds through hydrophobic interactions. These macromolecular systems preserve curcumin from degradation and enhance its absorption as well as its distribution [75]. Furthermore, liposomes modified with penetrating agents, including curcumin as well as other amyloids-targeting ligands, have been shown to facilitate the passage of the compound through the blood–brain barrier (BBB) and have been considered as suitable vehicle for the delivery of therapeutics in the central nervous system [79]. Recently, Giacomelli et al. developed a novel and advanced curcumin delivery system based on nanoparticles named lipid-core nano-capsules. As result of their studies, they found that curcumin loaded nano-capsules display a significantly higher neuroprotective effect against Aβ toxicity in a mouse model of AD as compared to free curcumin [80]. In addition, Yang et al. proposed a novel curcumin-loaded nanoparticle system made of chitosan and bovine serum albumin. Using this formulation, they observed an increased penetration of curcumin through the BBB and microglia activation with a subsequent increase of Aβ phagocytosis [81]. Cyclodextrins are also used as absorption enhancers in several pharmaceutical formulations. Li et al. demonstrated that α-cyclodextrin enhances intestinal absorption of curcumin via transcellular and paracellular mechanisms [82]. In recent years, the study and the analysis of several crystalline solid forms of curcumin have also been a focus of great interest due to the different physicochemical properties exhibited by these polymorphs [83,84]. In addition to these alternative formulations, Wang et al. suggested exosomes, membrane-bound extracellular vesicles, as potential delivery system of curcumin. Therefore, exosomes-derived from curcumin-treated cells were used as carrier to release selectively curcumin in the brain. This delivery system increases the percentage of curcumin crossing the BBB through receptor-mediated transcytosis. They observed a decreased phosphorylation of tau through inhibition of AKT/GSK pathway, following injection in an AD mice model [82,85].

## 4. Relationship between Structural Properties and Biological Activity of Curcumin Derivatives

The synthesis of novel curcumin derivatives represents an effective alternative to obtain curcumin analogs with a better solubility in biofluid in an effort to improve the pharmacokinetic profile of curcumin and its biological activity [48,86–88]. As mentioned above, curcumin acts as a neuroprotective agent blocking multiple mechanisms involved in neurodegeneration by interfering with the accumulation of misfolded aggregate proteins, including Aβ and tau, inflammation and oxidative stress. The modulation of each of these pathological pathways requires distinct structural feature of curcumin. Therefore, comprehensive structure–activity studies are extremely important to identify novel curcumin derivatives as potential therapeutic agents for neurodegenerative diseases.

In recent years, researchers have synthesized several compounds able to block Aβ fibrillogenesis. In this process, Aβ monomers aggregate to form oligomers, which then assemble to form insoluble aggregates [89]. This transformation is characterized by a structural transition from α-helix to β-sheet structure [90]. It is known that the short Aβ fragment, KLVFF (Aβ16-20) binds to full length Aβ and it is important for amyloid fibril formation [91]. A shared model hypothesizes that phenylalanine residue in the KLVFF sequence of Aβ peptides interact through Π-Π interactions during Aβ aggregation. Small molecules, such as curcumin, are able to block or break these interactions and could be valid candidates to revert amyloid formation [92].

Reinke and Gestwicki have created a library of compounds resembling curcumin structure to investigate and evaluate the effect of the three main features of curcumin on inhibition of amyloid aggregation [93]. The structural features contributing to the inhibitory potency of curcumin are the two aromatic rings, the substitution pattern of these phenyl groups, and the length and flexibility of the central linker region. To perform structural considerations and better understand which feature is critical for the inhibition of Aβ aggregation, Reinke and Gestwicki synthesized curcumin analogs by modifying only one structural feature at the time and retaining the other two. As a result of their studies, they found that compounds lacking one aromatic group are less active than curcumin, suggesting that both aromatic rings are essential to interact through hydrophobic interactions and hydrogen bonding with phenylalanine residue of Aβ monomers and inhibit amyloid formation [94]. Furthermore, hydroxyl substitution on the aromatic end group or other polar functional substituents are required for the inhibiting activity. In addition, Reinke and Gestwicki showed that both length and flexibility of the central linker region are key factors to take into consideration in the design of new Aβ aggregation inhibitors. Indeed, the inhibiting activity is negatively affected when the central linker region is too long, too short, or too flexible. The optimal length of the central linker is 8–16 Å and no more than one or two rotating sp3-hybridized carbons are required for an ideal flexibility.

It has been shown that the homeostasis of metal ions is critical for maintaining normal physiological functions. Some ions such as Al, Fe, Cu, and Zn have been observed in the brain of AD patients [95]. Their imbalance in the brain is closely related to the Aβ deposition and tau accumulation, suggesting that they play a role in the degenerative process of AD. The histidine residues of Aβ peptides (H13/H14) are good coordination sites for metal ions [96]. Curcumin can interact with metal ions forming strong complexes. Indeed, the α,β-unsaturated β-diketo moiety of curcumin has shown excellent chelating properties. Many studies reported the synthesis of stable metal-curcumin complex with a stoichiometry 2:1 (ligand:metal) [62]. Curcumin-metal complexes decrease Aβ plaques as well as suppress inflammatory processes by preventing metal induction of nuclear factor kappa B, NF-kB [97,98]; however, metal chelators can disrupt the normal brain homeostasis. Zhang et al. designed a novel curcumin derivative, named CRANAD-17, as a chelating agent to attenuate Aβ crosslinking induced by Cu [99].

Some curcumin derivatives exert their neuroprotective effects by promoting phagocytosis of Aβ fibrils. For example, it was demonstrated by Fiala et al. that bisdemethoxycurcumin (BDC) enhances macrophage-activated Aβ clearance and reduces the inflammation state [100]. Recently, Gagliardi et al. showed that the treatment of BDC derivatives in a human monocytic cell line, mimicking the peripheral blood mononuclear cells of AD, revealed overexpression of genes essential for macrophage function, including mannosylglycoprotein 4-beta-N-acetylglucosaminyltransferase and vitamin D receptor. BDC also showed a protective anti-inflammatory effect through downregulation of NF-kB and β-site APP cleaving enzyme 1 (BACE1) genes [101]. BACE 1 protein and γ-secretase enzyme cleaves APP to generate Aβ peptides, with the β-cleavage being the rate-limiting step of this sequential proteolytic pathway [102]. Inhibitors of BACE1 activity are, therefore, considered as a possible therapeutic approach and many BACE1 inhibitors have been synthesized. Two critical curcumin structural features associated with BACE 1 inhibitory activity are the phenolic rings and the unsaturated alkenyl linker between the aromatic rings. Derivatives with multiple hydroxy groups have been found to be more active than compounds with nonsubstituted phenyl groups or substituted with methoxy groups or halogen. When researchers replaced the phenol group with indole or a pyrrole ring, they produced more active compounds. These data suggest that inhibitor molecules interact with BACE 1 through hydrogen bonds [103]. Reduction products are not active against BACE 1. A planar structure is required to maintain the inhibitory activity and sp2 carbons give the optimal rigidity to the molecule. The substitution of 1,3-dicarbonyl moiety of curcumin by isosteric heterocycles, isoxazole, and pyrazole, resulted in the formation of potent inhibitors of γ-secretase enzyme [104].

Up to this point of our discussion, we have analyzed the structural aspects of curcuminoids that have been found to be important for their anti-Aβ aggregation activity. Curcumin and its derivatives also exert a protective role against misfolded tau aggregates. Unlike Aβ, tau lacks in hydrophobic residues and therefore its aggregation process does not lead to the formation of Π-Π interactions. However, under particular circumstances, the small degree of hydrophobicity, compared to other proteins, is sufficient to drive tau aggregation [105]. Tau aggregation inhibitors interact with tau by electrostatic interaction and hydrogen bonding. A recent study suggested two ruthenium-curcumin-bipyridine/phenanthroline complexes as inhibitors of tau aggregation. In these complexes, the metal ion is bound to the enol group of curcumin and to the nitrogen atoms of the ancillary ligands, bipyridine or phenanthroline. Curcumin inhibits aggregation at the nucleation stage while the positive charged ruthenium complex inhibits the elongation phase, reducing longer fibrils formation [106].

Oxidative damage plays an important role in neurodegeneration, therefore, to treat neurodegenerative disorders another pharmacological approach is to develop antioxidant compounds. The antioxidant property of curcumin is due to the abstractable phenolic hydrogen [107]. This group can reduce, for example, superoxide radicals to generate less reactive phenoxyl radicals that are resonance stabilized [108]. Ferrari et al. developed curcumin analogs substituted on the central carbon of the heptadienone linker and demonstrated that these complexes exhibit good metal chelating properties. However, these compounds showed less scavenging activity because of the presence of the substituent on central linker shifts the keto-enol tautomerism towards the di-keto form with less stabilization of phenoxyl radical [109].

## 5. Curcumin Derivatives and Hybrids Molecules

Given the large number of biologically active curcumin-like molecules that have been synthesized, we can divide them into different classes accordingly to the modified part of curcumin structure. Discussion on selected compounds is reported in the following subsections.

### 5.1. Monocarbonyl Analogs of Curcumin (MACs)

The monocarbonyl analogs of curcumin (MACs) belong to the group of compounds with a central core modification, as shown in Figure 1. Several researchers have proposed MACs as anticancer as well as anti-inflammatory agents. These compounds have been shown to exhibit a higher anticancer potency than curcumin in many cancer cell lines [110]. Recently, monocarbonyl derivatives have also been proposed for the treatment of AD.

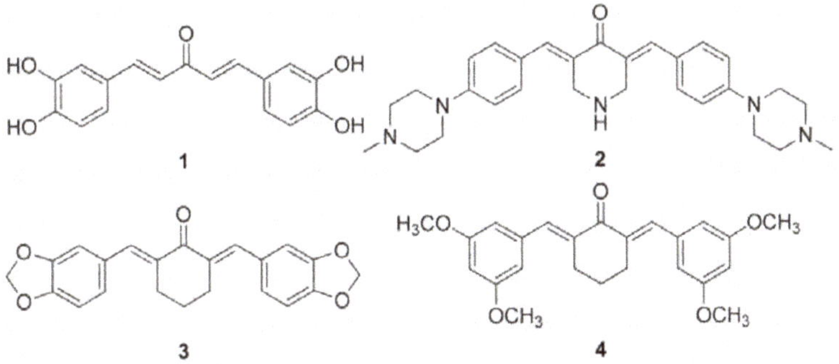

**Figure 1.** Structures of monocarbonyl analogs of curcumin (MACs).

The removal of the keto-enol motif, susceptible to hydrolysis, enhances the stability of MACs compared to curcumin; however, the presence of the enone group is important for the anti Aβ aggregation activity [111]. MACs can be divided into two main groups: acyclic (**1**) and cyclic MAC compounds (**2**, **3** and **4**) (Figure 1). In the cyclic MACs, the carbonyl group could also be part of a 5 or 6 membered heterocyclic ring containing NR, O, S or $SO_2$ groups [112]. In a general synthetic method reported by Ohori et al., MACs have been produced from aryl-aldehyde and acetone. To obtain cyclic MACs, acetone was substituted by cyclic ketone. The reaction is carried out in ethanol using sodium hydroxide and cetyltrimethylammonium bromide as catalysts [110].

Orlando et al. synthesized MAC derivatives with 5-carbon spacer between the aromatic rings. Compound **1** in Figure 1 showed a higher percentage of anti-Aβ aggregation activity compared to curcumin ($IC_{50}$ 0.8 μM vs. $IC_{50}$ 1.0 μM) [111]. In addition, newly synthesized monocarbonyl derivatives with a piperidone structure in the linker (**2**) are identified as potent inhibitor of Aβ fibrillation. Furthermore, substitution of a nitrogen atom within the piperidone ring with a carbon atom or N-methylation reduced the antiaggregation activity. The aliphatic linker gives the ideal flexibility, while the N-methylpiperazine groups on the two aromatic ends enhance hydrogen bond interactions with Aβ peptides. Compound **2** decreased the β-sheet structure and stabilized the α-helix content as assessed by circular dichroism spectroscopy (CD). In addition to the antiaggregating activity, compound **2** showed antioxidant and metal chelating properties [113]. MAC **3** was demonstrated to be more stable than curcumin at physiological pH. Furthermore, UV measurements of MAC **3** revealed that its spectra remained unchanged over time, while UV spectra of curcumin showed a decreased intensity and a shift towards the red. The protein hen egg white lysozyme (HEWL) was used as a model protein to study the inhibitory effect of MAC **3** on amyloid formation. MAC **3** also exhibits an optimal length of linker (8.84 Å) and it is more rigid than curcumin due to the absence of rotating sp3 carbon within the backbone. These structural features make it as an ideal inhibitor of Aβ aggregation. Fluorescence measurements using the molecular probe 8-anilinonaphatalene-sulphonate (ANS), showed decreased hydrophobic surface upon treatment with the curcumin analog MAC **3**. Docking studies demonstrated that the compound binds to the catalytic tryptophan (62 and 63) of HEWL with the carbonyl component pointing toward the hydrophilic residues of the active site [114]. The monocarbonyl-cyclohexanone derivative **4** was tested in vitro as an antioxidant agent and showed good scavenging activity for reactive oxygen species (ROS) [115]. MAC **4** exhibits antioxidant properties and protective effect against $H_2O_2$-induced cytotoxicity in PC12 cells. The compound was able to rescue the levels of glutathione (GSH) as well as the activity of superoxide dismutase and catalase. Moreover, compound **4** showed to increase mRNA expression of Nrf2, a key transcription factor of the antioxidant response [115].

*5.2. C4-Substituted Curcumin Derivatives*

Medicinal chemists have synthesized C4-substituted curcumin derivatives by modifying the central core of curcumin with the insertion of one or two alkyl substituents (Figure 2).

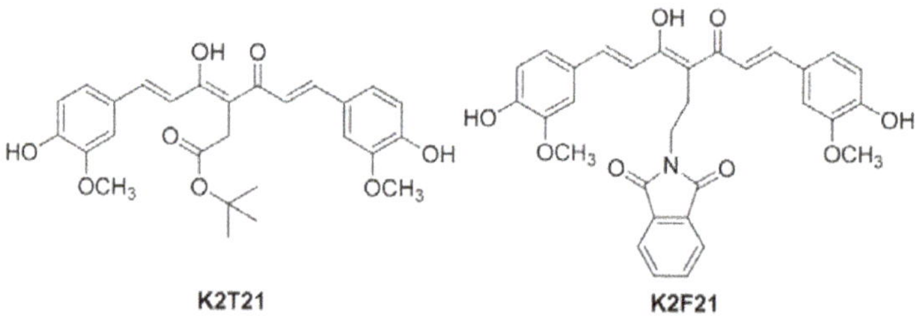

**Figure 2.** Structures of C4-substituted curcumin derivatives.

The synthetic pathway follows Pabon's route. In the first step, alkyl-substituents are inserted into an alkaline environment using acetyl-acetone and appropriate alkyl halides [116,117].

This modification as well as the synthesis of MACs, leads to the production of more stable compounds. Mono-substituted compounds have an acidic hydrogen within the linker and, therefore, retain the keto-enol tautomerism. The enolization of these derivatives is involved in the interaction with Aβ aggregates. Particularly, the anion of enol form has a reddish color while the other forms, including the neutral enol form and neutral or anion keto form, are yellow or colorless in solution. The same reddish color is observed when these molecules are incubated with Aβ aggregates, indicating an increase of the anion of the enol form when it is bound to Aβ aggregates. Notable, the interaction of the compound with Aβ monomer did not cause change in color. Therefore, this observation supports the involvement of the enol form in the binding to Aβ aggregates [118]. A decreased anti-Aβ inhibitory activity was observed for disubstituted compounds, including α,α-dimethylcurcumin. This compound lacks enol tautomer and planarity that are essential to interact with Aβ aggregates.

Ferrari et al. synthesized curcumin analogs, known as **K2T**, by introducing t-butyl ester in the C4 position [109]. **K2T** derivatives exhibit metal chelating properties towards gallium and copper ions and inhibit Aβ aggregation. The presence of alkyl substituent shifts the tautomeric equilibrium towards the di-keto tautomer and limits the radical scavenging ability. **K2T21** (Figure 2) is the best compound of this series with a good metal chelating property. In addition, the Cu(II):**K2T21** complex maintains a scavenger activity [109]. The derivative **K2F21** (Figure 2), functionalized with a phthalimide group in the α-position and vanillin-like structure on the aromatic portion, showed a higher stability, depolymerization, antioxidant and antiapoptotic activities [116]. Molecular docking simulations showed a high probability of van der Waals interactions of **K2F21** with $β_2$-site of Aβ1-40 fibrils. The $β_2$-binding site is located within the residues 31–40, which is a region known to be involved in modulating Aβ aggregation through the action of methionine 35 (Met35) [116].

*5.3. Heterocyclic Derivatives*

Several research groups designed and synthesized curcumin derivatives by replacing 1,3-dicarbonyl moiety with isosteric pyrazole and isoxazole rings. Isoxazole derivatives were synthesized at reflux starting from curcumin and hydroxylamine hydrochloride using pyridine and ethanol as solvents. Curcumin was converted into pyrazole and *N*-substituted pyrazole by reaction with corresponding hydrazines ($NH_2NH_2$ or $RNHNH_2$), using reaction conditions reported by Narlawar et al. Particularly, from their series, compound **5** and **6** (Figure 3) are the ones exhibiting the most interesting biological effects.

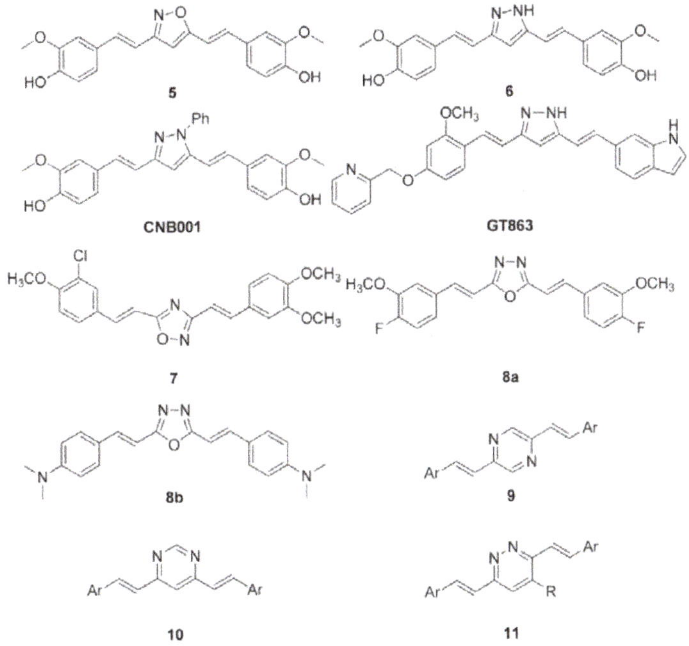

**Figure 3.** Structures of heterocyclic derivatives.

Both compounds interact with Aβ42 aggregates and can be used as an imaging agent for diagnostic purposes. In addition, compound **6**, at lower concentrations, demonstrated the ability to depolymerize tau aggregates, inhibit tau aggregation, and produce γ-secretase activity [104]. **CNB001** (Figure 3) is a pyrazole analog of curcumin that has been extensively studied because of its potential as reliable therapeutic candidate for the treatment of AD. **CNB001** was shown to improve memory and long-term potentiation and mitigate motor impairments in rats [119,120]. In addition, the compound showed anti-inflammatory activity through inhibition of proinflammatory mediators in LPS-induced microglia [121]. Another compound with curcumin-pyrazole structure is **GT863** (also named PE859, Figure 3). Evaluation of its anti-Aβ and tau aggregation activity revealed that substitution of the aromatic ring with a bicyclic system along with the protection of the phenolic group from metabolic reaction, may increase the inhibitory activity [122]. It was shown that **GT863** reduces the production of Aβ through alteration of nicastrin maturation, an essential glycoprotein component of the γ-secretase complex [123].

Heterocyclic derivatives of curcumin also include compounds with an oxadiazole ring instead of a β-diketone group. Our research group has synthesized a series of curcumin-like compounds with 1,2,4-oxadiazole or 1,3,4-oxadiazole motif. Compounds **7** and **8a** were tested as Aβ aggregation inhibitors using different biophysical techniques and both showed to affect the aggregation pattern of Aβ [124]. Induced Fit Docking (IFD) observations revealed that both compounds bind to Aβ in a saddle between Met35 and Val39 via hydrophobic interactions. In the presence of compound **7** was observed a perturbation of β-sheet content, while it was partially preserved in the presence of compound **8a**. The IFD results suggest that compound **8a** can interfere with Aβ aggregation by hampering the packing of oligomers along the fibril major axis. On the other hand, due to steric hindrance, compound **7** interferes with the formation of β-sheet structure, resulting in the formation of toxic off-pathway structures. Indeed, compound **7** showed to trigger less Aβ aggregation and enhance Aβ 1-40 toxicity, probably due to the higher presence of toxic oligomers in the medium [124]. Other newly synthesized curcumin derivatives demonstrated modulation of the aggregation pathway of preformed tau oligomers. Particularly, compound **8b** was found to convert toxic tau oligomers into more nontoxic tau aggregates and mitigated tau oligomer-associated toxicity in the human neuroblastoma cell line, SH-SY5Y, and primary neuronal cultures [87].

Novel pyrimidine **9**, pyrazine **10** and pyridazine **11** curcumin derivatives, with general structure reported in Figure 1, were efficiently synthesized and tested in vitro and in vivo as potential Aβ and tau imaging probes for the diagnosis of AD. These heterocyclic derivatives showed an excellent capacity to label Aβ as well as tau aggregates [125].

*5.4. Tetrahydrocurcumins (THCs)*

Hydrogenated curcuminoids attracted researcher's attention for their biological properties (Figure 4). These compounds lack the diketone bridge necessary to bind Aβ fibrils and to exert antioxidant activity.

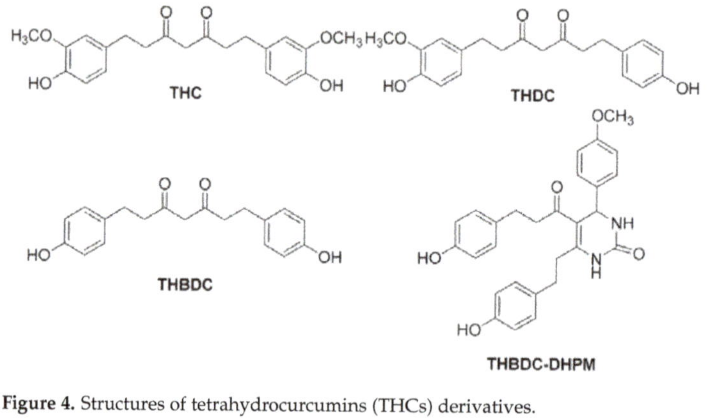

**Figure 4.** Structures of tetrahydrocurcumins (THCs) derivatives.

Tetrahydrocurcumin (**THC**) is a more stable metabolite of curcumin. Phenolic rings and methoxy groups, but not double bonds of curcumin, mediate the anti-inflammatory effect. **THC** has been shown to reduce neuroinflammation through reduction of IL1β in the brain and inhibition of LPS inducing the release of iNOS; however, it does not display any amyloidogenic inhibitor activity [126]. Tetrahydrodemethoxycurcumin (**THDMC**) and tetrahydrobisdemethoxycurcumin (**THBDMC**) are reported as inhibitors of acetyl cholinesterase activity (AChE). Particularly, the absence of the double bond and the methoxy group increases their inhibitory activity. In addition, **THCs** were conjugated with a dihydropyrimidinone, a known AChE inhibitor, to create a series of **THCs-DHPM** compounds. Compound **THBDC-DHPM** produced by **THBDMC** with methoxy group on phenyl group exhibits the lowest value of $IC_{50}$ against the enzymatic activity [127].

### 5.5. Curcumin-Like (CL) Compounds

To overcome the instability issues due to the β-di keto moiety, our research group synthesized a library of curcumin-like compounds without the α-carbon within the linker (Figure 5). In the synthetic method adopted, the diacetyl reacted in a double aldol condensation with the appropriate aromatic aldehyde. The resulting compounds **CL3** and **CL8** were found to modulate the aggregation state of recombinant toxic tau oligomers and disease-relevant tau oligomers [87,128]. Notably, **CL3** affected both the size and the surface hydrophobicity of brain-derived tau oligomers reducing their associated neurotoxicity [128].

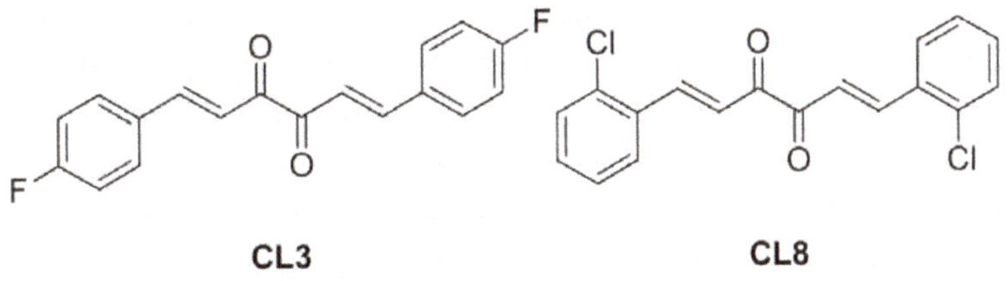

**Figure 5.** Structures of curcumin-like (CL) compounds.

### 5.6. Aromatic Ring Substitution: Methoxy and Hydroxy Groups

Aromatic rings of curcumin and curcumin-like compounds interact with Aβ aggregates by hydrophobic and hydrogen bonds. Therefore, chemical structure of curcumin containing two aromatic rings is optimal for inhibition of amyloidogenesis. Reinke and Gestwicki synthesized a series of curcumin analogs without an aromatic ring and evaluated their inhibitor activity on Aβ aggregation. These compounds did not show any effect on Aβ aggregation, even at higher concentrations (500 μM). Conversely, curcumin inhibits Aβ aggregation with an $IC_{50}$ value of 10 μM [93].

In the same study, they also evaluated the influence of aromatic substituent on the neuroprotective activity of curcumin and its derivatives. They showed that substituents capable of taking part in hydrogen bonding are essential for the activity.

Several structural–activity studies were performed to evaluate the effects of the position and number of methoxy and hydroxy group on the biological activity of the resulting derivatives (Figure 6).

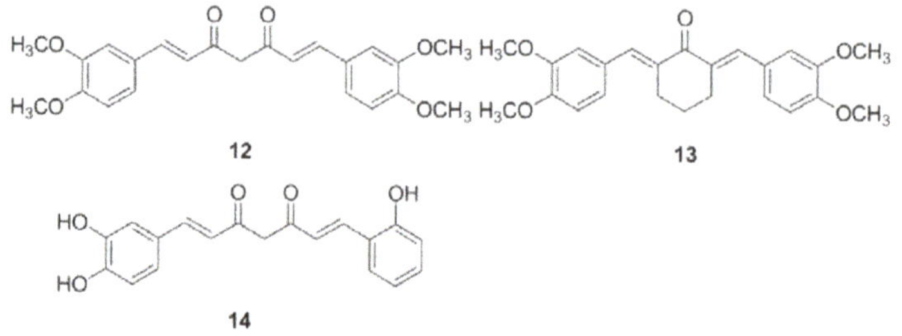

**Figure 6.** Structures of compounds with methoxy/hydroxy substituted aromatic rings.

Compounds with an anti-Aβ aggregation activity were obtained by maintaining methoxy and hydroxy group in para- and meta- positions, while orto-substitution did not improve the activity. Compound **12** was obtained from curcumin through the substitution of the para-hydroxy group with a methoxy group. Researchers observed a decreased polarity and an increased permeability across the BBB. Moreover, this substitution preserves the conjugation reaction of -OH groups with sulphate or glucuronide groups [111]. In addition, the mono-carbonyl compound **13** methoxy substituted showed an improved inhibitory activity on Aβ aggregation [114]. Hitoshi et al. showed the importance of the catechol motif for anti-Aβ aggregation activity. Particularly, they demonstrated that the o-phenol derivative **14** increases the water solubility as compared to para- and meta- phenol. Previous studies reported that an increased dihedral angle improved water solubility. In o-phenol compound hydroxyl and β-di keto groups are close and can interact by participation of water. This interaction causes a torsion of the molecule, which increases the angle between the phenol group and central linker and, thus, increases water solubility [129]. Compound **14** is a potent inhibitor of BACE1 enzyme. Computational studies suggest that the inhibitor interacts with BACE1 in the P3 pocket. It did not interact with the aspartic acid residues of active site (Asp32 and Asp228); hydroxy groups and ketone motif are involved in hydrogen bonds with Glu230 and Glu339 [103].

*5.7. Aromatic Ring Substitution: Halogenated and Prenylated Derivatives*

Chemists have made several efforts to synthesize new curcumin-like compounds that can be used as diagnostic tools to detect amyloid formation in the brain. They designed the compound **15** by the introduction of tri-fluomethoxy groups on the aromatic rings (Figure 7).

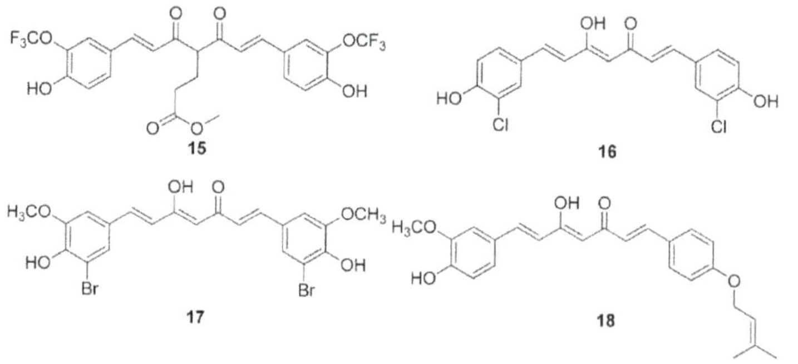

**Figure 7.** Structures of compounds with halogenated or prenylated aromatic rings.

This derivative passes through the BBB and reaches the brain, where it can be detected using fluorine 19 by MRI. Moreover, the trifluoromethoxy group is important for anti-Aβ aggregation activity [118]. Several studies reported other halogenated curcumin derivatives as biologically active compounds for the treatment of AD, including the chloro-substituted compound **16** [130]. In addition, the bromo-derivative **17** exhibits antioxidant properties [60]. Synthetic halogenated derivatives of curcumin have been identified as ligands for nuclear receptor of vitamin D as well as for nuclear receptor of retinoid (RXR and RAR) [131]. It was demonstrated that agonists of RXR stimulate Aβ clearance through induction of ApoE expression [132].

To increase the number of hydrogen bonding and electrostatic interactions between curcumin derivatives and Aβ peptide, a *N*-methylpiperazine group was introduced to the aromatic ring. Thus, a series of mono-carbonyl *N*-methylpiperazine substituted derivatives was synthesized and compound **2**, reported above (see Figure 1), showed the best inhibitory activity of Aβ aggregation [113]. Instead, prenylated curcumin analogs were prepared to enhance the hydrophobic contacts of curcumin with Aβ monomers. Compound **18** is the most active compound in term of antifibrillogenic and anti-inflammatory activities. It retains methoxy and hydroxy groups that are essential for H-bonds and the 4-prenyloxy group that is required to establish hydrophobic interactions with the nucleation core of Aβ peptides [133]. Indeed, the compound approaches to the self-recognition hydrophobic core, $^{16}$KLVFFA$^{21}$, which is known to be a nucleation site for the pathogenic aggregation of Aβ. In particular, **18** assumes an extended geometry by interacting with six different amyloid segments in the same residues, Leu18 and Lys16. Specifically, they form hydrophobic interactions with six Leu18 residues, which contact both the phenyl ring as well as the alkyl chain. In addition, they form H-bonds with six Lys16 residues, which approach the β-keto-enol central core and the substituents on phenyl rings. When the complexity of simulated amyloid structure increases, the interactions between compound **18** and the fibril structures are governed by hydrophobic interactions [133].

*5.8. Other Aromatic Rings*

Among lateral changes made to the structure of curcumin there is the substitution of one aromatic group with an indole moiety. The asymmetric compound **19** showed an inhibitory activity against the BACE1 enzyme and can be considered as anti-AD drug (Figure 8) [103,134]. In this compound, the substitution of phenol group with the indole motif improves the H-bonds with BACE1 enzyme.

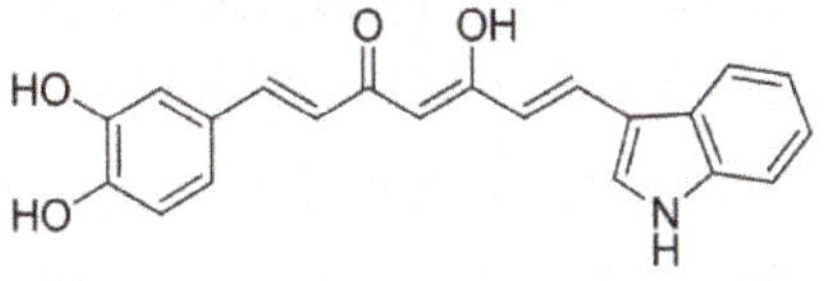

**Figure 8.** Structure of compound **19** with an indole aromatic ring.

The pyrazole curcumin derivative **GT863** (Figure 3) also presents an indole ring on the lateral part of the molecule. It inhibits both Aβ and tau aggregation. This compound is more stable than curcumin due to the presence of the pyrazole moiety and the protection of the phenolic hydroxyl group that is prone to metabolic reaction [122].

*5.9. Hemi-Curcuminoids*

Hemi-curcuminoid β-diketones are another class of asymmetric curcumin-like compounds that can be considered the start point for the development of new neuroprotective agents (Figure 9).

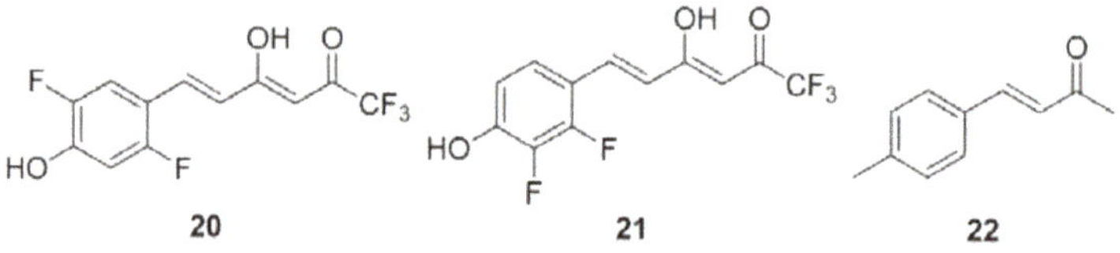

Figure 9. Structures of hemi-curcuminoids.

These derivatives were prepared following Pabon's method starting from substituted benzaldehydes and di-ketonic compounds. Compounds **20** and **21** display metal chelating properties and scavenger activity against ROS. The para-hydroxy group is considered a required structural feature to exert the antioxidant effect [135].

Claisen–Schmidt Aldol condensation of the aromatic aldehyde with acetone under basic conditions generated a series of hemi-curcuminoid compounds [87]. These compounds were tested as a modulator of the aggregation state of preformed tau oligomers. Compound **22** showed interaction with tau oligomers promoting the formation of larger, less hydrophobic and nontoxic tau aggregates as assessed in human SH-SY5Y neuroblastoma cells [87].

*5.10. Calebin A Derivatives*

Darrik and colleagues isolated Calebin A from Curcuma Longa and synthesized it for the first time [136]. After evaluating the protective role of Calebin A against Aβ associated toxicity in neuronal cells, several Calebin A derivatives have been synthesized (Figure 10).

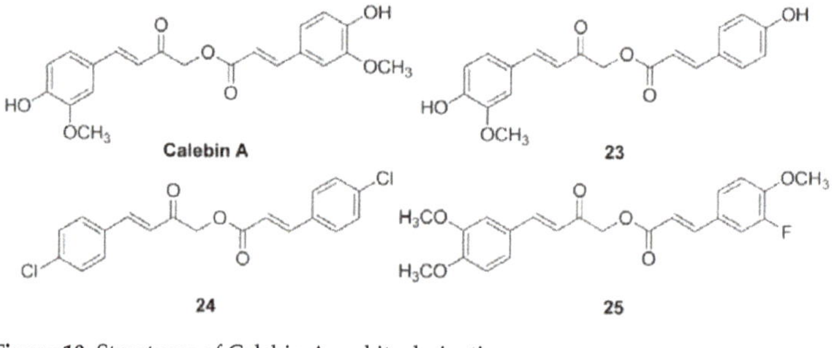

Figure 10. Structures of Calebin A and its derivatives.

Compound **23** showed that the hydroxyl group is important to protect cells from Aβ25-35 associated toxicity [137]. Calebin A derivatives are usually obtained by protecting the aromatic substituents [138]. Compounds **24** and **25** were synthesized following an alternative synthetic procedure, by substitution reaction of a cinnamic acid derivative on iodoketone in basic conditions. Both compounds were shown to protect neuronal cultures from tau oligomer-associated neurotoxicity by promoting the formation of larger nontoxic tau aggregates [87].

*5.11. Hybrid Compounds*

The bibliography about curcumin and curcumin-like compounds reports several studies on the design and biological evaluation of hybrid molecules. These compounds comprise curcumin fused with other biological active entities to enhance its biological and pharmaceutical properties (Figure 11).

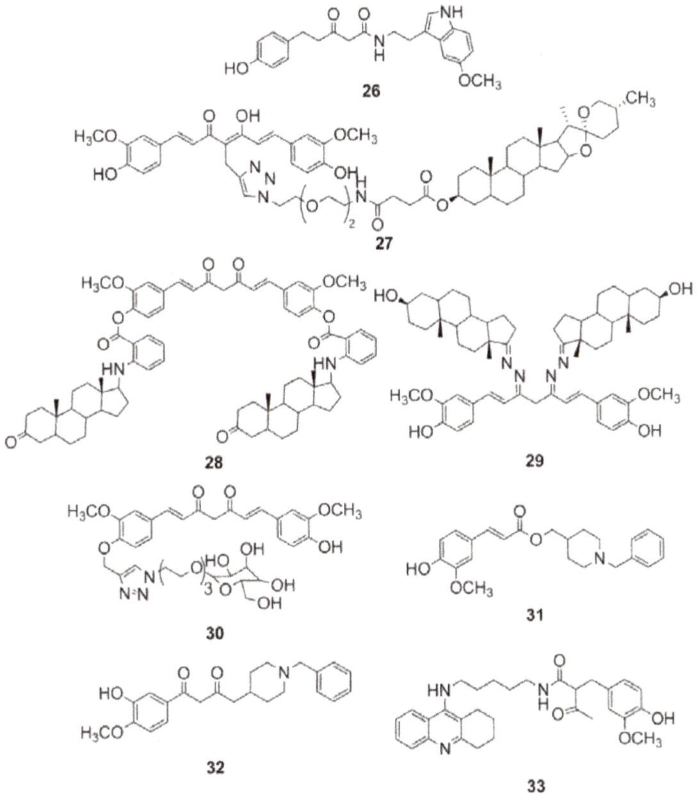

**Figure 11.** Curcumin hybrid molecules.

Curcumin-melatonin hybrids were discovered as neuroprotective agents and have the potential to become new therapeutic strategies to treat AD. Melatonin as well as curcumin exhibit antioxidant, anti-inflammatory, and anti-Aβ aggregation activity [139]. Moreover, clinical studies have revealed that AD patients experience circadian dysfunctions due to the decreased melatonin levels in cerebrospinal fluid [140].

The presence of the methoxy group and the acetamide moiety is believed to be crucial for the neuroprotective activity of melatonin and its hybrids. Curcumin-melatonin hybrids without the p-hydroxy group of curcumin exhibited reduced neuroprotection. Contrarily, the double bound and conjugation of the β-diketone group with a phenyl ring is not necessary for the activity. The compound **26** inhibited the formation of Aβ oligomers and showed neuroprotective effects on MC65 cells [141].

Bivalent compounds were created by binding curcumin to the steroidal compound diosgenin using linkers with different lengths. The steroidal part acts as an anchor to localize curcumin into membrane lipid raft where ROS and Aβ oligomers are produced. Compound **27** with steroid moiety attached to the α-carbon of curcumin showed better neuroprotective property than those with a different position attachment. In addition, it exhibited antioxidant and anti-Aβ aggregation inhibitor activities [142]. Steroidal compounds **28** and **29** increased acetylcholine in the brain through inhibition of AChE activity and overexpression of choline acetyl transferase levels. Moreover, both compounds exert an antioxidant effect due to the phenolic groups combined to the methylene group of β-diketone group. The steroid portion can be involved in an interaction with the estrogen receptors and modulate the expression of antioxidant enzymes via intracellular pathway. Additionally, the increased levels of GSH may have a decisive role in the antioxidant effects observed.

Both compounds exhibit an antiapoptotic activity as a result of the overexpression of the antiapoptotic factor Bcl2 in the brain of AD mice model [143]. Therefore, these hybrid molecules can be considered as an alternative approach to reverse the oxidative stress in neurodegeneration [143]. Additionally, bioconjugates of curcumin with demethylenated piperic acid, valine or glutamic acid display a protective effect against GSH depletion in dopaminergic neuronal cells and, therefore, may exert their antioxidant activities in the treatment of Parkinson's disease [144]. To increase curcumin water solubility, a sugar moiety was attached to the phenol residues. The hydroxyl groups of sugar can act as β-sheet breakers through competitive hydrogen bonding with amyloids fibrils. Sugar-curcumin conjugate **30** was shown to inhibit Aβ and tau aggregation [145].

To date, acetylcholinesterase inhibitors, such as Tacrine or Donepezil, are used in the treatment of Alzheimer's disease. Recently, new curcumin-hybrids were created by fusion of curcumin with these known drugs. Donepezil-curcumin hybrids **31** and **32** have a potent AChE inhibitor effect and both compounds showed metal chelating properties for $Cu^{2+}$. Compound **31** also showed antioxidant activity in neuronal SH-SY5H cells. The phenyl group of the compound **31** interacts by stacking type interactions with Trp86 and the nitrogen atom binds to Tyr337 through cation-Π interaction. The carbonyl group forms a hydrogen bond with the main chain NH group of Phe295. On the other hand, compound **32** interacts with both catalytic site (CAS) and anionic site (PAS) of AChE. The two phenyl groups and the hydroxyl group interact with the active site. The hydroxyl forms an H-bond with the carbonyl group of Ser286 and Arg289, while the phenyl ring on the piperidine part formed Π-Π interactions with Trp84. The piperidine ring is located on the aromatic pocket connecting PAS and CAS sites [146,147]. Tacrine-curcumin hybrid **33** has been evaluated as an AChE inhibitor and it showed a higher potency than Tacrine [148]. Indeed, docking simulations showed that the benzene ring binds to the catalytic site of AChE, while the Tacrine motif interacts with the anionic site. The carbonyl group forms an H-bond with the Tyr121 thus stabilizing the complex. Therefore, due to the ability to inhibit both the catalytic as well as the anionic sites, compound **33** exhibited the most potent activity. Moreover, the curcumin moiety is responsible for the antioxidant properties, while the β-diketone moiety confers remarkable ion-chelating ability [148].

Biological activities of compounds discussed in this paragraph are presented in Table 1.

**Table 1.** Summary of biological activities of compounds showed in Figures 1–11.

| Compound | Activity | Reference |
|---|---|---|
| MAC 1 (Figure 1) | Aβ oligomerization inhibitor | [111] |
| MAC 2 (Figure 1) | Aβ aggregation inhibitor<br>Antioxidant<br>Metal chelating | [113] |
| MAC 3 (Figure 1) | Aβ aggregation inhibitor<br>Protection against Aβ oligomers toxicity<br>Stabilization of proteins in the native state | [114] |
| MAC 4 (Figure 1) | Antioxidant | [115] |
| K2T21 (Figure 2) | Cu (II)-chelating<br>Antiradical | |
| K2F21 (Figure 2) | Depolymerizing activity of Aβ (1–40) fibrils<br>Antioxidant<br>Antiapoptotic | [116] |

Table 1. Cont.

| Compound | Activity | Reference |
|---|---|---|
| 5 (Figure 3) | Interaction with Aβ aggregates | [104] |
| 6 (Figure 3) | Depolymerizing activity of tau aggregates<br>Tau aggregation inhibitor<br>γ-secretase activity inhibitor | [104] |
| CNB001 (Figure 3) | Anti-inflammatory | [121] |
| GT863 (Figure 3) | Aβ aggregation inhibitor<br>Tau aggregation inhibitor<br>Inhibitor of glycation of Nicastrin | [123] |
| 7–8a (Figure 3) | Aβ aggregation modulator | [124] |
| 8b (Figure 3) | Tau oligomers modulator | [87] |
| 9–10–11 (Figure 3) | Interaction with Aβ and tau aggregates | [125] |
| THC (Figure 4) | Anti-inflammatory | [126] |
| THDC<br>THBDC<br>THBDC DHPM<br>(Figure 4) | Acetyl cholinesterase inhibitor | [127] |
| CL3–CL8 (Figure 5) | Tau oligomers modulator | [87,128] |
| 12–13 (Figure 6) | Aβ aggregation inhibitor | [111–114] |
| 14 (Figure 6) | BACE1 inhibitor | [129] |
| 15 (Figure 7) | Aβ aggregation inhibitor<br>Diagnostic tool to detect Aβ amyloid | [118] |
| 16 (Figure 7) | Aβ aggregation inhibitor | [130] |
| 17 (Figure 7) | Antioxidant | [60] |
| 18 (Figure 7) | Aβ fibrillation inhibitor | [133] |
| 19 (Figure 8) | BACE1 inhibitor | [103,134] |
| 20–21 (Figure 9) | Metal chelating<br>Scavenger activity against ROS | [135] |
| 22 (Figure 9)<br>24–25 (Figure 10) | Modulators of tau oligomers | [87] |
| 23 (Figure 10) | Protection against Aβ (25–35) toxicity | [137] |
| 26 (Figure 11) | Aβ oligomerization inhibitor<br>Antioxidant | [141] |
| 27 (Figure 11) | Aβ aggregation inhibitor<br>Antioxidant | [142] |
| 28–29 (Figure 11) | Increase of acetyl choline levels<br>Increase of GSH levels<br>Antiapoptotic | [143] |
| 30 (Figure 11) | Aβ aggregation inhibitor<br>Tau-aggregation inhibitor | [145] |
| 31–32–33 (Figure 11) | Acetyl cholinesterase inhibitor<br>Antioxidant<br>Metal chelating | [146,147] |

## 6. Conclusions

After more than two centuries from the first discovery of curcumin, its clinical applications are still under investigation. Many potential applications of this compound are envisioned but its administration and metabolic fate need to be still deeply investigated.

To overcome some issues related to curcumin use as a drug candidate and address its low bioavailability, many curcumin derivatives were synthesized and tested. The field of neuroprotective compounds accounts for hundreds of different derivatives and many of them are promising drugs for the treatment of AD and related diseases. In the next years, the clinical development of these compounds will assess the real effectiveness of curcumin as a lead compound for the synthesis of novel neuroprotective drugs.

**Author Contributions:** All authors contributed to paper selection and discussion. All authors have read and agreed to the published version of the manuscript.

**Funding:** This research and APC were funded by MIUR, within the "FIRB-Futuro in Ricerca 2012" Program-Grant Project RBFR12SIPT. Mitchell Center for Neurodegenerative Diseases, and National Institute of Health grants: R01AG054025, R01NS094557 (R.K.).

**Institutional Review Board Statement:** Not applicable.

**Informed Consent Statement:** Not applicable.

**Data Availability Statement:** Not applicable.

**Conflicts of Interest:** The authors declare no conflict of interest.

## References

1. Newman, D.J.; Cragg, G.M. Natural Products as Sources of New Drugs from 1981 to 2014. *J. Nat. Prod.* **2016**, *79*, 629–661. [CrossRef] [PubMed]
2. Vogel, A.; Pelletier, J. Examen chimique de la racine de Curcuma. *J. Pharm.* **1815**, *1*, 289–300.
3. Ravindran, P.N.; Babu, K.N.; Sivaraman, K. *Turmeric: The Genus Curcuma*; Taylor & Francis: Boca Raton, FL, USA, 2007.
4. Wilken, R.; Veena, M.S.; Wang, M.B.; Srivatsan, E.S. Curcumin: A review of anti-cancer properties and therapeutic activity in head and neck squamous cell carcinoma. *Mol. Cancer* **2011**, *10*, 12. [CrossRef] [PubMed]
5. Nishiyama, T.; Mae, T.; Kishida, H.; Tsukagawa, M.; Mimaki, Y.; Kuroda, M.; Sashida, Y.; Takahashi, K.; Kawada, T.; Nakagawa, K.; et al. Curcuminoids and sesquiterpenoids in turmeric (*Curcuma longa* L.) suppress an increase in blood glucose level in type 2 diabetic KK-Ay mice. *J. Agric. Food Chem.* **2005**, *53*, 959–963. [CrossRef]
6. Prasad, S.; Aggarwal, B.B. Turmeric, the Golden Spice: From Traditional Medicine to Modern Medicine. In *Herbal Medicine: Biomolecular and Clinical Aspects*; Benzie, I.F.F., Wachtel-Galor, S., Eds.; Taylor and Francis Group, LLC.: Boca Raton, FL, USA, 2011.
7. Hatami, M.; Abdolahi, M.; Soveyd, N.; Djalali, M.; Togha, M.; Honarvar, N.M. Molecular Mechanisms of Curcumin in Neuroinflammatory Disorders: A Mini Review of Current Evidences. *Endocr. Metab. Immune Disord. Drug Targets* **2019**, *19*, 247–258. [CrossRef] [PubMed]
8. Sharma, O.P. Antioxidant activity of curcumin and related compounds. *Biochem. Pharmacol.* **1976**, *25*, 1811–1812. [CrossRef]
9. Bagheri, H.; Ghasemi, F.; Barreto, G.E.; Rafiee, R.; Sathyapalan, T.; Sahebkar, A. Effects of curcumin on mitochondria in neurodegenerative diseases. *Biofactors (Oxf. Engl.)* **2020**, *46*, 5–20. [CrossRef]
10. Lakey-Beitia, J.; Berrocal, R.; Rao, K.S.; Durant, A.A. Polyphenols as therapeutic molecules in Alzheimer's disease through modulating amyloid pathways. *Mol. Neurobiol.* **2015**, *51*, 466–479. [CrossRef]
11. Maiti, P.; Dunbar, G.L. Use of Curcumin, a Natural Polyphenol for Targeting Molecular Pathways in Treating Age-Related Neurodegenerative Diseases. *Int. J. Mol. Sci.* **2018**, *19*, 1637. [CrossRef]
12. World Health Organization. Dementia. 21 September 2020. Available online: https://www.who.int/news-room/fact-sheets/detail/dementia (accessed on 9 February 2021).
13. Hardy, J.; Allsop, D. Amyloid deposition as the central event in the aetiology of Alzheimer's disease. *Trends Pharm. Sci.* **1991**, *12*, 383–388. [CrossRef]
14. Citron, M. Alzheimer's disease: Treatments in discovery and development. *Nat. Neurosci.* **2002**, *5*, 1055–1057. [CrossRef]
15. Tarawneh, R.; Holtzman, D.M. The clinical problem of symptomatic Alzheimer disease and mild cognitive impairment. *Cold Spring Harb. Perspect. Med.* **2012**, *2*, a006148. [CrossRef] [PubMed]
16. Jahn, H. Memory loss in Alzheimer's disease. *Dialogues Clin. Neurosci.* **2013**, *15*, 445–454.
17. Mesulam, M.M.; Thompson, C.K.; Weintraub, S.; Rogalski, E.J. The Wernicke conundrum and the anatomy of language comprehension in primary progressive aphasia. *Brain A J. Neurol.* **2015**, *138*, 2423–2437. [CrossRef] [PubMed]
18. Walker, L.C.; LeVine, H. The cerebral proteopathies. *Mol. Neurobiol.* **2000**, *21*, 83–95. [CrossRef]
19. Nedelsky, N.B.; Todd, P.K.; Taylor, J.P. Autophagy and the ubiquitin-proteasome system: Collaborators in neuroprotection. *Biochim. Biophys. Acta* **2008**, *1782*, 691–699. [CrossRef]
20. Sweeney, P.; Park, H.; Baumann, M.; Dunlop, J.; Frydman, J.; Kopito, R.; McCampbell, A.; Leblanc, G.; Venkateswaran, A.; Nurmi, A.; et al. Protein misfolding in neurodegenerative diseases: Implications and strategies. *Transl. Neurodegener.* **2017**, *6*, 6. [CrossRef] [PubMed]
21. Selkoe, D.J. Alzheimer's disease: A central role for amyloid. *J. Neuropathol. Exp. Neurol.* **1994**, *53*, 438–447. [CrossRef]

22. Chiti, F.; Dobson, C.M. Protein Misfolding, Amyloid Formation, and Human Disease: A Summary of Progress Over the Last Decade. *Annu. Rev. Biochem.* **2017**, *86*, 27–68. [CrossRef]
23. Glabe, C.G.; Kayed, R. Common structure and toxic function of amyloid oligomers implies a common mechanism of pathogenesis. *Neurology* **2006**, *66*, S74–S78. [CrossRef] [PubMed]
24. Kayed, R.; Head, E.; Thompson, J.L.; McIntire, T.M.; Milton, S.C.; Cotman, C.W.; Glabe, C.G. Common structure of soluble amyloid oligomers implies common mechanism of pathogenesis. *Science* **2003**, *300*, 486–489. [CrossRef]
25. Lesné, S.; Koh, M.T.; Kotilinek, L.; Kayed, R.; Glabe, C.G.; Yang, A.; Gallagher, M.; Ashe, K.H. A specific amyloid-beta protein assembly in the brain impairs memory. *Nature* **2006**, *440*, 352–357. [CrossRef] [PubMed]
26. Naseri, N.N.; Wang, H.; Guo, J.; Sharma, M.; Luo, W. The complexity of tau in Alzheimer's disease. *Neurosci. Lett.* **2019**, *705*, 183–194. [CrossRef] [PubMed]
27. Alonso, A.; Zaidi, T.; Novak, M.; Grundke-Iqbal, I.; Iqbal, K. Hyperphosphorylation induces self-assembly of tau into tangles of paired helical filaments/straight filaments. *Proc. Natl. Acad. Sci. USA* **2001**, *98*, 6923–6928. [CrossRef]
28. Cook, C.; Stankowski, J.N.; Carlomagno, Y.; Stetler, C.; Petrucelli, L. Acetylation: A new key to unlock tau's role in neurodegeneration. *Alzheimer's Res. Ther.* **2014**, *2*, 29. [CrossRef]
29. Alonso, A.D.; Cohen, L.S.; Corbo, C.; Morozova, V.; ElIdrissi, A.; Phillips, G.; Kleiman, F.E. Hyperphosphorylation of Tau Associates with Changes in Its Function Beyond Microtubule Stability. *Front. Cell. Neurosci.* **2018**, *12*, 338. [CrossRef]
30. Kadavath, H.; Hofele, R.V.; Biernat, J.; Kumar, S.; Tepper, K.; Urlaub, H.; Mandelkow, E.; Zweckstetter, M. Tau stabilizes microtubules by binding at the interface between tubulin heterodimers. *Proc. Natl. Acad. Sci. USA* **2015**, *112*, 7501–7506. [CrossRef] [PubMed]
31. Strang, K.H.; Croft, C.L.; Sorrentino, Z.A.; Chakrabarty, P.; Golde, T.E.; Giasson, B.I. Distinct differences in prion-like seeding and aggregation between Tau protein variants provide mechanistic insights into tauopathies. *J. Biol. Chem.* **2018**, *293*, 2408–2421. [CrossRef]
32. Von Bergen, M.; Friedhoff, P.; Biernat, J.; Heberle, J.; Mandelkow, E.M.; Mandelkow, E. Assembly of tau protein into Alzheimer paired helical filaments depends on a local sequence motif ((306)VQIVYK(311)) forming beta structure. *Proc. Natl. Acad. Sci. USA* **2000**, *97*, 5129–5134. [CrossRef]
33. Belostozky, A.; Richman, M.; Lisniansky, E.; Tovchygrechko, A.; Chill, J.H.; Rahimipour, S. Inhibition of tau-derived hexapeptide aggregation and toxicity by a self-assembled cyclic d,l-alpha-peptide conformational inhibitor. *Chem. Commun. (Camb. Engl.)* **2018**, *54*, 5980–5983. [CrossRef]
34. Gomez-Isla, T.; Hollister, R.; West, H.; Mui, S.; Growdon, J.H.; Petersen, R.C.; Parisi, J.E.; Hyman, B.T. Neuronal loss correlates with but exceeds neurofibrillary tangles in Alzheimer's disease. *Ann. Neurol.* **1997**, *41*, 17–24. [CrossRef] [PubMed]
35. Terry, R.D. Do neuronal inclusions kill the cell? *J. Neural Transm. Suppl.* **2000**, *59*, 91–93. [PubMed]
36. Van De Nes, J.A.; Nafe, R.; Schlote, W. Non-tau based neuronal degeneration in Alzheimer's disease – an immunocytochemical and quantitative study in the supragranular layers of the middle temporal neocortex. *Brain Res.* **2008**, *1213*, 152–165. [CrossRef]
37. Maeda, S.; Sahara, N.; Saito, Y.; Murayama, S.; Ikai, A.; Takashima, A. Increased levels of granular tau oligomers: An early sign of brain aging and Alzheimer's disease. *Neurosci. Res* **2006**, *54*, 197–201. [CrossRef]
38. Lasagna-Reeves, C.A.; Castillo-Carranza, D.L.; Sengupta, U.; Sarmiento, J.; Troncoso, J.; Jackson, G.R.; Kayed, R. Identification of oligomers at early stages of tau aggregation in Alzheimer's disease. *FASEB J.* **2012**. [CrossRef] [PubMed]
39. Patterson, K.R.; Remmers, C.; Fu, Y.; Brooker, S.; Kanaan, N.M.; Vana, L.; Ward, S.; Reyes, J.F.; Philibert, K.; Glucksman, M.J.; et al. Characterization of prefibrillar Tau oligomers in vitro and in Alzheimer disease. *J. Biol. Chem.* **2011**, *286*, 23063–23076. [CrossRef] [PubMed]
40. Gerson, J.E.; Castillo-Carranza, D.L.; Kayed, R. Advances in therapeutics for neurodegenerative tauopathies: Moving toward the specific targeting of the most toxic tau species. *ACS Chem. Neurosci.* **2014**, *5*, 752–769. [CrossRef]
41. Gerson, J.E.; Kayed, R. Formation and propagation of tau oligomeric seeds. *Front. Neurol.* **2013**, *4*, 93. [CrossRef] [PubMed]
42. Usenovic, M.; Niroomand, S.; Drolet, R.E.; Yao, L.; Gaspar, R.C.; Hatcher, N.G.; Schachter, J.; Renger, J.J.; Parmentier-Batteur, S. Internalized Tau Oligomers Cause Neurodegeneration by Inducing Accumulation of Pathogenic Tau in Human Neurons Derived from Induced Pluripotent Stem Cells. *J. Neurosci. Off. J. Soc. Neurosci.* **2015**, *35*, 14234–14250. [CrossRef]
43. Mayeux, R.; Sano, M. Treatment of Alzheimer's disease. *N. Engl. J. Med.* **1999**, *341*, 1670–1679. [CrossRef]
44. Reisberg, B.; Doody, R.; Stöffler, A.; Schmitt, F.; Ferris, S.; Möbius, H.J. Memantine in moderate-to-severe Alzheimer's disease. *N. Engl. J. Med.* **2003**, *348*, 1333–1341. [CrossRef]
45. Yang, F.; Lim, G.P.; Begum, A.N.; Ubeda, O.J.; Simmons, M.R.; Ambegaokar, S.S.; Chen, P.P.; Kayed, R.; Glabe, C.G.; Frautschy, S.A.; et al. Curcumin inhibits formation of amyloid beta oligomers and fibrils, binds plaques, and reduces amyloid in vivo. *J. Biol. Chem.* **2005**, *280*, 5892–5901. [CrossRef]
46. Necula, M.; Kayed, R.; Milton, S.; Glabe, C.G. Small molecule inhibitors of aggregation indicate that amyloid beta oligomerization and fibrillization pathways are independent and distinct. *J. Biol. Chem.* **2007**, *282*, 10311–10324. [CrossRef]
47. Thapa, A.; Jett, S.D.; Chi, E.Y. Curcumin Attenuates Amyloid-β Aggregate Toxicity and Modulates Amyloid-β Aggregation Pathway. *ACS Chem. Neurosci.* **2016**, *7*, 56–68. [CrossRef] [PubMed]
48. Ma, Z.; Wang, N.; He, H.; Tang, X. Pharmaceutical strategies of improving oral systemic bioavailability of curcumin for clinical application. *J. Control. Release Off. J. Control. Release Soc.* **2019**, *316*, 359–380. [CrossRef] [PubMed]

49. Rane, J.S.; Bhaumik, P.; Panda, D. Curcumin Inhibits Tau Aggregation and Disintegrates Preformed Tau Filaments in vitro. *J. Alzheimer's Dis. JAD* **2017**, *60*, 999–1014. [CrossRef] [PubMed]
50. Pandey, N.; Strider, J.; Nolan, W.C.; Yan, S.X.; Galvin, J.E. Curcumin inhibits aggregation of alpha-synuclein. *Acta Neuropathol.* **2008**, *115*, 479–489. [CrossRef]
51. Wang, M.S.; Boddapati, S.; Emadi, S.; Sierks, M.R. Curcumin reduces α-synuclein induced cytotoxicity in Parkinson's disease cell model. *BMC Neurosci.* **2010**, *11*, 57. [CrossRef]
52. Liu, Z.; Yu, Y.; Li, X.; Ross, C.A.; Smith, W.W. Curcumin protects against A53T alpha-synuclein-induced toxicity in a PC12 inducible cell model for Parkinsonism. *Pharmacol. Res.* **2011**, *63*, 439–444. [CrossRef]
53. Kim, G.Y.; Kim, K.H.; Lee, S.H.; Yoon, M.S.; Lee, H.J.; Moon, D.O.; Lee, C.M.; Ahn, S.C.; Park, Y.C.; Park, Y.M. Curcumin inhibits immunostimulatory function of dendritic cells: MAPKs and translocation of NF-kappa B as potential targets. *J. Immunol.* **2005**, *174*, 8116–8124. [CrossRef] [PubMed]
54. Baum, L.; Ng, A. Curcumin interaction with copper and iron suggests one possible mechanism of action in Alzheimer's disease animal models. *J. Alzheimer's Dis. JAD* **2004**, *6*, 367–377. [CrossRef]
55. Lampe, V.; Milobedzka, J. Studien über Curcumin. *Ber. Der Dtsch. Chem. Ges.* **2006**, *46*, 2235–2240. [CrossRef]
56. Pabon, H.J.J. A synthesis of curcumin and related compounds. *Recueil Travaux Chimiques Pays-Bas* **1964**, *83*, 379–386. [CrossRef]
57. Krackov, M.H.; Bellis, H.E. Process for the Synthesis of Curcumin Related Compounds. US Patent 5,679,864, 21 October 1997.
58. Babu, K.V.D.; Rajasekharan, K.N. Simplified condition for synthesis of Curcumin I and other curcuminoids. *Org. Prep. Proced. Int.* **1994**, *26*, 674–677. [CrossRef]
59. Rao, E.V.; Sudheer, P. Revisiting curcumin chemistry part I: A new strategy for the synthesis of curcuminoids. *Indian J. Pharm. Sci.* **2011**, *73*, 262–270. [CrossRef]
60. Venkateswarlu, S.; Ramachandra, M.S.; Subbaraju, G.V. Synthesis and biological evaluation of polyhydroxycurcuminoids. *Bioorg. Med. Chem.* **2005**, *13*, 6374–6380. [CrossRef]
61. Buadonpri, W.; Wichitnithad, W.; Rojsitthisak, P.; Towiwat, P. Synthetic Curcumin Inhibits Carrageenan-Induced Paw Edema in Rats. *J. Health Res.* **2018**, *23*, 11–16.
62. Priyadarsini, K.I. The chemistry of curcumin: From extraction to therapeutic agent. *Molecules* **2014**, *19*, 20091–20112. [CrossRef]
63. Jovanovic, S.V.; Steenken, S.; Boone, C.W.; Simic, M.G. H-Atom Transfer Is A Preferred Antioxidant Mechanism of Curcumin. *J. Am. Chem. Soc.* **1999**, *121*, 9677–9681. [CrossRef]
64. Basnet, P.; Skalko-Basnet, N. Curcumin: An anti-inflammatory molecule from a curry spice on the path to cancer treatment. *Molecules* **2011**, *16*, 4567–4598. [CrossRef]
65. Lee, W.-H.; Loo, C.-Y.; Bebawy, M.; Luk, F.; Mason, R.S.; Rohanizadeh, R. Curcumin and its derivatives: Their application in neuropharmacology and neuroscience in the 21st century. *Curr. Neuropharmacol.* **2013**, *11*, 338–378. [CrossRef]
66. Parimita, S.P.; Ramshankar, Y.V.; Suresh, S.; Guru Row, T.N. Redetermination of curcumin: (1E,4Z,6E)-5-hydroxy-1,7-bis(4-hydroxy-3-methoxyphenyl)hepta-1,4,6-trien-3-one. *Acta Crystallogr. Sect. E* **2007**, *63*, o860–o862. [CrossRef]
67. Balasubramanian, K. Molecular Orbital Basis for Yellow Curry Spice Curcumin's Prevention of Alzheimer's Disease. *J. Agric. Food Chem.* **2006**, *54*, 3512–3520. [CrossRef] [PubMed]
68. Chignell, C.F.; Bilski, P.; Reszka, K.J.; Motten, A.G.; Sik, R.H.; Dahl, T.A. Spectral and photochemical properties of curcumin. *Photochem. Photobiol.* **1994**, *59*, 295–302. [CrossRef] [PubMed]
69. Yang, K.Y.; Lin, L.C.; Tseng, T.Y.; Wang, S.C.; Tsai, T.H. Oral bioavailability of curcumin in rat and the herbal analysis from *Curcuma longa* by LC-MS/MS. *J. Chromatogr. BAnal. Technol. Biomed. Life Sci.* **2007**, *853*, 183–189. [CrossRef] [PubMed]
70. Prasad, S.; Tyagi, A.K.; Aggarwal, B.B. Recent developments in delivery, bioavailability, absorption and metabolism of curcumin: The golden pigment from golden spice. *Cancer Res. Treat. Off. J. Korean Cancer Assoc.* **2014**, *46*, 2–18. [CrossRef]
71. Vareed, S.K.; Kakarala, M.; Ruffin, M.T.; Crowell, J.A.; Normolle, D.P.; Djuric, Z.; Brenner, D.E. Pharmacokinetics of curcumin conjugate metabolites in healthy human subjects. *Cancer Epidemiol. Biomark. Prev.* **2008**, *17*, 1411–1417. [CrossRef] [PubMed]
72. Sun, J.; Bi, C.; Chan, H.M.; Sun, S.; Zhang, Q.; Zheng, Y. Curcumin-loaded solid lipid nanoparticles have prolonged in vitro antitumour activity, cellular uptake and improved in vivo bioavailability. *Coll. Surf. B Biointerfaces* **2013**, *111*, 367–375. [CrossRef]
73. Asai, A.; Miyazawa, T. Occurrence of orally administered curcuminoid as glucuronide and glucuronide/sulfate conjugates in rat plasma. *Life Sci.* **2000**, *67*, 2785–2793. [CrossRef]
74. Nelson, K.M.; Dahlin, J.L.; Bisson, J.; Graham, J.; Pauli, G.F.; Walters, M.A. The Essential Medicinal Chemistry of Curcumin. *J. Med. Chem.* **2017**, *60*, 1620–1637. [CrossRef]
75. Priyadarsini, K.I. Photophysics, photochemistry and photobiology of curcumin: Studies from organic solutions, bio-mimetics and living cells. *J. Photochem. Photobiol. C Photochem. Rev.* **2009**, *10*, 81–95. [CrossRef]
76. Khurana, A.; Ho, C.-T. High Performance Liquid Chromatographic Analysis of Curcuminoids and Their Photo-oxidative Decomposition Compounds in *Curcuma longa*, L. *J. Liq. Chromatogr.* **1988**, *11*, 2295–2304. [CrossRef]
77. Ringman, J.M.; Frautschy, S.A.; Teng, E.; Begum, A.N.; Bardens, J.; Beigi, M.; Gylys, K.H.; Badmaev, V.; Heath, D.D.; Apostolova, L.G.; et al. Oral curcumin for Alzheimer's disease: Tolerability and efficacy in a 24-week randomized, double blind, placebo-controlled study. *Alzheimer's Res. Ther.* **2012**, *4*, 43. [CrossRef] [PubMed]
78. Andrade, S.; Ramalho, M.J.; Loureiro, J.A.; Pereira, M.d.C. Natural Compounds for Alzheimer's Disease Therapy: A Systematic Review of Preclinical and Clinical Studies. *Int. J. Mol. Sci.* **2019**, *20*, 2313. [CrossRef] [PubMed]

79. Ross, C.; Taylor, M.; Fullwood, N.; Allsop, D. Liposome delivery systems for the treatment of Alzheimer's disease. *Int. J. Nanomed.* **2018**, *13*, 8507–8522. [CrossRef]
80. Giacomeli, R.; Izoton, J.C.; Dos Santos, R.B.; Boeira, S.P.; Jesse, C.R.; Haas, S.E. Neuroprotective effects of curcumin lipid-core nanocapsules in a model Alzheimer's disease induced by β-amyloid 1-42 peptide in aged female mice. *Brain Res.* **2019**, *1721*, 146325. [CrossRef] [PubMed]
81. Yang, R.; Zheng, Y.; Wang, Q.; Zhao, L. Curcumin-loaded chitosan-bovine serum albumin nanoparticles potentially enhanced Aβ 42 phagocytosis and modulated macrophage polarization in Alzheimer's disease. *Nanoscale Res. Lett.* **2018**, *13*, 330. [CrossRef]
82. Li, X.; Uehara, S.; Sawangrat, K.; Morishita, M.; Kusamori, K.; Katsumi, H.; Sakane, T.; Yamamoto, A. Improvement of intestinal absorption of curcumin by cyclodextrins and the mechanisms underlying absorption enhancement. *Int. J. Pharm.* **2018**, *535*, 340–349. [CrossRef]
83. Suresh, K.; Nangia, A. Curcumin: Pharmaceutical solids as a platform to improve solubility and bioavailability. *CrystEngComm* **2018**, *20*, 3277–3296. [CrossRef]
84. Sanphui, P.; Bolla, G. Curcumin, a Biological Wonder Molecule: A Crystal Engineering Point of View. *Cryst. Growth Des.* **2018**, *18*, 5690–5711. [CrossRef]
85. Wang, H.; Sui, H.; Zheng, Y.; Jiang, Y.; Shi, Y.; Liang, J.; Zhao, L. Curcumin-primed exosomes potently ameliorate cognitive function in AD mice by inhibiting hyperphosphorylation of the Tau protein through the AKT/GSK-3β pathway. *Nanoscale* **2019**, *11*, 7481–7496. [CrossRef]
86. Farkhondeh, T.; Samarghandian, S.; Pourbagher-Shahri, A.M.; Sedaghat, M. The impact of curcumin and its modified formulations on Alzheimer's disease. *J. Cell. Physiol.* **2019**, *234*, 16953–16965. [CrossRef] [PubMed]
87. Lo Cascio, F.; Puangmalai, N.; Ellsworth, A.; Bucchieri, F.; Pace, A.; Palumbo Piccionello, A.; Kayed, R. Toxic Tau Oligomers Modulated by Novel Curcumin Derivatives. *Sci. Rep.* **2019**, *9*, 19011. [CrossRef] [PubMed]
88. Pithadia, A.S.; Bhunia, A.; Sribalan, R.; Padmini, V.; Fierke, C.A.; Ramamoorthy, A. Influence of a curcumin derivative on hIAPP aggregation in the absence and presence of lipid membranes. *Chem. Commun. (Camb. Engl.)* **2016**, *52*, 942–945. [CrossRef] [PubMed]
89. Murphy, R.M. Kinetics of amyloid formation and membrane interaction with amyloidogenic proteins. *Biochim. Biophys. Acta* **2007**, *1768*, 1923–1934. [CrossRef] [PubMed]
90. Fändrich, M.; Schmidt, M.; Grigorieff, N. Recent progress in understanding Alzheimer's β-amyloid structures. *Trends Biochem. Sci.* **2011**, *36*, 338–345. [CrossRef] [PubMed]
91. Tjernberg, L.O.; Näslund, J.; Lindqvist, F.; Johansson, J.; Karlström, A.R.; Thyberg, J.; Terenius, L.; Nordstedt, C. Arrest of beta-amyloid fibril formation by a pentapeptide ligand. *J. Biol. Chem.* **1996**, *271*, 8545–8548. [CrossRef] [PubMed]
92. Belluti, F.; Rampa, A.; Gobbi, S.; Bisi, A. Small-molecule inhibitors/modulators of amyloid-β peptide aggregation and toxicity for the treatment of Alzheimer's disease: A patent review (2010–2012). *Expert Opin. Ther. Pat.* **2013**, *23*, 581–596. [CrossRef]
93. Reinke, A.A.; Gestwicki, J.E. Structure-activity relationships of amyloid beta-aggregation inhibitors based on curcumin: Influence of linker length and flexibility. *Chem. Biol. Drug Des.* **2007**, *70*, 206–215. [CrossRef]
94. Buchete, N.-V.; Hummer, G. Structure and dynamics of parallel beta-sheets, hydrophobic core, and loops in Alzheimer's A beta fibrils. *Biophys. J.* **2007**, *92*, 3032–3039. [CrossRef]
95. Miller, L.M.; Wang, Q.; Telivala, T.P.; Smith, R.J.; Lanzirotti, A.; Miklossy, J. Synchrotron-based infrared and X-ray imaging shows focalized accumulation of Cu and Zn co-localized with beta-amyloid deposits in Alzheimer's disease. *J. Struct. Biol.* **2006**, *155*, 30–37. [CrossRef]
96. Huang, X.; Atwood, C.S.; Moir, R.D.; Hartshorn, M.A.; Tanzi, R.E.; Bush, A.I. Trace metal contamination initiates the apparent auto-aggregation, amyloidosis, and oligomerization of Alzheimer's Aβ peptides. *JBIC J. Biol. Inorg. Chem.* **2004**, *9*, 954–960. [CrossRef]
97. Liu, Y.; Nguyen, M.; Robert, A.; Meunier, B. Metal Ions in Alzheimer's Disease: A Key Role or Not? *Acc. Chem. Res.* **2019**, *52*, 2026–2035. [CrossRef]
98. Aggarwal, B.B.; Harikumar, K.B. Potential therapeutic effects of curcumin, the anti-inflammatory agent, against neurodegenerative, cardiovascular, pulmonary, metabolic, autoimmune and neoplastic diseases. *Int. J. Biochem. Cell Biol.* **2009**, *41*, 40–59. [CrossRef] [PubMed]
99. Zhang, X.; Tian, Y.; Li, Z.; Tian, X.; Sun, H.; Liu, H.; Moore, A.; Ran, C. Design and Synthesis of Curcumin Analogues for in Vivo Fluorescence Imaging and Inhibiting Copper-Induced Cross-Linking of Amyloid Beta Species in Alzheimer's Disease. *J. Am. Chem. Soc.* **2013**, *135*, 16397–16409. [CrossRef] [PubMed]
100. Fiala, M.; Liu, P.T.; Espinosa-Jeffrey, A.; Rosenthal, M.J.; Bernard, G.; Ringman, J.M.; Sayre, J.; Zhang, L.; Zaghi, J.; Dejbakhsh, S.; et al. Innate immunity and transcription of MGAT-III and Toll-like receptors in Alzheimer's disease patients are improved by bisdemethoxycurcumin. *Proc. Natl. Acad. Sci. USA* **2007**, *104*, 12849–12854. [CrossRef]
101. Gagliardi, S.; Franco, V.; Sorrentino, S.; Zucca, S.; Pandini, C.; Rota, P.; Bernuzzi, S.; Costa, A.; Sinforiani, E.; Pansarasa, O.; et al. Curcumin and Novel Synthetic Analogs in Cell-Based Studies of Alzheimer's Disease. *Front. Pharmacol.* **2018**, *9*, 1404. [CrossRef] [PubMed]
102. Das, U.; Wang, L.; Ganguly, A.; Saikia, J.M.; Wagner, S.L.; Koo, E.H.; Roy, S. Visualizing APP and BACE-1 approximation in neurons yields insight into the amyloidogenic pathway. *Nat. Neurosci.* **2016**, *19*, 55–64. [CrossRef]

103. Konno, H.; Endo, H.; Ise, S.; Miyazaki, K.; Aoki, H.; Sanjoh, A.; Kobayashi, K.; Hattori, Y.; Akaji, K. Synthesis and evaluation of curcumin derivatives toward an inhibitor of beta-site amyloid precursor protein cleaving enzyme 1. *Bioorganic Med. Chem. Lett.* **2014**, *24*, 685–690. [CrossRef] [PubMed]
104. Narlawar, R.; Pickhardt, M.; Leuchtenberger, S.; Baumann, K.; Krause, S.; Dyrks, T.; Weggen, S.; Mandelkow, E.; Schmidt, B. Curcumin-derived pyrazoles and isoxazoles: Swiss army knives or blunt tools for Alzheimer's disease? *ChemMedChem* **2008**, *3*, 165–172. [CrossRef] [PubMed]
105. Avila, J.; Jiménez, J.S.; Sayas, C.L.; Bolós, M.; Zabala, J.C.; Rivas, G.; Hernández, F. Tau Structures. *Front. Aging Neurosci.* **2016**, *8*, 262. [CrossRef]
106. Liu, W.; Hu, X.; Zhou, L.; Tu, Y.; Shi, S.; Yao, T. Orientation-Inspired Perspective on Molecular Inhibitor of Tau Aggregation by Curcumin Conjugated with Ruthenium(II) Complex Scaffold. *J. Phys. Chem. B* **2020**, *124*, 2343–2353. [CrossRef]
107. Priyadarsini, K.I.; Maity, D.K.; Naik, G.H.; Kumar, M.S.; Unnikrishnan, M.K.; Satav, J.G.; Mohan, H. Role of phenolic O-H and methylene hydrogen on the free radical reactions and antioxidant activity of curcumin. *Free Radic. Biol. Med.* **2003**, *35*, 475–484. [CrossRef]
108. Mishra, B.; Priyadarsini, K.I.; Bhide, M.K.; Kadam, R.M.; Mohan, H. Reactions of superoxide radicals with curcumin: Probable mechanisms by optical spectroscopy and EPR. *Free Radic. Res.* **2004**, *38*, 355–362. [CrossRef]
109. Ferrari, E.; Benassi, R.; Saladini, M.; Orteca, G.; Gazova, Z.; Siposova, K. In vitro study on potential pharmacological activity of curcumin analogues and their copper complexes. *Chem. Biol. Drug Des.* **2017**, *89*, 411–419. [CrossRef]
110. Ohori, H.; Yamakoshi, H.; Tomizawa, M.; Shibuya, M.; Kakudo, Y.; Takahashi, A.; Takahashi, S.; Kato, S.; Suzuki, T.; Ishioka, C.; et al. Synthesis and biological analysis of new curcumin analogues bearing an enhanced potential for the medicinal treatment of cancer. *Mol. Cancer Ther.* **2006**, *5*, 2563–2571. [CrossRef] [PubMed]
111. Orlando, R.A.; Gonzales, A.M.; Royer, R.E.; Deck, L.M.; Vander Jagt, D.L. A Chemical Analog of Curcumin as an Improved Inhibitor of Amyloid Abeta Oligomerization. *PLoS ONE* **2012**, *7*, e31869. [CrossRef] [PubMed]
112. Shetty, D.; Kim, Y.J.; Shim, H.; Snyder, J.P. Eliminating the heart from the curcumin molecule: Monocarbonyl curcumin mimics (MACs). *Molecules* **2014**, *20*, 249–292. [CrossRef] [PubMed]
113. Chen, S.-Y.; Chen, Y.; Li, Y.-P.; Chen, S.-H.; Tan, J.-H.; Ou, T.-M.; Gu, L.-Q.; Huang, Z.-S. Design, synthesis, and biological evaluation of curcumin analogues as multifunctional agents for the treatment of Alzheimer's disease. *Bioorganic Med. Chem.* **2011**, *19*, 5596–5604. [CrossRef] [PubMed]
114. Ramshini, H.; mohammad-zadeh, M.; Ebrahim-Habibi, A. Inhibition of amyloid fibril formation and cytotoxicity by a chemical analog of Curcumin as a stable inhibitor. *Int. J. Biol. Macromol.* **2015**, *78*, 396–404. [CrossRef]
115. Ao, G.-Z.; Chu, X.-J.; Ji, Y.-Y.; Wang, J.-W. Antioxidant properties and PC12 cell protective effects of a novel curcumin analogue (2E,6E)-2,6-bis(3,5- dimethoxybenzylidene)cyclohexanone (MCH). *Int. J. Mol. Sci.* **2014**, *15*, 3970–3988. [CrossRef]
116. Orteca, G.; Tavanti, F.; Bednarikova, Z.; Gazova, Z.; Rigillo, G.; Imbriano, C.; Basile, V.; Asti, M.; Rigamonti, L.; Saladini, M.; et al. Curcumin derivatives and Aβ-fibrillar aggregates: An interactions' study for diagnostic/therapeutic purposes in neurodegenerative diseases. *Bioorganic Med. Chem.* **2018**, *26*, 4288–4300. [CrossRef] [PubMed]
117. Pedersen, U.; Rasmussen, P.B.; Lawesson, S.-O. Synthesis of Naturally Occurring Curcuminoids and Related Compounds. *Liebigs Ann. Der Chem.* **1985**, *1985*, 1557–1569. [CrossRef]
118. Yanagisawa, D.; Shirai, N.; Amatsubo, T.; Taguchi, H.; Hirao, K.; Urushitani, M.; Morikawa, S.; Inubushi, T.; Kato, M.; Kato, F.; et al. Relationship between the tautomeric structures of curcumin derivatives and their Abeta-binding activities in the context of therapies for Alzheimer's disease. *Biomaterials* **2010**, *31*, 4179–4185. [CrossRef]
119. Jayaraj, R.L.; Elangovan, N.; Dhanalakshmi, C.; Manivasagam, T.; Essa, M.M. CNB-001, a novel pyrazole derivative mitigates motor impairments associated with neurodegeneration via suppression of neuroinflammatory and apoptotic response in experimental Parkinson's disease mice. *Chem. Biol. Interact.* **2014**, *220*, 149–157. [CrossRef] [PubMed]
120. Maher, P.; Akaishi, T.; Schubert, D.; Abe, K. A pyrazole derivative of curcumin enhances memory. *Neurobiol. Aging* **2010**, *31*, 706–709. [CrossRef]
121. Akaishi, T.; Abe, K. CNB-001, a synthetic pyrazole derivative of curcumin, suppresses lipopolysaccharide-induced nitric oxide production through the inhibition of NF-κB and p38 MAPK pathways in microglia. *Eur. J. Pharmacol.* **2018**, *819*, 190–197. [CrossRef] [PubMed]
122. Okuda, M.; Hijikuro, I.; Fujita, Y.; Teruya, T.; Kawakami, H.; Takahashi, T.; Sugimoto, H. Design and synthesis of curcumin derivatives as tau and amyloid β dual aggregation inhibitors. *Bioorganic Med. Chem. Lett.* **2016**, *26*, 5024–5028. [CrossRef] [PubMed]
123. Urano, Y.; Takahachi, M.; Higashiura, R.; Fujiwara, H.; Funamoto, S.; Imai, S.; Futai, E.; Okuda, M.; Sugimoto, H.; Noguchi, N. Curcumin Derivative GT863 Inhibits Amyloid-Beta Production via Inhibition of Protein N-Glycosylation. *Cells* **2020**, *9*, 349. [CrossRef] [PubMed]
124. Battisti, A.; Palumbo Piccionello, A.; Sgarbossa, A.; Vilasi, S.; Ricci, C.; Ghetti, F.; Spinozzi, F.; Marino Gammazza, A.; Giacalone, V.; Martorana, A.; et al. Curcumin-like compounds designed to modify amyloid beta peptide aggregation patterns. *RSC Adv.* **2017**, *7*, 31714–31724. [CrossRef]
125. Boländer, A.; Kieser, D.; Voss, C.; Bauer, S.; Schön, C.; Burgold, S.; Bittner, T.; Hölzer, J.; Heyny-Von Haußen, R.; Mall, G.; et al. Bis(arylvinyl)pyrazines, -pyrimidines, and -pyridazines As Imaging Agents for Tau Fibrils and β-Amyloid Plaques in Alzheimer's Disease Models. *J. Med. Chem.* **2012**, *55*, 9170–9180. [CrossRef] [PubMed]

126. Begum, A.N.; Jones, M.R.; Lim, G.P.; Morihara, T.; Kim, P.; Heath, D.D.; Rock, C.L.; Pruitt, M.A.; Yang, F.; Hudspeth, B.; et al. Curcumin structure-function, bioavailability, and efficacy in models of neuroinflammation and Alzheimer's disease. *J. Pharmacol. Exp. Ther.* **2008**, *326*, 196–208. [CrossRef] [PubMed]
127. Arunkhamkaew, S.; Athipornchai, A.; Apiratikul, N.; Suksamrarn, A.; Ajavakom, V. Novel racemic tetrahydrocurcuminoid dihydropyrimidinone analogues as potent acetylcholinesterase inhibitors. *Bioorg. Med. Chem. Lett.* **2013**, *23*, 2880–2882. [CrossRef]
128. Lo Cascio, F.; Garcia, S.; Montalbano, M.; Puangmalai, N.; McAllen, S.; Pace, A.; Palumbo Piccionello, A.; Kayed, R. Modulating Disease-Relevant Tau Oligomeric Strains by Small Molecules. *J. Biol. Chem.* **2020**. [CrossRef]
129. Endo, H.; Nikaido, Y.; Nakadate, M.; Ise, S.; Konno, H. Structure activity relationship study of curcumin analogues toward the amyloid-beta aggregation inhibitor. *Bioorg. Med. Chem. Lett.* **2014**, *24*, 5621–5626. [CrossRef]
130. Cashman, J.R.; Fiala, M. Diagnostic Methods And genetic Markers for Alzheimer Disease. U.S. Patent Application No. 12/407,756, 22 October 2009.
131. Batie, S.; Lee, J.H.; Jama, R.A.; Browder, D.O.; Montano, L.A.; Huynh, C.C.; Marcus, L.M.; Tsosie, D.G.; Mohammed, Z.; Trang, V.; et al. Synthesis and biological evaluation of halogenated curcumin analogs as potential nuclear receptor selective agonists. *Bioorg. Med. Chem.* **2013**, *21*, 693–702. [CrossRef] [PubMed]
132. Cramer, P.E.; Cirrito, J.R.; Wesson, D.W.; Lee, C.Y.; Karlo, J.C.; Zinn, A.E.; Casali, B.T.; Restivo, J.L.; Goebel, W.D.; James, M.J.; et al. ApoE-directed therapeutics rapidly clear β-amyloid and reverse deficits in AD mouse models. *Science* **2012**, *335*, 1503–1506. [CrossRef]
133. Bisceglia, F.; Seghetti, F.; Serra, M.; Zusso, M.; Gervasoni, S.; Verga, L.; Vistoli, G.; Lanni, C.; Catanzaro, M.; De Lorenzi, E.; et al. Prenylated Curcumin Analogues as Multipotent Tools to Tackle Alzheimer's Disease. *ACS Chem. Neurosci.* **2019**, *10*, 1420–1433. [CrossRef]
134. Kumar, B.; Singh, V.; Shankar, R.; Kumar, K.; Rawal, R.K. Synthetic and Medicinal Prospective of Structurally Modified Curcumins. *Curr. Top. Med. Chem.* **2017**, *17*, 148–161. [CrossRef]
135. Nieto, C.I.; Cornago, M.P.; Cabildo, M.P.; Sanz, D.; Claramunt, R.M.; Torralba, M.C.; Torres, M.R.; Martínez Casanova, D.; Sánchez-Alegre, Y.R.; Escudero, E.; et al. Evaluation of the Antioxidant and Neuroprotectant Activities of New Asymmetrical 1,3-Diketones. *Molecules* **2018**, *23*, 1837. [CrossRef] [PubMed]
136. Park, S.Y.; Kim, D.S. Discovery of natural products from *Curcuma longa* that protect cells from beta-amyloid insult: A drug discovery effort against Alzheimer's disease. *J. Nat. Prod.* **2002**, *65*, 1227–1231. [CrossRef]
137. Kim, D.S.; Kim, J.Y. Total synthesis of Calebin-A, preparation of its analogues, and their neuronal cell protectivity against beta-amyloid insult. *Bioorg. Med. Chem. Lett.* **2001**, *11*, 2541–2543. [CrossRef]
138. Majeed, M.; Nagabhushanam, K.; Majeed, A.; Thomas, S.M. Synthesis of Calebin-A and its Biologically Active Analogs. U.S. Patent No. 9,365,486, 14 June 2016.
139. Rosales-Corral, S.A.; Acuña-Castroviejo, D.; Coto-Montes, A.; Boga, J.A.; Manchester, L.C.; Fuentes-Broto, L.; Korkmaz, A.; Ma, S.; Tan, D.-X.; Reiter, R.J. Alzheimer's disease: Pathological mechanisms and the beneficial role of melatonin. *J. Pineal Res.* **2012**, *52*, 167–202. [CrossRef] [PubMed]
140. Zhou, J.N.; Liu, R.Y.; Kamphorst, W.; Hofman, M.A.; Swaab, D.F. Early neuropathological Alzheimer's changes in aged individuals are accompanied by decreased cerebrospinal fluid melatonin levels. *J. Pineal Res.* **2003**, *35*, 125–130. [CrossRef] [PubMed]
141. Chojnacki, J.E.; Liu, K.; Yan, X.; Toldo, S.; Selden, T.; Estrada, M.; Rodríguez-Franco, M.I.; Halquist, M.S.; Ye, D.; Zhang, S. Discovery of 5-(4-Hydroxyphenyl)-3-oxo-pentanoic Acid [2-(5-Methoxy-1H-indol-3-yl)-ethyl]-amide as a Neuroprotectant for Alzheimer's Disease by Hybridization of Curcumin and Melatonin. *ACS Chem. Neurosci.* **2014**, *5*, 690–699. [CrossRef]
142. Chojnacki, J.E.; Liu, K.; Saathoff, J.M.; Zhang, S. Bivalent ligands incorporating curcumin and diosgenin as multifunctional compounds against Alzheimer's disease. *Bioorg. Med. Chem.* **2015**, *23*, 7324–7331. [CrossRef] [PubMed]
143. Elmegeed, G.A.; Ahmed, H.H.; Hashash, M.A.; Abd-Elhalim, M.M.; El-kady, D.S. Synthesis of novel steroidal curcumin derivatives as anti-Alzheimer's disease candidates: Evidences-based on in vivo study. *Steroids* **2015**, *101*, 78–89. [CrossRef]
144. Harish, G.; Venkateshappa, C.; Mythri, R.B.; Dubey, S.K.; Mishra, K.; Singh, N.; Vali, S.; Bharath, M.M.S. Bioconjugates of curcumin display improved protection against glutathione depletion mediated oxidative stress in a dopaminergic neuronal cell line: Implications for Parkinson's disease. *Bioorg. Med. Chem.* **2010**, *18*, 2631–2638. [CrossRef] [PubMed]
145. Dolai, S.; Shi, W.; Corbo, C.; Sun, C.; Averick, S.; Obeysekera, D.; Farid, M.; Alonso, A.; Banerjee, P.; Raja, K. "Clicked" Sugar–Curcumin Conjugate: Modulator of Amyloid-β and Tau Peptide Aggregation at Ultralow Concentrations. *ACS Chem. Neurosci.* **2011**, *2*, 694–699. [CrossRef]
146. Yan, J.; Hu, J.; Liu, A.; He, L.; Li, X.; Wei, H. Design, synthesis, and evaluation of multitarget-directed ligands against Alzheimer's disease based on the fusion of donepezil and curcumin. *Bioorg. Med. Chem.* **2017**, *25*, 2946–2955. [CrossRef]
147. Dias, K.S.; De Paula, C.T.; Dos Santos, T.; Souza, I.N.; Boni, M.S.; Guimarães, M.J.; Da Silva, F.M.; Castro, N.G.; Neves, G.A.; Veloso, C.C.; et al. Design, synthesis and evaluation of novel feruloyl-donepezil hybrids as potential multitarget drugs for the treatment of Alzheimer's disease. *Eur. J. Med. Chem.* **2017**, *130*, 440–457. [CrossRef] [PubMed]
148. Liu, Z.; Fang, L.; Zhang, H.; Gou, S.; Chen, L. Design, synthesis and biological evaluation of multifunctional tacrine-curcumin hybrids as new cholinesterase inhibitors with metal ions-chelating and neuroprotective property. *Bioorg. Med. Chem.* **2017**, *25*. [CrossRef] [PubMed]

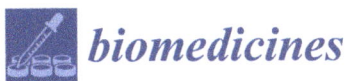 

*Review*

# Critical Molecular and Cellular Contributors to Tau Pathology

Liqing Song, Evan A. Wells and Anne Skaja Robinson *

Department of Chemical Engineering, Carnegie Mellon University, Pittsburgh, PA 15213, USA; liqing@cmu.edu (L.S.); eawells@andrew.cmu.edu (E.A.W.)
* Correspondence: anne.robinson@cmu.edu; Tel.: (+1)-412-268-7673

**Abstract:** Tauopathies represent a group of neurodegenerative diseases including Alzheimer's disease (AD) that are characterized by the deposition of filamentous tau aggregates in the brain. The pathogenesis of tauopathies starts from the formation of toxic 'tau seeds' from hyperphosphorylated tau monomers. The presence of specific phosphorylation sites and heat shock protein 90 facilitates soluble tau protein aggregation. Transcellular propagation of pathogenic tau into synaptically connected neuronal cells or adjacent glial cells via receptor-mediated endocytosis facilitate disease spread through the brain. While neuroprotective effects of glial cells—including phagocytotic microglial and astroglial phenotypes—have been observed at the early stage of neurodegeneration, dysfunctional neuronal-glial cellular communication results in a series of further pathological consequences as the disease progresses, including abnormal axonal transport, synaptic degeneration, and neuronal loss, accompanied by a pro-inflammatory microenvironment. Additionally, the discovery of microtubule-associated protein tau (*MAPT*) gene mutations and the strongest genetic risk factor of tauopathies—an increase in the presence of the ε2 allele of apolipoprotein E (*ApoE*)—provide important clues to understanding tau pathology progression. In this review, we describe the crucial signaling pathways and diverse cellular contributors to the progression of tauopathies. A systematic understanding of disease pathogenesis provides novel insights into therapeutic targets within altered signaling pathways and is of great significance for discovering effective treatments for tauopathies.

**Keywords:** tauopathies; Alzheimer's disease; prion-like propagation; tau self-aggregation; endocytosis; neuron-glial communication; neuroinflammation; apolipoprotein E

Citation: Song, L.; Wells, E.A.; Robinson, A.S. Critical Molecular and Cellular Contributors to Tau Pathology. *Biomedicines* **2021**, *9*, 190. https://doi.org/10.3390/biomedicines9020190

Academic Editor: Lorenzo Falsetti

Received: 18 January 2021
Accepted: 11 February 2021
Published: 14 February 2021

**Publisher's Note:** MDPI stays neutral with regard to jurisdictional claims in published maps and institutional affiliations.

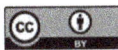

**Copyright:** © 2021 by the authors. Licensee MDPI, Basel, Switzerland. This article is an open access article distributed under the terms and conditions of the Creative Commons Attribution (CC BY) license (https:// creativecommons.org/licenses/by/ 4.0/).

## 1. Introduction

Intraneuronal accumulation of neurofibrillary tangles (NFT) made of abnormally hyperphosphorylated tau is centrally involved in the pathogenesis of primary tauopathies, such as supranuclear palsy (PSP), corticobasal degeneration (CBD), Pick's disease (PiD), and frontotemporal dementia with Parkinsonism linked to chromosome 17 (FTDP-17), and secondary tauopathies such as Alzheimer's disease (AD) [1]. The development of tau pathology has been postulated to follow spatiotemporal patterns, starting from the dissociation of phosphorylated tau from microtubules and followed by the formation of toxic tau species via self-aggregation [2]. Even though polyanionic molecules are normally required for inducing tau aggregation in vitro, modifications to tau, such as site-specific mutations and site-specific phosphorylation, have driven spontaneous seeding and self-aggregation of tau in vivo under pathological situation [3]. Physiologically, extracellular tau is present in brain interstitial fluid (ISF) and then passes into the cerebrospinal fluid (CSF) [4,5]; however, the elevated concentrations of tau found in the brain ISF of human P301S tau transgenic mice has suggested that cellular tau release may be a part of disease progression [6]. Additionally, soluble tau concentrations in brain homogenates decrease with the deposition of intracellular insoluble tau, suggesting that transcellular tau propagation requires cellular internalization of extracellular tau, which has also been found to mediate the progression of neurodegeneration [6–8]. The cellular pathways for internalizing tau species are regulated by both heparan sulfate proteoglycan (HSPG)-mediated cellular uptake and specific receptor-mediated endocytosis, which are highly dependent on the isoform being internalized [8–10].

Extensive experimental data have demonstrated that transcellular propagation of soluble tau species occurs mainly through synaptic connections, leading to neuronal dysfunction characterized by the breakdown of cytoskeletal integrity, abnormal axonal transport, and synapse loss [9,10]. In particular, glial cells, activated microglia, and reactive astrocytes are also involved in the progression of tau pathology by directly affecting the homeostasis of the neuronal microenvironment or indirectly exerting inflammatory effects across multiple tauopathies [11,12]. For example, the degree of glial cell activation correlates with the severity of neurodegeneration in AD, in terms of the degeneration of synapses, neuronal loss, the formation of NFTs, or even cognitive impairment [13]. Alternatively, dysfunctional neuron-glial communication has been widely observed in AD patients and has recently developed in vitro tau pathology animal models [14,15]. Abnormal neuron-glial crosstalk strongly impairs neuronal homeostasis including neuronal metabolism, synaptogenesis, neurotransmission, and neuromodulation, contributing to the progression of neurodegeneration [14,16]. The investigation of critical molecular and cellular contributors to tau pathology provides a comprehensive understanding of tau pathogenesis that will accelerate the discovery of novel therapeutic targets and the development of drugs for treating tauopathies.

The purpose of this review is to summarize the factors that contribute to the formation of tau aggregates, tau cell-to-cell propagation, and glial contributions in tauopathies, by using the scientific evidence published in the last decade that bring promising insights into the therapeutic development for tau protein pathology. Keywords for this topic, such as tauopathies, Alzheimer's disease, prion-like propagation, tau self-aggregation, endocytosis, neuron-glial communication, neuroinflammation, and apolipoprotein E were first chosen, and searches conducted in PubMed, Google Scholar, and Web of Science. The results of these searches were then refined and categorized into cellular contributors at the early stage and later stage of neurodegeneration, based on the characterized Braak-like spatiotemporal staging scheme for tau pathology. Lastly, the combined keywords search strategy was used for searching for potential treatments for tauopathies such as using the affected signaling pathway and tau phosphorylation together. The pathological roles of phosphorylation sites, Hsp90 and site-specific mutations in tau aggregation, the roles of CX3CR1/fractalkine signaling in microglia and neurons, the roles of the glutamate-glutamine cycle between astrocyte and neurons in the progression of tau pathologies, and the possible therapeutic role of NLR3 inflammasome in the treatment of tauopathies are the major focus of this review. A list of the abbreviations used in this review is provided in Table 1.

**Table 1.** Table of abbreviations used in this review.

| Abbreviation | Explanation |
|---|---|
| AD | Alzheimer's disease |
| MAPT | Microtubule-associated protein tau |
| ApoE | Apolipoprotein E |
| NFT | Neurofibrillary tangles |
| PSP | Supranuclear palsy |
| CBD | Corticobasal degeneration |
| PiD | Pick's disease |
| FTDP-17 | Frontotemporal dementia with Parkinsonism linked to chromosome 17 |
| CNS | Central nervous system |
| MBD | Microtubule-binding domain |
| Aβ | Amyloid β |
| PRR | Proline-rich region |
| PHF | Paired helical filaments |
| ISF | Interstitial fluid |
| CSF | Cerebrospinal fluid |

Table 1. Cont.

| Abbreviation | Explanation |
|---|---|
| HSPG | Heparan sulfate proteoglycans |
| ALP | Autophagy-lysosomal pathway |
| NMDA | N-methyl-D-aspartate |
| TFEB | Transcription factor EB |
| LTP | Long-term potentiation |
| LTD | Long-term depression |

## 2. Factors Involved in the Formation of Tau Seeds

The formation of NFTs from soluble tau is a multistep process. This process begins with the dimerization of two conformationally altered monomers and is followed by the formation of intermediate soluble oligomers with varying higher-order conformations and degrees of phosphorylation. Tau oligomers have been implicated as toxic 'tau seeds' capable of seeding new aggregates by recruiting normal monomers. Despite evidence of tau trimers being the minimal unit of spontaneous cellular uptake and intracellular fibrillary structure formation in vivo [17], the folding potency of monomer could be much more critical in initiating the early nucleation process of tau aggregation (Figure 1).

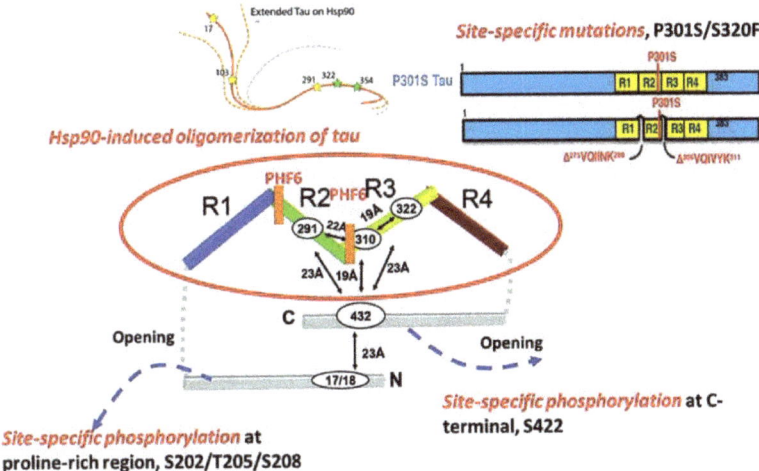

Figure 1. The molecular mechanisms involved in tau aggregation. Molecular factors such as site-specific phosphorylation, site-specific mutations on MAPT, and specific chaperones (Hsp90) are associated with tau aggregation.

### 2.1. Site-Specific Phosphorylation-Mediated Tau Self-Aggregation

Previous work details that although tau itself is intrinsically disordered, proteins in solution possess a 'paperclip-like' conformation where the N- and C-terminal ends of tau fold over in proximity to the center of the repeat domains [18]. Site-specific phosphorylation directly influences the conformation of monomeric tau and affects the stability of a folded conformation, contributing to the propensity for tau to aggregate [19]. Two hexapeptides, known as PHF6s, $^{275}$VQIINK$^{280}$, and $^{306}$VQIVYK$^{311}$, are located at the beginning of the second and third repeat domains of the MBDs, and appear to drive β-sheet structure formation during the tau aggregation process. The accessibility of residues in the two PHF6s defines the structural differences between inert (Mi) and seed-competent (Ms) tau monomer, meaning that the inert (Mi) tau monomer has less inter-chain accessibility to these residues compared with that in the seed-competent (Ms) monomer [2]. Phosphorylation outside of, but proximal to, these regions is relevant to the formation of

NFTs. A previous study systematically investigated the effects of different phosphorylation sites on tau self-aggregation, using a series of in vitro pseudo-phosphorylated tau proteins [20]. Phosphorylation sites T175/T176/T181 within N-terminal, recognized by AT270 antibody, mainly suppress tau aggregation [21]. In addition, phosphorylation at three sites, S202/T205/S208, within the proline-rich region (PRR) is enough to induce tau self-aggregation without any exogenous aggregation inducer [22]. The monoclonal antibody AT8 that specifically recognizes tau phosphorylation at the S202/T205 site has been established as a valid biochemical marker for identifying abnormally phosphorylated tau as well as the paired helical filament form. Moreover, phosphorylation sites near the C-terminus have been found to preferentially promote tau self-aggregation. For example, pseudo-phosphorylated S396, specifically recognized by PHF-1 antibody [21], has led to increased tau aggregation in the presence of metal ion inducer. In particular, the strong effect on aggregation has been seen in pS422 tau protein, which showed increased aggregation in the presence of both metal ions and heparin inducers [20], which may be related to the conversion of tau monomer from inert to seed-competent form, due to increased accessibility of these residues [3], as shown in Figure 1. By performing a comprehensive electrochemiluminescence ELISA assay, Ercan-Herbst et al. [23] found that specific phosphorylation events (pS198, pS199, and pS416) correlated with increased oligomerization in all brain regions, which implies that phospho-sites regulate tau aggregation during the progression of AD neurodegeneration. Collectively, phosphorylation plays a major role in tau self-aggregation by altering the charge and conformations of physiological tau.

### 2.2. Hsp90-Mediated Tau Aggregation

Tau phosphorylation and aggregation that lead to conformational changes could involve molecular chaperones, which regulate protein folding, degradation, and accumulation. The protective effect of Hsp70 and Hsp104 in tauopathies has been described in previous studies [24]. Hsp70 inhibits the aggregation of tau protein by forming a complex with tau oligomer or fibril tau, preventing toxic effects or further seeding of tau aggregation [25,26]. Despite the recognition of its disaggregase activity for many aggregates, a distinct mechanism of Hsp104 in preventing tau aggregation is related to its holdase activity on soluble amyloid tau through the small subdomain of nucleotide-binding domain 2 (ssNBD2) [27].

In contrast to the preventative functions of Hsp70 and Hsp104, heat shock protein 90 (Hsp90), one of the major tau-binding chaperones, has been found to drive the aggregation of tau species [28]. Although Hsp90 is normally thought to act as cellular protection during stress, Hsp90 binding to tau at the VQIVYK motif facilitates a conformational change that results in its phosphorylation by glycogen synthase kinase 3, which further promotes tau aggregation [28]. Additionally, a recent study found that Hsp90 binding to tau uncovered the repeat domains by conformationally opening the 'paper-clip' structure of tau, suggesting that the formation of tau oligomers was caused by the conversion of tau monomers from inert to aggregation-prone forms [29].

### 2.3. Site-Specific Mutations and Tau Aggregation

Abnormal tau mutants related to FTDP-17 possess distinct structures leading to a differential aggregation propensity [30–32]. Recently, Strang and coworkers demonstrated that the susceptibility of FTDP-17-associated mutants to aggregate with seeded, exogenous fibrillar tau depended highly on site-specific mutations and their surrounding amino acid sequences [33]. Robust aggregation with exogenous tau fibril seeds, both homotypic and heterotypic, has been seen in FTDP-17 mutations at sites P301 and S320. In particular, the unique property of the P301L variant in regulating the aggregation propensity of tau has been demonstrated by mutating individual proline residues into leucine residues within conserved PGGG motifs in each of the four MTBDs in tau [33]. Only P301L showed a propensity to aggregate when seeded with exogenous fibrillar tau. In contrast, other FTDP-17-associated variants near the PHF6 site showed no propensity to aggregate when seeded. Double mutants at P301L/S320F and P301S/S320F have been shown to facilitate aggregation. For these P301L/S320F and P301S/S320F tau protein variants, robust aggregation was observed in vivo without exogenous fibrillar tau seeding [33]. A possible underlying cause of this enhanced aggregation propensity is altered conformation with higher accessibility to PHF6, that converts the inert monomer into aggregation-prone monomer; alternatively, more frequent interactions with chaperones may be required to stabilize a folded conformation for these variants. In either case, further investigation is needed to identify the mechanism.

### 3. Molecular Mechanisms of Tau Cellular Uptake

Transcellular tau propagation has been implicated in tauopathies following a 'prion-like' transmission pattern [34], suggesting that the internalization of extracellular tau by recipient cells is mediated mainly by endocytosis. Recent studies showing distinct features of prion-like propagation of tau species under diverse cell and animal models are summarized in Table 2. Endocytosis can be divided generally into clathrin-dependent and -independent internalization, of which the latter can be further divided into caveolin-dependent, -independent endocytosis, and actin-dependent macropinocytosis. Previous studies highlighted cellular internalization pathways associated with tau including bulk endocytosis [35], heparin sulfate proteoglycan (HSPG)-associated macropinocytosis [8], and clathrin-mediated endocytosis [35].

The majority of extracellular tau consists of soluble oligomers and monomers, while a minority of tau species exist in truncated forms cleaved by various proinflammatory cytokines in AD brains [6]. The size and conformation of tau species determine the cellular mechanisms for extracellular tau uptake, which may not be restricted to one particular pathway [8,36]. For instance, smaller sized tau aggregates enter neurons in a dynamin-dependent endocytosis pathway that is independent of actin polymerization [35]. For larger tau aggregates, actin-dependent macropinocytosis has been identified as the main pathway for internalization by neuronal cells [37]. However, the cellular entry pathways of monomeric tau are highly dependent on the specific conformation and isoform. A recent study demonstrated that monomeric tau could enter human neurons via both the dynamin-dependent endocytosis process and through actin-dependent macropinocytosis, which could be regulated by HSPGs [35].

*3.1. The Effects of HSPGs on the Cellular Uptake of Tau Seeds*

HSPGs are highly expressed on the cell surface and have been identified as critical cell-surface endocytosis receptors for tau internalization in various studies. Most recent research has focused on understanding the interaction of heparan sulfate (HS) with tau protein at the structural level, which would provide a mechanistic understanding of how tau-HS interaction regulates tau internalization during the progression of tau pathologies. HS-tau interactions appear to be driven mainly by electrostatic forces between negatively charged sulfo groups on HS and positively charged lysines or arginines on tau protein [38]. Even though electrostatic interactions between tau and HS are relatively nonspecific, a few studies have also identified the importance of specific HS sulfation patterns on the tau-HS interaction. Prior works demonstrated the crucial role of the 6-O-sulfation of HSPGs in the tau-HS interaction by performing an SPR competition assay [39]. Moreover, 6-O-desulfated heparin showed the weakest competitive effect on tau binding to heparin immobilized on a chip among a variety of HS derivatives tested, including N-desulfated and 2-O-desulfated HS derivatives. NMR mapping showed that HS derivatives bound the second repeat motif (R2) in tau. Consistently, a knockout of 6-O-sulfotransferase also significantly reduced tau uptake by HEK293 cells [40]. Reduced intracellular tau uptake and tau cell surface binding in a 3-O-sulfotransferase knockout cell line compared with the wild-type cells suggest that tau protein is capable of recognizing the less common 3-O-sulfation site of HS [41]. The importance of sulfation was further validated in competition assays performed by Zhao and coworkers—3-O-sulfated low molecular weight HS (LMWHS) oligosaccharides had higher inhibitory effects on the tau-HS interaction compared with those without sulfation in an SPR competition assay, further validating the specific role of 3-O-sulfation in tau-heparin interactions. Furthermore, 3-O-sulfation is rare and minor sulfation is found on HS chains, which is likely not responsible for any charge effects in HS chains. More likely, HS interacts with tau via a specific 3-O-sulfation of HS recognized by both the PRR2 and R2 regions of tau instead of non-specific electrostatic interactions. The tau-heparin interaction has also been found to be chain size-dependent due to enhanced electrostatic interactions [40]. Knockouts of extension enzymes of the HSPG biosynthetic pathway, such as extension enzymes exostosin 1 (*EXT1*), exostosin 2 (*EXT2*), and exostosin-like 3 (*EXTL3*) in HEK293T cells significantly reduced the uptake of tau oligomers [36].

HSPGs can be considered as the natural receptors for the uptake of macromolecules, such as larger tau fibrils, through the micropinocytosis pathway; nevertheless, the exact role of HSPGs in the uptake of tau species dominated by the clathrin-mediated pathway needs further investigation within specific systems. Key questions include whether HSPGs are part of a multi-receptor complex or merely an initial attachment site during tau uptake. Moreover, HS-modifying enzyme expression patterns show cell-type-specific patterns, resulting in enormous HS diversity because of the many different cell types in the brain. Because of the heterogeneity of HS-expression, the specific role of HSPGs in tau internalization should be investigated on a cell type-specific basis.

Table 2. A summary of recent tau transmission models.

| Forms of Tau | Animal/Cell Model | Conformation/Characteristics | 'Prion-Like' Transmission | Reference |
|---|---|---|---|---|
| 2N4R tau monomer | Mouse primary hippocampal and cortical neurons | Wild-type tau-paperclip like | Internalized by non-neuronal cells, MLECs 3-O-sulfation is required for HSPG-mediated tau monomer internalization | [41,42] |
| 2N4R tau oligomers | Non-neuronal cells including HEK293, Hela, MC17, and MLECs | Spherical structure Diameters ranging from 10 nm to 30 nm | Dynamin-dependent endocytosis Bulk endocytosis | |
| Heparin-induced tau short fibrils (2N4R) | | Helical twist Varied length, from 40 nm to 250 nm | Tau species in endosome transported in neurons anterogradely and retrogradely | |
| Tau filaments purified from rTg4510 mouse brain | Primary neurons Hela cells P301L tau expressing mice | Fibrillary structure | Internalized by neuronal cells, but not non-neuronal cells 1-week post-injection, NFTs were detected by immunostaining against MC1 at the tau aggregates injection site | |
| Heparin-induced tau long fibrils (2N4R) | Primary neurons Hela cells | Helical twist Varied length, from 200 nm to 1600 nm | No internalization detected in both neuronal cells and non-neuronal cells | |
| 2N4R tau monomer | Human neuroglioma, H4 cells Human SH-SY5Y hiPSC-derived neurons | Size averaged at 5.7 nm | Internalized by neuronal cells rapidly HSPG-dependent internalization | [36] |
| Heparin-induced oligomer (2N4R) | | Helical filaments/19 nm | Tau monomer interacts with 6-O-sulfation on the HSPGs, but not N-sulfation | |
| Short fibrils (2N4R) | | Helical fragments/33nm | | |
| Heparin-induced fibrils (2N4R) | | Helical filaments/80 nm | Less internalization detected in both cell lines | |
| Tau RD monomers | | Wild-type tau repeat domain | No internalization detected | |
| Heparin-induced tau fibrils (both RD and WT 2N4R) | Mouse NPCs, C17.2 Primary neurons | Fibrillary structure | Tau fibrils require HSPGs for neurons 6-O- and N-sulfation are required for tau aggregates internalization HSPG mediated intracellular tau seeding Actin-dependent macropinocytosis Clathrin- or dynamin-independent endocytosis | [8,40] |
| Tau P301S monomer | hiPSCs-derived cortical neurons | Seeding-prone form | Actin-dependent macropinocytosis Dynamin-dependent endocytosis | [35] |
| Heparin-induced tau fibrils (Tau P301S) | | Fibrillary structure | Dynamin-dependent endocytosis Actin-independent endocytosis | |
| Tau oligomers | Mouse primary neuronal cells HEK293 CHO cells | Spherical structure | Muscarinic receptor-mediated endocytosis of tau by neuronal and HEK293 cells, but not by CHO cells Muscarinic receptor highly expressed by neuronal cells | [43] |
| Soluble tau oligomers derived from AD patient | Mouse primary neuronal cells | Spherical structure | Muscarinic receptor-mediated endocytosis of tau | |
| 2N4R tau monomer, oligomers, and fibrils | H4 neuroglioma hiPSCs-derived neuronal cells | Spherical structure Filaments | Receptor-mediated tau endocytosis Knockdown of *LRP1* blocks soluble tau uptake including tau monomers/oligomers, but only reduce tau fibrils uptake | [36] |

## 3.2. Receptor-Mediated Endocytosis of Tau

Apart from HSPG-dependent uptake, cellular internalization of tau is also regulated by specific receptor-mediated endocytosis, as suggested by several previous studies [35,44]. Rapid dynamin-dependent endocytosis of tau species would typically require one or more receptors, the identities of which are still under investigation. Muscarinic receptors M1/M3 have been found to regulate monomeric tau internalization by neurons [43]. Glial cells including microglia and astrocytes also take up tau efficiently. CX3CR1 has been demonstrated to mediate monomeric tau uptake in microglia [45]. For astrocytes, monomeric tau was internalized in a non-HSPG dependent pathway [46]; further study is still needed to identify specific receptors responsible for rapid dynamin-dependent endocytosis of monomeric tau in astrocytes (Figure 2). Low-density lipoprotein receptor-related protein-1 (LRP1) represents a promiscuous endocytosis receptor for macromolecular ligands, including ApoE and Aβ, and delivers these ligands to the endosomal/lysosomal compartments. Knockdown of LRP1 abolished uptake of various forms of tau, including monomers, oligomers, and fibrils in H4 neuroglioma cells, suggesting that it may serve as a master regulator of tau uptake [44]. Additionally, knocking down LRP1 also prevented tau transmission within human tau transgenic mice. Once associated with specific ligands, LRP1 is also involved in the activation of signaling pathways including MAPK, by assisting the assembly of the intracellular protein complex [47]. LRP1 is also abundantly expressed by radial glia, microglia, and astrocytes, and involved in the clearance of Aβ [47,48]. Further studies are still needed to identify whether and how LRP1 is involved in tau endocytosis by glial cells, and whether the tau-LRP1 interaction alters the immune response of glial cells.

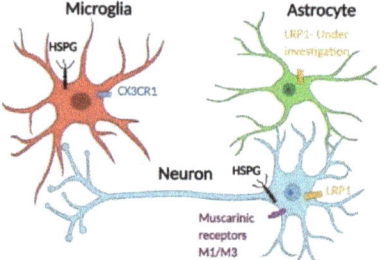

**Figure 2.** Receptor-mediated endocytosis of tau species is facilitated by several receptors. Central nervous system cells actively internalize monomeric tau via receptor-mediated endocytosis in addition to the HSPG-dependent pathway. Monomeric tau is internalized by muscarinic receptors M1 and M3 in neurons [43]. CX3CR1 mediates monomeric tau uptake in microglia [45]. For astrocytes, monomeric tau can be internalized in a non-HSPG dependent pathway [46]. Further work should be focused on identifying specific receptors of tau endocytosis. Additionally, LRP1 has recently been identified as a major regulator of tau spread in the brain [44]; LRP1 is abundantly expressed by microglia, astrocytes, and neuronal cells [47,48].

## 4. Cellular Contributors to Tau Pathology

In 1991, the work of Braak proposed the sequence of progression of Alzheimer's disease neuropathology, demonstrating that soluble hyperphosphorylated tau first appears in the locus coeruleus (LC) neurons and subsequently appears along LC axons to their terminals in the entorhinal cortex (EC) [49,50]. Transgenic mice models that display human tau pathology have been established to recapitulate the development of neurodegeneration and diverse pathological phenotypes, including gliosis, synaptic loss, tangles, and neuronal loss (Figure 3A). These models also demonstrate the involvement of diverse cellular contributors, including neuronal cells, microglia, and astrocytes, to the progression and spread of tauopathies (Figure 3B).

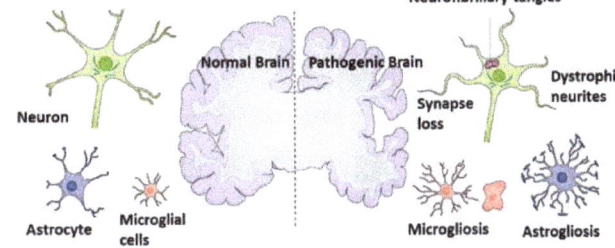

**Figure 3.** The interplay between different cell types including neurons, microglia, and astrocytes, in tauopathy progression. (**A**) A representative human tau pathology model: PS19 transgenic mice express mutant human *MAPT* with a P301S mutation and display a series of pathological features of tauopathies, such as gliosis, synaptic loss, tangles, and neuronal loss over their lifetimes. Adapted from [51,52]. Note that in this model, no plaques were found; LTP, long-term potentiation; LTD, long-term depression. (**B**) Both microgliosis and astrogliosis are involved in the progression of tauopathies and abnormal neuronal activities, as indicated by phenotypic characterization of human tau pathology models [53]. Copyright © 2021, John Wiley and Sons.

As described in detail in the following sections, the development of tau-related pathologies has been postulated to follow spatiotemporal patterns and is characterized by multiple progressive stages, each with pathological features in the form of differential cellular behaviors and distinguished phenotypes (Figure 4). At the earliest stage, tau seeds formed by phosphorylated tau dissociate from microtubules spread along a transsynaptic pathway, involving the release of tau species in the synaptic cleft, with subsequent internalization by post-synaptic neurons [54]. Glial cells, on the other hand, adapt a neuroprotective phenotype with microglia classically activated to engulf tau species in a CX3CR1-dependent way [55], and astrocytes actively involved in clearing tau species with an exacerbated autophagy-lysosomal pathway (ALP) [56]. As the disease progresses, astrocytes display a 'loss-of-function' phenotype by exhibiting a decreased level of glutamate transporters, leading to neuronal excitotoxicity and upregulated tau release [57]. Additionally, microglia develop an alternative pro-inflammatory phenotype after responding to diverse pro-inflammatory stimuli, including higher concentrations of tau protein and the presence of reactive oxygen species [11]. These activated microglia continue to produce proinflammatory cytokines, such as TNF-α and IL-1β, which are necessary and sufficient to convert inactive astrocytes into reactive astrocytes, resulting in further neuroinflammatory cytokine release [58].

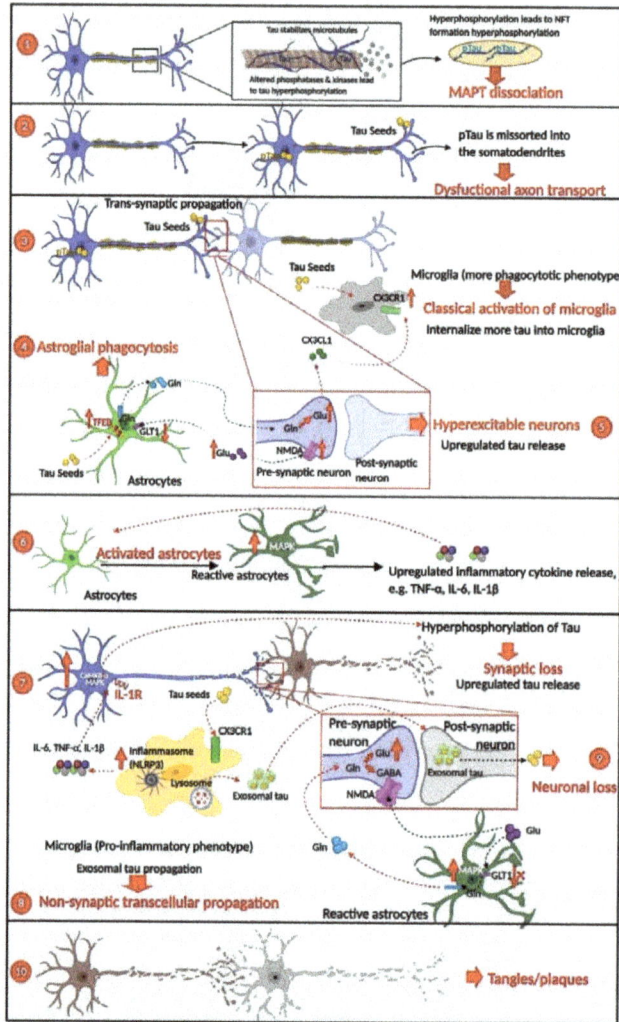

**Figure 4.** Cellular contributors to tau-dependent degeneration. The development of tau-related pathogenesis has characteristic stages, starting from the formation of tau species consisting of phosphorylated tau dissociated from microtubules ①. Abbreviation: pTau, phosphorylated tau. Hyperphosphorylation of tau incorrectly sorts tau into the somatodendritic compartment, which is linked to dysfunctional axonal transport ②, one of the earliest pathological features of tauopathies. Glial cells adapt a more neuroprotective phenotype with microglia classically activated ③ and astrocytes actively phagocytosing tau species ④. As disease progresses, astrocytes transform into a loss-of-function phenotype via lower-level expression of astrocyte-specific transporters, leading to neuronal excitotoxicity and upregulated tau release. Additionally, alternatively activated microglia in a pro-inflammatory phenotype are necessary and sufficient to induce reactive astrocytes with the capability of releasing neuroinflammatory cytokines ⑥. At the later stages of disease progression, the microglial-exosomal pathway acts as the essential tau propagation pathway ⑧ as an alternative to transsynaptic transduction, due to extensive synaptic degeneration and neuronal death ⑨. The formation of neuronal and glial tau plaques is the most important hallmark of tauopathies ⑩. Red arrows indicate pathological consequences of change. Created in BioRender.com.

Activation of the NLRP3 inflammasome in microglia has been demonstrated to facilitate the progression of tau pathologies, mainly through intensifying neuronal tau hyperphosphorylation in an IL-1 receptor-dependent way [59]. At the late stage of disease progression, dysfunctional synaptic transmission caused by synaptic loss and neuronal death leads to microglia-exosomal tau transmission that takes precedence over transsynaptic tau transmission [60]. Finally, neuronal and glial tau plaques are formed, which are the most important hallmarks of tauopathies [9].

Overexpression of the ε4 allele of apolipoprotein (*ApoE4*) in multiple cell types shows cell-type-specific effects; overexpression in neuronal cells upregulates neurotransmitter release while enhancing inflammatory signaling of microglia. For astrocytes, ApoE4 overexpression downregulates phagocytosis of pathogenic proteins and disrupts lipid transport and metabolism. Taken together, ApoE4 serves as a common genetic risk in AD and primary tauopathies, and can worsen tau pathology, indicating an overlap between ApoE4 and tau pathogenesis. LRP1, as a major receptor of tau species and ApoE, may play an intermediate role between ApoE and tau species, which could point to a therapeutic potential for treating tauopathies via LRP1 interaction.

*4.1. The Involvement of Neuronal Activity in the Spreading of Pathogenic Tau*

Under physiological conditions, tau is crucial for microtubule stabilization and is located mainly in axons [61]. Immunoblot analysis with phosphorylation-dependent antibodies revealed that phosphorylated tau is missorted into the somatodendritic compartment during the early stages of AD progression [62]. Missorted tau results in axonal transport deficits and loss of synaptic functions and is more prone to forming toxic tau oligomers if seeded [62].

The progression of tau pathology follows a defined hierarchical pattern, starting from the EC, then advancing into anatomically connected neurons downstream in the synaptic circuit, such as the dentate gyrus (DG), the hippocampus, and the neocortex, as demonstrated by tau transgenic animal models [54,63]. Despite the identification of the physiological role of neurons in regulating synaptic tau release and translocation [5], the specific neuronal activities resulting in the propagation of tau pathologies are still under investigation. Amyloid precursor protein (*APP*) transgenic mouse models show that endogenous tau in CSF increases during the progression of amyloid plaque formation, accompanied by hyperexcitable neurons [64,65]. A key question is whether the hyperexcitable neurons are essential for the release of pathogenic tau, independent of Aβ. Indeed, tau pathology mouse models combined with novel neuronal stimulation approaches showed that neuronal hyperexcitability and accelerated synaptic tau release are critically linked and independent of Aβ toxicity [66]. Using an optogenetic activation approach, the stimulated side of the hippocampus of the rTg4510 mice line tended to accumulate more human tau protein, along with increased evidence of neuronal atrophy [66]. Additionally, tau pathology spread from the stimulated-EC to the synaptically connected DG region, suggesting that the propagation of tau pathology accelerates through synaptic circuits.

Abnormal extracellular glutamate levels have been proposed as one of several mechanisms that account for an excitotoxic microenvironment in AD [67]. Notably, alterations in synaptic glutamate homeostasis caused by dysfunctional astrocytes can be deleterious to neuronal cells. To some extent, the activities of reactive astrocytes correlate with the reduction in astroglial glutamate transporters, which in turn elevates the extracellular glutamate level. Accumulation of excess glutamate contributes to neuronal excitability through activating NMDA (N-methyl-D-aspartate) receptors. NMDA receptors, present in glutamatergic neurons, respond to the glutamate levels via binding to their GluN2 subunit that activates increased calcium flux in the neurons [57]. Sequentially, activation of extrasynaptic NMDA receptors has been linked to tau-induced neuronal cell death mediated by calpain I and ERK/MAPK activation [68]. Therefore, alteration of astroglial glutamate transporters and overstimulation of extrasynaptic NMDA receptors of neuronal cells may have an overlapping role in neuronal hyperexcitability, and these actions have been implicated in the progression of tau pathology along with synaptic connections [69].

*4.2. Glial Cells Are Involved in the Progression of Tau Pathology*

Even though tau is expressed primarily by neurons, most primary tauopathies are characterized by the presence of both neuronal and glial tau pathologies [12]. Glial cells adopt immune functions and closely interact with neuronal cells for maintaining brain development and homeostasis [70]. Most glial tau pathologies have been observed in astrocytes and oligodendrocytes, and in some cases, tau pathologies have also been seen in microglia. Moreover, both primary tauopathies and AD are characterized by microgliosis and astrogliosis, along with a significant increase in the pro-inflammatory cytokines [6,71]. Glial cell dysfunction has also been implicated in the progression of neurodegenerative diseases [51]. This part of the review aims to highlight the role of dysfunctional neuronal-glial communication in the spreading and propagation of pathological tau during the progression of tauopathies.

4.2.1. Microgliosis in Tauopathies
Neuroprotective Effects of CX3CL1/CX3CR1 Signaling

Microglia are the innate immune cells of the CNS and account for 5–20% of total neural cells in the functional tissue of the brain [72,73]. They have two main CNS functions: immune defense and maintenance and promoting programmed cell death during development [72,73]. Recently, microglia-induced neuroinflammation has been linked to tau hyperphosphorylation, suggesting that microglia play an important role in the progression of tau-related neuropathogenesis [74]. As discussed previously, extensive studies have demonstrated that tau pathology predominantly spreads along with synaptic connections. Physiologically, microglia control and regulate synaptic plasticity through pruning of inactive synapses via phagocytosis during CNS development [75]. Among the key factors emerging as potential regulators of neuronal-microglial interaction, chemokine ligand 1 (CX3CL1) secreted by neurons plays an essential role in regulating phagocytic capability of microglia by binding to CX3CR1 [76], a key receptor that maintains the normal synaptic pruning ability of microglia [77]. Altered CX3CL1/CX3CR1 signaling has been demonstrated to regulate the pathological changes in both animal models of tauopathies and AD patients [78,79]. Single-cell RNA-seq of microglia in AD-transgenic mouse brains shows that CX3CR1 is upregulated as part of the initial innate immune response [80], which facilitates the internalization of tau by microglia to enhance the clearance of extracellular Tau [55].

However, at the later stages of AD, CX3CR1, among many other genes, is downregulated [80]. The downregulation of CX3CR1 has also been observed in human brain tissue from AD patients, showing that CX3CR1 levels decrease as microglial phagocytic phenotypes are reduced [55]. Microglia have been found to phagocytose extracellular tau oligomers directly via the tau-CX3CR1 interaction, which is impaired by the loss of CX3CR1 at the later stages of AD. The deletion of CX3CR1 in models of tau pathology has accelerated tau phosphorylation and exacerbated neurodegeneration [55,81]. This CX3CR1 deficiency led to elevated levels of tau phosphorylation on the AT8 (pS202), AT180 (pT231), and PHF1 (pS396/S404) epitopes [58], which is mediated by neuronal IL-1 and TLR-4 receptors triggered by the microglial release of proinflammatory cytokines [82]. Indeed, the deletion of CX3CR1 in the hAPP-transgenic mice model exacerbates microglial inflammation and neurotoxicity by upregulating the secretion of proinflammatory cytokines [78]. Similarly, CX3CL1 overexpression in the human tau transgenic mouse model rTg4510 significantly reduced neurodegeneration and microglial activation [83]. Therefore, the investigation of CX3CR1-CX3CL1 signaling has provided novel insights for treating tauopathies.

The Role of NLRP3-ASC Inflammasome Activation in Tau Phosphorylation

Extracellular fibrillary Aβ-induced microgliosis has been linked to NOD-like receptor family, pyrin domain containing 3 (NLRP3) inflammasome activation, which further exacerbates Aβ pathology [84]. The role of microglia and NLRP3-caspase recruitment domain (ASC) inflammasome activation has been demonstrated recently in Aβ-independent tau pathology [59]. Phagocytosis of fibrillar Aβ induced the assembly of the NLRP3 inflammasome consisting of NLRP3, ASC, and pro-caspase 1, which led to the caspase 1-dependent release of pro-inflammatory cytokines such as IL-1β and IL-18 [85]. Stancu and colleagues [86] demonstrated that aggregated tau was capable of activating the NLRP3 inflammasome, which further exacerbated the tau aggregate seeding and increased the secretion of proinflammatory cytokines. The importance of NLRP3 on the progression of tau pathology also was demonstrated in tau transgenic mice models deficient for NLRP3 or ASC. A significantly lower level of tau phosphorylation was observed in the hippocampal samples of the transgenic mice deficient for NLRP3 or ASC compared with wild-type mice [86]. Additionally, templated seeding of tau pathology was reduced in tau transgenic mice with an ASC deficiency.

Reduced activities of GSK-3β and CaMKII-α, but not p38/MAPK and Cdk5, were correlated with the deficiency of NLRP3 or ASC, suggesting the potential role of the NLRP3 inflammasome in regulating tau kinases in neuronal cells [86]. To understand how the NLRP3 inflammasome regulates tau phosphorylation, conditioned medium collected from LPS-activated microglia induced an increased level of tau phosphorylation in neuronal cells, along with the activation of CaMKII-α [59]. However, once the neuronal IL-1 receptor was inhibited, the effects on CaMKII-α were abolished, suggesting that the activation of the NLRP3 inflammasome in microglia promotes neuronal tau hyperphosphorylation in an IL-1 receptor-dependent manner via the regulation of multiple tau kinases (Figure 5). Potential therapeutic interventions targeting the NLRP3 inflammasome have been attempted for treating AD in mouse models [87]. By increasing *ASC* and *NLRP3* gene expression in Tau22 transgenic mice, the formation of tau aggregates was attenuated, as determined by thioflavin T staining and reduced tau phosphorylation at serine 416, due to diminished CaMKIIα activity [87]. Pharmacological NLRP3 inhibition using the molecular inhibitor MCC50 also significantly decreased tau-seed induced tau aggregates, as determined by AT8 detection, in tau transgenic mice [86].

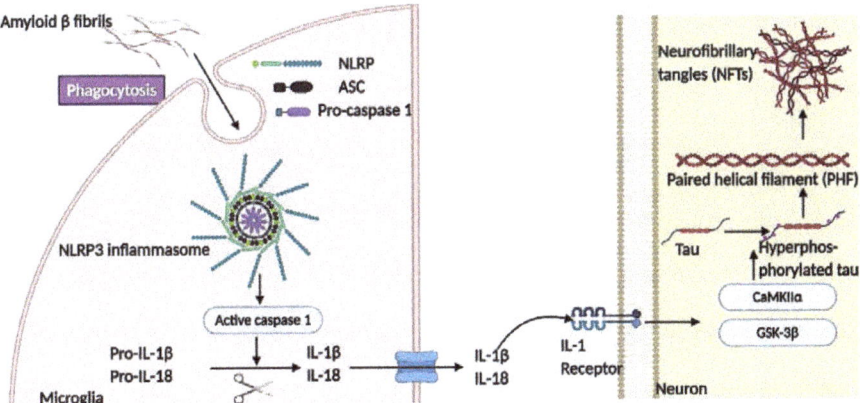

**Figure 5.** The role of the NLRP3-ASC inflammasome in tau pathogenesis. Either fibrillary Aβ or tau species in the form of monomers or oligomers are sufficient to induce the assembly of the NLRP3 inflammasome, consisting of NLRP3, ASC, and pro-caspase 1, which further leads to caspase 1-dependent release of the pro-inflammatory cytokines IL-1β and IL-18 [85]. The activation of the NLRP3 inflammasome in microglia has been demonstrated to promote neuronal tau hyperphosphorylation in an IL-1 receptor-dependent manner via the regulation of multiple tau kinases, like GSK-3β and CaMKII-α.

Even though these studies demonstrate the involvement of neuroinflammation and altered CX3CR1-CX3CL1 signaling in the spreading of tau pathology, further investigation is still needed to uncover the interplay between neuroinflammation induced by extracellular tau aggregates and disrupted phagocytosis caused by impaired CX3CR1-CX3CL1 signaling. Most likely, the relationship between inflammation and phagocytosis will demonstrate the crucial role of microglia in the development of tau pathology.

Non-Transsynaptic Tau Propagation-Microglial and Exosomal Spreading of Tau Species as an Alternative Pathway

In addition to the important role of CX3CR1-CX3CL1 signaling and the NLRP3 inflammasome in tau pathogenesis via the crosstalk between neurons and microglia, exosomes are another key mediator between glial-neuronal communication for both synaptic pruning in the healthy brain as well as neuroinflammation under pathological conditions [88,89]. Physiologically, neuronal exosomes stimulate microglial phagocytosis under selective elimination of synaptic connections. Microglia-derived exosomes play a major role in hierarchical tau transmission [60], despite pathogenic tau readily propagating from neuron to neuron in the form of free-floating fibrils [34] and interconnected neuronal contacts [90], as well as neuronal exosomes [4].

Recently, a tau rapid-propagation mouse model was created with adeno-associated viral (AAV)-tau injection into the EC [60]. This model exhibits rapid tau pathology, as demonstrated by the spreading of human tau from EC to the DG within 1 month, recapitulating the perforant diffusion pathway of AD progression in the human brain [91]. Moreover, inhibition of exosome synthesis or depletion of microglia in this AAV-GFP/tau injection mouse model led to a dramatic reduction of AT8+ tau detected in the DG without changing the tau expressed in the injection site, indicating the important role of microglia-derived exosomes in the spreading of tau pathology. Pharmacologic inhibition of exosome synthesis in microglia not only dramatically reduced secretion of the tau-containing exosomes but also decreased the capabilities of exosomes to deliver hTau, as observed in co-cultured primary neurons [60]. As the synaptic connection becomes less functional throughout disease progression, the microglial and exosomal transmission pathways become the primary means of tau propagation [9], suggesting exosomal transmission as a potential therapeutic target.

4.2.2. Astrogliosis in Tauopathies

The concept of astroglial excitability—activation of membrane ion receptors in response to stimulation—facilitates the bidirectional communication between neurons and astrocytes mediated by a 'tripartite synapse' [92]. The close physical proximity between synapses and astrocytes and resulting efficient neurotransmission explain why astrocytes are key regulators in maintaining essential neuronal functions, including synaptic plasticity and neurodevelopment [57]. Besides their crucial role in supporting neuronal functions in the CNS, astrocytes represent the largest group of glial cells that interact closely with microglia for maintaining efficient immune surveillance of the CNS [92]. Like microglia, astrocytes also express genes involved in phagocytosis [93], and eliminate synaptic debris [94], and protein aggregates, as seen by the clearance of Aβ [95]. In recent years, the involvement of astrocytes in the progression of tau pathology has drawn much attention because of their widely demonstrated role in the progression of neurodegeneration in tauopathies [11,57]. For example, reactive astrocytes induced by microglial activation have been observed to precede tangle formation in P301S tau transgenic mice models (PS19) [51].

Reactive Astrocyte Phagocytosis Has a Neuroprotective Effect

Under pathological conditions, astrocytes develop more neurotoxic features by transforming into reactive astrocytes (A1 subtype), induced by activated microglia and neuroinflammation in various human neurodegenerative disorders [16]. The phagocytic ability of reactive astrocytes appears to be enhanced in tau transgenic mouse models [96]. Astrocyte activation is accompanied by upregulated expression of transcription factor EB (TFEB), the key regulator of the autophagy-lysosomal pathway (ALP). When compared with wild-type counterparts, two widely used tau pathology mouse models, rTg4510 and PS19, showed increased expression of TFEB and lysosomal protein LAMP1 [56]. In particular, astrocytes of rTg4510 mice (transgenic mice expressing human P301L tau protein) showed much higher nuclear localization of TFEB in GFAP-expressing astrocytes compared with the wild-type mice [96]. However, overexpression of astrocytic TFEB in rTg4510 showed minimal effects on neuronal activities. In vitro, TFEB overexpression in primary astrocytes led to enhanced cellular uptake of tau fibrils by stimulating lysosomal biogenesis. In contrast, the TFEB-transduced PS19 tau pathology mouse model showed reduced tau pathogenesis and reduced tau transmission compared to the rTg4510 mouse model. These data demonstrated that the neuroprotective effects of astroglial activation took place primarily at the early stage of tauopathies by enhancing endocytosis and subsequently, triggering intensive lysosomal-mediated degradation of abnormal tau species. The effects of ALP on regulating phagocytic properties of reactive astrocytes may be one of the mechanisms that explains why tau protein enters astrocytes more efficiently than neurons, as observed in prior work [97] and has been implicated in the glial inclusions, as seen in most of the primary tauopathies, including PSP, CBD, and PiD [97].

Neuroinflammatory Microenvironment Induced by Reactive Astrocytes

Reactive microglia secrete inflammatory cytokines such as IL-1a, TNF-a, C1q, and IL-1β [16,97]. These cytokines themselves are necessary and sufficient to induce the A1 subtype of astrocytes, which further stimulates inactive astrocytes in proximity. Reactive astrocytes lose their ability to promote neuronal survival, synaptogenesis, and phagocytosis. Enhanced release of inflammatory cytokines from activated glial cells can induce active neuronal p38 MAPK by interacting with multiple receptors, such as TNFR1, and lead to enhanced phosphorylation and aggregation of tau, which precedes the progression of tau pathology [98]. Thus, reactive astrocytes also play a role in neuroinflammation-induced tau pathology.

Dysfunctional Neuronal-Astroglial Communication

Reactive astrocytes also exhibit neurotoxicity by impairing glutamate transport between neurons and astrocytes and disturbing the synaptic neurotransmitter balance via direct contact [57,99]. Astrocytes are key regulators for maintaining homeostasis of major neurotransmitters like glutamate (Glu) and γ-aminobutyric acid (GABA) via the glutamine-glutamate/GABA cycle [99]. The rapid uptake of tau species by reactive astrocytes disrupts intracellular $Ca^{2+}$ signaling, leading to a significant reduction in the release of gliotransmitters such as glutamate, glutamine, and serine, and formation of synaptic vesicles [97]. Moreover, it has also been reported that conditioned medium (CM) collected from primary astrocyte cultures isolated from P301S mice decreased the expression of synaptic neuronal markers in cultured cortical neurons, while CM from control astrocytes enhanced these markers in co-cultured neurons [100]. Taken together, reactive astrocytes appear to affect neuronal tau pathologies by impairing the neuronal synaptic transmission as well as synaptic plasticity.

The glutamine (Gln)/glutamate (Glu) cycle (GGC) is critical for maintaining homeostasis of the major neurotransmitters Glu and γ-aminobutyric acid (GABA), which is a key metabolic interaction between neurons and astrocytes [57,101]. Astrocytes uptake excess Glu released by glutamatergic neurons in the synaptic cleft via glutamate transporter-1 (GLT1) receptor (see Figure 4). Glu is then converted into Gln by astrocyte-specific enzymes, and released into the extracellular space. Subsequently, Gln is taken up by neurons and metabolized into Glu by neuron-related enzymes. Recent studies have reported that the dysfunctional neuronal-astroglial communication via the GGC may contribute to tau protein pathology [57]. For instance, reduced expression of astrocytic glutamate transporters, such as GLT1, has been found to coincide with tau inclusion pathology, as well as neuromuscular weakness in the spinal cord and the brainstem, as seen in both tau transgenic mouse models and CBD patients [99]. The reduction of glutamate transporters in astrocytes also elevates extracellular glutamate levels that then further overstimulate glutamatergic receptors (NMDA receptors), causing increased calcium flux and more neuronal excitotoxicity [62]. Subsequently, activation of NMDA receptors has led to tau phosphorylation at specific sites, the most efficient being Ser-396, mediated by p38/MAPK activation [102]. The mechanistic effects of tau pathology on the downregulation of glutamate transporters and reduction of GLT1 in glial cells are unknown, but investigations on the involvement of astrocytes in the progression of tauopathies have provided novel insights for treating glial tau pathology.

*4.3. ApoE4 Plays a Cell-Type Dependent Role in Tau Pathology*

ApoE protein serves as a major cholesterol carrier in the brain, as well as helping to clear Aβ plaques. Among the three alleles for ApoE, the presence of ApoE4 is considered an important genetic risk factor for Alzheimer's disease, leading to tau hyperphosphorylation in an Aβ-dependent manner [103]. However, a key question is whether ApoE4 influences tau pathology in primary tauopathies, such as PSD, in which tau pathology is not accompanied by Aβ. Using a P301S transgenic mouse model, Shi et al. [104] have demonstrated ApoE4-induced tau pathology independent of Aβ pathology, suggesting the crucial role of cholesterol in the tau pathogenesis of primary tauopathies.

ApoE4 expressed by different cell types has been shown to affect tau pathologies in a cell type-dependent manner. ApoE4 toxicity has been observed in multiple cell types, including neurons, as demonstrated in human iPSCs-derived cell types [105] despite ApoE4 being primarily produced by microglia and astrocytes in the CNS. ApoE4-expressing neurons exhibited tau hyperphosphorylation, while ApoE4 glial cells had reduced capacity for neuronal homeostasis and thus contributed to the pathogenesis of tau pathology. For instance, Wang and colleagues [106] showed that ApoE4-expressing neuronal cultures derived from human iPSCs expressed higher levels of the synaptic proteins SYN1 and PSD95, alongside an elevated release of neurotransmitters, compared with ApoE3-expressing neurons. Additionally, ApoE4 cerebral organoids exhibited an elevated level of phosphorylated tau (p-S202/T205) compared with ApoE3 organoids. ApoE4-expressing astrocytes had impaired lipid metabolism/transport and phagocytosis, while ApoE4-expressing microglia exhibited intensive immune reactivities upon LPS stimulation compared with wild-type microglia.

Neurons co-cultured with ApoE knockout glial cells displayed the greatest neuronal viability with the lowest level of TNF-α secretion [104]. Analogously, co-culturing P301S tau-expressing neurons with ApoE4-expressing microglia resulted in markedly reduced neuronal viability and a significantly high level of TNF-α secretion. Similarly, Friedberg and colleagues have demonstrated that inflammatory profiles of AD-associated microglia that regulate tau pathologies are highly dependent on the presence of ApoE4 [107]. These data have suggested that ApoE4 plays a crucial intermediate role between microglia inflammatory signaling and tau pathology. Furthermore, LRP1, a major receptor for ApoE and tau, has been shown to mediate the inflammatory responses of microglia via the regulation of the JNK and NF-κB signaling pathways [47]. ApoE may facilitate the assembly of the tau-LRP1 complex to exacerbate the pro-inflammatory signaling pathways on microglia.

## 5. Therapeutic Approaches Targeting Molecular/Cellular Signaling Pathways

A comprehensive understanding of cellular and molecular contributors to tau pathogenesis provides novel insights for discovering therapeutics for human tauopathies, including AD. Extensive investigations have demonstrated that HSPGs play a crucial role in the transcellular spreading of tau pathogenesis; therefore, HS-based therapeutics hold great potential for treating tau pathologies. Small molecules or anti-HS peptides interfering with HS-tau interaction are of therapeutic potential for the treatment of tauopathies, which have been reviewed previously [108]. Glycan-based compounds targeting 3-O-sulfated motifs on HS recognized by tau seeds represent a novel therapy for tauopathies [41].

NLRP3 inflammasome activation has been linked to the development of multiple inflammatory diseases, such as atherosclerosis, type II diabetes, and Alzheimer's disease, as well as various cancers [109]. The inhibition of NLRP3 inflammasome activity has been demonstrated to decrease tau phosphorylation and aggregation via attenuated neuronal GSK-3β and CaMKIIα activities. Antagonizing purinoreceptor (P2×7R) to prevent the assembly of an active NLRP3 inflammasome in microglia has been suggested as one of the best approaches to control neuroinflammation caused by microglial activation and has therapeutic potential for treating tauopathies [109,110].

Hsp90 directly binds to tau species [110], and Hsp90 inhibitors have been considered as promising therapeutics for treating tauopathies. However, disappointing clinical results due to poor blood–brain barrier permeability and toxicity of all tested drugs have led researchers to alternatives to Hsp90, such as Hsp90 co-chaperones, including ATPase homolog 1 (Aha1), a small 38-kDa cochaperone that binds to the N-terminal and middle domains of Hsp90. The role of Aha1 in tau pathogenesis via interactions with Hsp90 has been demonstrated in a transgenic tau mouse model, rTg4510 [111]. Overexpression of Aha1 led to an increased level of sarkosyl-insoluble tau, as well as the tau with T22 reactivity (anti-oligomer antibody). Treatment with KU-177, which binds specifically to Aha1, reduced the accumulation of insoluble P301L tau in cultured cells, suggesting that Aha1 may be a promising therapeutic target for tauopathies by directly reducing tau aggregation [111].

The autophagy-lysosomal pathway (ALP) shows beneficial effects on tau clearance in reactive astrocytes during the early stages of tau pathogenesis. Because of this, activation of TFEB, a key regulator of this pathway, could be considered as a promising treatment for tauopathies [96]. The therapeutic role of a novel TFEB activator named curcumin analog C1 has been studied using three AD animal models [56]. Treatment with curcumin analog C1 has significantly reduced the levels of Aβ42/Aβ40 in brain lysates from 5×FAD mice models, and phospho-tau epitopes (AT8+ and PHF1+) in a P301S mice model. In addition, curcumin analog C1 attenuated both APP and tau pathology in a 3×Tg AD mice model, accompanied by TFEB activation, increased autophagy, and lysosomal activity.

Neuroprotective effects of CX3CR1-CX3CL1 signaling in tau clearance through microglia phagocytosis has been suggested at an early stage of tau pathogenesis, revealing that the enhancement of this signaling at an early stage of disease progression could be beneficial for disease treatment. Indeed, soluble CX3CL1 overexpression by adenoviral transformation in the Tg4510 mouse model has rescued tau pathology by regulating microglial activation [83]. An alternative approach by Fan et al. [112] via neuronal CX3CL1 overexpression reduced neuronal loss and improved cognitive function in a P19 tauopathy model by enhancing neurogenesis through the CX3CL1–TGF-β2/3–Smad2 pathway. Taken together, CX3CL1 overexpression could be considered a key therapeutic target for treating AD by either promoting neurogenesis for neuronal loss recovery or attenuating microglia-induced neuroinflammation.

Given the overlapping effects on neuronal excitotoxicity by overstimulation of NMDA receptors and decreased expression of astrocyte-specific glutamate receptors observed in multiple neurodegenerative disorders, both NMDA receptors and reactive astrocytes have been implicated as therapeutic targets for treating tau pathology including AD. NMDA receptor-dependent excitotoxicity has been shown to depend on the extrasynaptic GluN2B-containing NMDA receptors rather than synaptic GluN2A-containing NMDA receptors. Antagonists selectively inhibiting extrasynaptic NMDA receptors may have neuroprotective effects [113]. Recently, a new NMDA receptor blocker, RL-208, has been tested on a mouse model of late-onset AD, showing cognitive function improvement in terms of increased synaptic protein density, increased phosphorylation of NMDA2B, reduced protein-related apoptosis, as well as decreased phosphorylated tau levels [114]. This study points out that this novel neuroprotective drug may be valuable for treating AD.

Ameliorating dysfunctional neuronal-astrocyte communication via reducing reactive astrocytes may pose an additional therapeutic target for neurodegenerative disorders.

Decreased levels of astrocyte-specific glutamate transporters have been associated with the pathogenesis of tau pathology [115]. For instance, small molecule LDN/OSU-0212320 has been shown to upregulate the expression of EAAT2, a glutamate transporter, in astrocytes via translational activation. Thus, LDN/OSU-0212320 treatment has attenuated glutamate-induced cytotoxicity in neuron and astrocyte coculture, as indicated by the greatest neuronal survival compared to untreated cells. Furthermore, significantly ameliorated symptoms and prolonged lifespan upon the treatment with LDN/OSU-0212320 have been demonstrated in an ALS transgenic mice model [116]. Similar studies are still warranted to determine the drug efficacy for AD models.

*ApoE4* is the most recognized genetic risk factor of AD and is thus considered an important therapeutic target for treating AD. Despite the incomplete understanding of the mechanisms underlying the effects of *ApoE4*, the conversion of *ApoE4* to less-toxic isoforms of *ApoE*—either *ApoE3* or *ApoE2*—may hold promising therapeutic potential. For instance, gene editing to convert *ApoE4* to *ApoE3* or the addition of a 'structural corrector' on *ApoE4*-expressing culture to refold *ApoE4* into more *ApoE3*-like conformation has rescued *ApoE4* neurons from AD pathology [106]. Additionally, an AAV-mediated *ApoE2* expression vector targeting the *ApoE4* gene of AD patients to transform the ApoE4 homozygote to an *ApoE2*-*ApoE4* heterozygote for treating AD is currently in clinical trials [117]. A summary of therapeutic approaches targeting altered molecular and cellular signaling pathways in tauopathies is presented in Table 3.

Table 3. Potential therapeutic targets for the treatment of tauopathies.

| Signaling Targets | Therapeutics | Settings/Organisms | Outcomes/Affected Functional Effects | Affected Phosphorylated Sites | State of Process | Reference |
|---|---|---|---|---|---|---|
| Interfering HSPG-tau interaction | HS oligosaccharide containing two 3-O-sulfo group | Mouse lung endothelial cells (MLECs) | • Blocking tau cell surface binding and internalization | NA | Research stage | [41] |
| Intervening the formation of NLRP3 inflammasome | Cias1 and *Pycard* gene dysfunction | FTD mice model, ACS- or NLRP3-deficient Tau22 mice | • Attenuating the level of tau hyperphosphorylation (AT8) in hippocampus<br>• Decreasing level of GSK-3β and CaMKII-α activities | pS416 | Research stage | [59,87] |
| Hsp90 cochaperones, Aha1 | KU-177 | Inducible HEK-P301L cells transfected with Aha1 | • Reduced insoluble tau | pS396/404 | Research stage | [111] |
| Promoting the autophagy-lysosomal pathway (ALP) | Curcumin analog C1 | Transgenic mice models, 5×FAD, P301S, and 3×Tg | • Attenuating both APP and tau pathology<br>• Activating autophagy-lysosomal pathway (ALP) | pS396/404<br>pS202/T205 | Research stage | [56] |
| Promoting CX3CL1 regulated signaling | CX3CL1 overexpression | P19 tau pathology mice model | • Reducing neurodegeneration and improving cognitive function with increased neurogenesis | NA | Research stage | [112] |
| Inhibiting extra-synaptic NMDA receptor | RL-208 | A mice model of late-onset AD (LOAD) | • Reduced apoptosis-related proteins, caspase-3 and calpain-1<br>• Increased phosphorylation level of NMDA2B<br>• Decreased kinase activity of Cdk5/p25 accompanied by a reduced level of p-tau | pS396 | Research stage | [114] |
| GLT1 upregulation | LDN/OSU-0212320 | Neuron and astrocyte coculture | • Upregulating the expression of EAAT2 in primary astrocytes<br>• Preventing neurons from glutamate-induced cytotoxicity in a neuronal-astrocytic coculture | NA | Research stage | [116] |
| ApoE4 gene therapy | AAV ApoE2-expressing vector targeting CNS/CSF ApoE4 | AD patients | • Targeting to transform ApoE4 in CNS/CSF of AD patients into ApoE2, which is less toxic | NA | Phase I | [117] |

## 6. Conclusions

Tauopathies are characterized by multiple pathological features, including the transcellular propagation of pathogenic tau seeds, neuronal loss, neuroinflammation, and neurofibrillary tangles. HSPGs and LRP1 have been identified as major receptors for transneuronal propagation of pathogenic tau. Altered neuronal tau kinases contribute to hyperphosphorylated tau, which is further exacerbated by intracellular oxidative stress, microglial NLRP3 inflammasome activation, and dysfunctional astroglial-dominant glutamate transport and metabolism. Neuronal loss is the consequence of both neuronal excitotoxicity and pathological tau toxicity, mainly manifested by dysfunctional axonal transport, synaptic degeneration, and upregulated levels of pro-inflammatory cytokines. As pathological phenotypes continue to develop, tau inclusions become increasingly evident and severe, which gives further rise to the pathogenic tauopathy diagnosis. The NLRP3 inflammasome, the autophagy-lysosomal pathway, CX3CL1 signaling pathway, and ApoE4 are all therapeutic targets that could yield potential new treatments for tauopathies. Interventions of tau self-aggregation via disease-specific antibodies or Hsp90 inhibitor provide one novel tool for tau pathology at an early stage of neurodegeneration. Because of the neuroprotective effect of the CX3CR1/CX3CL1 signaling pathway between microglial and neuronal communication, CX3CL1 or CX3CR1 overexpression may protect neuronal cells from toxic tau by enhancing neurogenesis, as well as internalizing more soluble tau from the extracellular matrix. As a link between amyloid deposition and neurofibrillary tangle formation, targeting the activation of the NLRP3 inflammasome provides a promising approach for the development of therapies for AD via inhibiting two hallmarks of AD simultaneously. Translational activation of glutamate transporters shows the advantageous effects on rescuing the dysfunctional GGC between astrocyte and neurons, as well as ameliorating the neurotoxicity caused by the high level of extracellular glutamate.

**Author Contributions:** Conceptualization and project administration, A.S.R.; writing—original draft preparation, L.S., A.S.R.; writing—revision and editing; A.S.R., E.A.W.; preparation of tables and figures, L.S. All authors have read and agreed to the published version of the manuscript.

**Funding:** This research received no external funding.

**Institutional Review Board Statement:** Not applicable.

**Informed Consent Statement:** Not applicable.

**Conflicts of Interest:** The authors declare no conflict of interest.

## References

1. Hock, E.M.; Polymenidou, M. Prion-like propagation as a pathogenic principle in frontotemporal dementia. *J. Neurochem.* **2016**, *138* (Suppl. 1), 163–183. [CrossRef]
2. Mirbaha, H.; Chen, D.; Morazova, O.A.; Ruff, K.M.; Sharma, A.M.; Liu, X.; Goodarzi, M.; Pappu, R.V.; Colby, D.W.; Mirzaei, H.; et al. Inert and seed-competent tau monomers suggest structural origins of aggregation. *eLife* **2018**. [CrossRef] [PubMed]
3. Liu, F.; Li, B.; Tung, E.J.; Grundke-Iqbal, I.; Iqbal, K.; Gong, C.X. Site-specific effects of tau phosphorylation on its microtubule assembly activity and self-aggregation. *Eur. J. Neurosci.* **2007**, *26*, 3429–3436. [CrossRef]
4. Wang, Y.; Balaji, V.; Kaniyappan, S.; Kruger, L.; Irsen, S.; Tepper, K.; Chandupatla, R.; Maetzler, W.; Schneider, A.; Mandelkow, E.; et al. The release and trans-synaptic transmission of Tau via exosomes. *Mol. Neurodegenerat.* **2017**, *12*, 5. [CrossRef] [PubMed]
5. Pooler, A.M.; Phillips, E.C.; Lau, D.H.W.; Noble, W.; Hanger, D.P. Physiological release of endogenous tau is stimulated by neuronal activity. *EMBO Rep.* **2013**, *14*, 389–394. [CrossRef] [PubMed]
6. Dal Pra, I.; Chiarini, A.; Gui, L.; Chakravarthy, B.; Pacchiana, R.; Gardenal, E.; Whitfield, J.F.; Armato, U. Do astrocytes collaborate with neurons in spreading the "infectious" abeta and Tau drivers of Alzheimer's disease? *Neuroscientist* **2015**, *21*, 9–29. [CrossRef]
7. Yamada, K.; Cirrito, J.R.; Stewart, F.R.; Jiang, H.; Finn, M.B.; Holmes, B.B.; Binder, L.I.; Mandelkow, E.M.; Diamond, M.I.; Lee, V.M.Y.; et al. In Vivo Microdialysis Reveals Age-Dependent Decrease of Brain Interstitial Fluid Tau Levels in P301S Human Tau Transgenic Mice. *J. Neurosci.* **2011**, *31*, 13110–13117. [CrossRef] [PubMed]
8. Holmes, B.B.; DeVos, S.L.; Kfoury, N.; Li, M.; Jacks, R.; Yanamandra, K.; Ouidja, M.O.; Brodsky, F.M.; Marasa, J.; Bagchi, D.P.; et al. Heparan sulfate proteoglycans mediate internalization and propagation of specific proteopathic seeds. *Proc. Natl. Acad. Sci. USA* **2013**, *110*, E3138–E3147. [CrossRef] [PubMed]

9. Mudher, A.; Colin, M.; Dujardin, S.; Medina, M.; Dewachter, I.; Alavi Naini, S.M.; Mandelkow, E.M.; Mandelkow, E.; Buee, L.; Goedert, M.; et al. What is the evidence that tau pathology spreads through prion-like propagation? *Acta Neuropathol. Commun.* **2017**, *5*, 99. [CrossRef]
10. Ozcelik, S.; Sprenger, F.; Skachokova, Z.; Fraser, G.; Abramowski, D.; Clavaguera, F.; Probst, A.; Frank, S.; Muller, M.; Staufenbiel, M.; et al. Co-expression of truncated and full-length tau induces severe neurotoxicity. *Mol. Psychiatry* **2016**, *21*, 1790–1798. [CrossRef] [PubMed]
11. Leyns, C.E.G.; Holtzman, D.M. Glial contributions to neurodegeneration in tauopathies. *Mol. Neurodegenerat.* **2017**, *12*, 50. [CrossRef]
12. Kahlson, M.A.; Colodner, K.J. Glial Tau Pathology in Tauopathies: Functional Consequences. *J. Exp. Neurosci.* **2015**, *9*, 43–50. [CrossRef] [PubMed]
13. Parachikova, A.; Agadjanyan, M.G.; Cribbs, D.H.; Blurton-Jones, M.; Perreau, V.; Rogers, J.; Beach, T.G.; Cotman, C.W. Inflammatory changes parallel the early stages of Alzheimer disease. *Neurobiol. Aging* **2007**, *28*, 1821–1833. [CrossRef] [PubMed]
14. Chun, H.; Marriott, I.; Lee, C.J.; Cho, H. Elucidating the Interactive Roles of Glia in Alzheimer's Disease Using Established and Newly Developed Experimental Models. *Front. Neurol.* **2018**, *9*, 797. [CrossRef]
15. Cagnin, A.; Brooks, D.J.; Kennedy, A.M.; Gunn, R.N.; Myers, R.; Turkheimer, F.E.; Jones, T.; Banati, R.B. In-vivo measurement of activated microglia in dementia. *Lancet* **2001**, *358*, 461–467. [CrossRef]
16. Liddelow, S.A.; Guttenplan, K.A.; Clarke, L.E.; Bennett, F.C.; Bohlen, C.J.; Schirmer, L.; Bennett, M.L.; Munch, A.E.; Chung, W.S.; Peterson, T.C.; et al. Neurotoxic reactive astrocytes are induced by activated microglia. *Nature* **2017**, *541*, 481–487. [CrossRef]
17. Mirbaha, H.; Holmes, B.B.; Sanders, D.W.; Bieschke, J.; Diamond, M.I. Tau trimers are the minimal propagation unit spontaneously internalized to seed intracellular aggregation. *J. Biol. Chem.* **2015**. [CrossRef]
18. Jeganathan, S.; von Bergen, M.; Brutlach, H.; Steinhoff, H.J.; Mandelkow, E. Global hairpin folding of tau in solution. *Biochemistry* **2006**, *45*, 2283–2293. [CrossRef]
19. Tenreiro, S.; Eckermann, K.; Outeiro, T.F. Protein phosphorylation in neurodegeneration: Friend or foe? *Front. Mol. Neurosci.* **2014**, *7*, 42. [CrossRef] [PubMed]
20. Haase, C.; Stieler, J.; Arendt, T.; Holzer, M. Pseudophosphorylation of tau protein alters its ability for self-aggregation. *J. Neurochem.* **2004**, *88*, 1509–1520. [CrossRef] [PubMed]
21. Šimić, G.; Babić Leko, M.; Wray, S.; Harrington, C.; Delalle, I.; Jovanov-Milošević, N.; Bažadona, D.; Buée, L.; De Silva, R.; Di Giovanni, G. Tau protein hyperphosphorylation and aggregation in Alzheimer's disease and other tauopathies, and possible neuroprotective strategies. *Biomolecules* **2016**, *6*, 6. [CrossRef]
22. Despres, C.; Byrne, C.; Qi, H.; Cantrelle, F.X.; Huvent, I.; Chambraud, B.; Baulieu, E.E.; Jacquot, Y.; Landrieu, I.; Lippens, G.; et al. Identification of the Tau phosphorylation pattern that drives its aggregation. *Proc. Natl. Acad. Sci. USA* **2017**, *114*, 9080–9085. [CrossRef] [PubMed]
23. Ercan-Herbst, E.; Ehrig, J.; Schöndorf, D.C.; Behrendt, A.; Klaus, B.; Ramos, B.G.; Oriol, N.P.; Weber, C.; Ehrnhoefer, D.E. A post-translational modification signature defines changes in soluble tau correlating with oligomerization in early stage Alzheimer's disease brain. *Acta Neuropathol. Commun.* **2019**, *7*, 1–19. [CrossRef]
24. Glover, J.R.; Lindquist, S. Hsp104, Hsp70, and Hsp40: A novel chaperone system that rescues previously aggregated proteins. *Cell* **1998**, *94*, 73–82. [CrossRef]
25. Kundel, F.; De, S.; Flagmeier, P.; Horrocks, M.H.; Kjaergaard, M.; Shammas, S.L.; Jackson, S.E.; Dobson, C.M.; Klenerman, D. Hsp70 inhibits the nucleation and elongation of tau and sequesters tau aggregates with high affinity. *ACS Chem. Biol.* **2018**, *13*, 636–646. [CrossRef]
26. Patterson, K.R.; Ward, S.M.; Combs, B.; Voss, K.; Kanaan, N.M.; Morfini, G.; Brady, S.T.; Gamblin, T.C.; Binder, L.I. Heat shock protein 70 prevents both tau aggregation and the inhibitory effects of preexisting tau aggregates on fast axonal transport. *Biochemistry* **2011**, *50*, 10300–10310. [CrossRef]
27. Zhang, X.; Zhang, S.; Zhang, L.; Lu, J.; Zhao, C.; Luo, F.; Li, D.; Li, X.; Liu, C. Heat shock protein 104 (HSP104) chaperones soluble Tau via a mechanism distinct from its disaggregase activity. *J. Biol. Chem.* **2019**, *294*, 4956–4965. [CrossRef] [PubMed]
28. Tortosa, E.; Santa-Maria, I.; Moreno, F.; Lim, F.; Perez, M.; Avila, J. Binding of Hsp90 to tau promotes a conformational change and aggregation of tau protein. *J. Alzheimers Dis.* **2009**, *17*, 319–325. [CrossRef]
29. Weickert, S.; Wawrzyniuk, M.; John, L.H.; Rudiger, S.G.D.; Drescher, M. The mechanism of Hsp90-induced oligomerizaton of Tau. *Sci. Adv.* **2020**, *6*, eaax6999. [CrossRef]
30. Kaufman, S.K.; Sanders, D.W.; Thomas, T.L.; Ruchinskas, A.J.; Vaquer-Alicea, J.; Sharma, A.M.; Miller, T.M.; Diamond, M.I. Tau Prion Strains Dictate Patterns of Cell Pathology, Progression Rate, and Regional Vulnerability In Vivo. *Neuron* **2016**, *92*, 796–812. [CrossRef] [PubMed]
31. Rossi, G.; Bastone, A.; Piccoli, E.; Mazzoleni, G.; Morbin, M.; Uggetti, A.; Giaccone, G.; Sperber, S.; Beeg, M.; Salmona, M.; et al. New mutations in MAPT gene causing frontotemporal lobar degeneration: Biochemical and structural characterization. *Neurobiol. Aging* **2012**, *33*, 834.e1–834.e6. [CrossRef] [PubMed]
32. Stein, K.C.; True, H.L. Extensive diversity of prion strains is defined by differential chaperone interactions and distinct amyloidogenic regions. *PLoS Genet.* **2014**, *10*, e1004337. [CrossRef]
33. Strang, K.H.; Croft, C.L.; Sorrentino, Z.A.; Chakrabarty, P.; Golde, T.E.; Giasson, B.I. Distinct differences in prion-like seeding and aggregation between Tau protein variants provide mechanistic insights into tauopathies. *J. Biol. Chem.* **2018**, *293*, 4579. [CrossRef]

34. Holmes, B.B.; Diamond, M.I. Prion-like properties of Tau protein: The importance of extracellular Tau as a therapeutic target. *J. Biol. Chem.* **2014**, *289*, 19855–19861. [CrossRef] [PubMed]
35. Evans, L.D.; Wassmer, T.; Fraser, G.; Smith, J.; Perkinton, M.; Billinton, A.; Livesey, F.J. Extracellular Monomeric and Aggregated Tau Efficiently Enter Human Neurons through Overlapping but Distinct Pathways. *Cell Rep.* **2018**, *22*, 3612–3624. [CrossRef]
36. Rauch, J.N.; Chen, J.J.; Sorum, A.W.; Miller, G.M.; Sharf, T.; See, S.K.; Hsieh-Wilson, L.C.; Kampmann, M.; Kosik, K.S. Tau Internalization is Regulated by 6-O Sulfation on Heparan Sulfate Proteoglycans (HSPGs). *Sci. Rep.* **2018**, *8*. [CrossRef]
37. Jacks, R.L. Spreading the Seeds of Neurodegeneration: Tau Fibrils Enter Cells by Macroendocytosis. Ph.D. Thesis, University of California, San Francisco, CA, USA, 2010.
38. Fichou, Y.; Vigers, M.; Goring, A.K.; Eschmann, N.A.; Han, S. Correction: Heparin-induced tau filaments are structurally heterogeneous and differ from Alzheimer's disease filaments. *Chem. Commun.* **2018**, *54*, 8653. [CrossRef] [PubMed]
39. Zhao, J.; Huvent, I.; Lippens, G.; Eliezer, D.; Zhang, A.; Li, Q.; Tessier, P.; Linhardt, R.J.; Zhang, F.; Wang, C. Glycan Determinants of Heparin-Tau Interaction. *Biophys. J.* **2017**, *112*, 921–932. [CrossRef] [PubMed]
40. Stopschinski, B.E.; Holmes, B.B.; Miller, G.M.; Manon, V.A.; Vaquer-Alicea, J.; Prueitt, W.L.; Hsieh-Wilson, L.C.; Diamond, M.I. Specific glycosaminoglycan chain length and sulfation patterns are required for cell uptake of tau versus alpha-synuclein and beta-amyloid aggregates. *J. Biol. Chem.* **2018**, *293*, 10826–10840. [CrossRef]
41. Zhao, J.; Zhu, Y.; Song, X.; Xiao, Y.; Su, G.; Liu, X.; Wang, Z.; Xu, Y.; Liu, J.; Eliezer, D.; et al. 3-O-Sulfation of Heparan Sulfate Enhances Tau Interaction and Cellular Uptake. *Angew. Chem. Int. Ed. Engl.* **2020**, *59*, 1818–1827. [CrossRef] [PubMed]
42. Wu, J.W.; Herman, M.; Liu, L.; Simoes, S.; Acker, C.M.; Figueroa, H.; Steinberg, J.I.; Margittai, M.; Kayed, R.; Zurzolo, C.; et al. Small misfolded Tau species are internalized via bulk endocytosis and anterogradely and retrogradely transported in neurons. *J. Biol. Chem.* **2013**, *288*, 1856–1870. [CrossRef] [PubMed]
43. Morozova, V.; Cohen, L.S.; Makki, A.E.; Shur, A.; Pilar, G.; El Idrissi, A.; Alonso, A.D. Normal and Pathological Tau Uptake Mediated by M1/M3 Muscarinic Receptors Promotes Opposite Neuronal Changes. *Front. Cell Neurosci.* **2019**, *13*, 403. [CrossRef]
44. Rauch, J.N.; Luna, G.; Guzman, E.; Audouard, M.; Challis, C.; Sibih, Y.E.; Leshuk, C.; Hernandez, I.; Wegmann, S.; Hyman, B.T.; et al. LRP1 is a master regulator of tau uptake and spread. *Nature* **2020**, *580*, 381–385. [CrossRef]
45. Bolos, M.; Llorens-Martin, M.; Jurado-Arjona, J.; Hernandez, F.; Rabano, A.; Avila, J. Direct Evidence of Internalization of Tau by Microglia In Vitro and In Vivo. *J. Alzheimers Dis.* **2016**, *50*, 77–87. [CrossRef] [PubMed]
46. Perea, J.R.; López, E.; Díez-Ballesteros, J.C.; Ávila, J.; Hernández, F.; Bolós, M. Extracellular Monomeric Tau Is Internalized by Astrocytes. *Front. Neurosci.* **2019**, *13*, 442. [CrossRef]
47. Yang, L.; Liu, C.C.; Zheng, H.; Kanekiyo, T.; Atagi, Y.; Jia, L.; Wang, D.; N'Songo, A.; Can, D.; Xu, H.; et al. LRP1 modulates the microglial immune response via regulation of JNK and NF-kappaB signaling pathways. *J. Neuroinflam.* **2016**, *13*, 304. [CrossRef]
48. Liu, C.C.; Hu, J.; Zhao, N.; Wang, J.; Wang, N.; Cirrito, J.R.; Kanekiyo, T.; Holtzman, D.M.; Bu, G. Astrocytic LRP1 Mediates Brain Abeta Clearance and Impacts Amyloid Deposition. *J. Soc. Neurosci.* **2017**, *37*, 4023–4031. [CrossRef]
49. Braak, H.; Braak, E. Neuropathological stageing of Alzheimer-related changes. *Acta Neuropathol.* **1991**, *82*, 239–259. [CrossRef]
50. Ghosh, A.; Torraville, S.E.; Mukherjee, B.; Walling, S.G.; Martin, G.M.; Harley, C.W.; Yuan, Q. An experimental model of Braak's pretangle proposal for the origin of Alzheimer's disease: The role of locus coeruleus in early symptom development. *Alzheimer's Res. Ther.* **2019**, *11*, 59. [CrossRef]
51. Yoshiyama, Y.; Higuchi, M.; Zhang, B.; Huang, S.M.; Iwata, N.; Saido, T.C.; Maeda, J.; Suhara, T.; Trojanowski, J.Q.; Lee, V.M. Synapse loss and microglial activation precede tangles in a P301S tauopathy mouse model. *Neuron* **2007**, *53*, 337–351. [CrossRef] [PubMed]
52. Sasner, M. Tau P301S (Line PS19). Available online: https://www.alzforum.org/research-models/tau-p301s-line-ps19 (accessed on 4 January 2021).
53. Congdon, E.E.; Sigurdsson, E.M. Tau-targeting therapies for Alzheimer disease. *Nat. Rev. Neurol.* **2018**, *14*, 399–415. [CrossRef]
54. Liu, L.; Drouet, V.; Wu, J.W.; Witter, M.P.; Small, S.A.; Clelland, C.; Duff, K. Trans-synaptic spread of tau pathology in vivo. *PLoS ONE* **2012**, *7*, e31302. [CrossRef]
55. Bolos, M.; Llorens-Martin, M.; Perea, J.R.; Jurado-Arjona, J.; Rabano, A.; Hernandez, F.; Avila, J. Absence of CX3CR1 impairs the internalization of Tau by microglia. *Mol. Neurodegener.* **2017**, *12*, 59. [CrossRef]
56. Song, J.X.; Malampati, S.; Zeng, Y.; Durairajan, S.S.K.; Yang, C.B.; Tong, B.C.; Iyaswamy, A.; Shang, W.B.; Sreenivasmurthy, S.G.; Zhu, Z.; et al. A small molecule transcription factor EB activator ameliorates beta-amyloid precursor protein and Tau pathology in Alzheimer's disease models. *Aging Cell* **2020**, *19*, e13069. [CrossRef]
57. Sidoryk-Wegrzynowicz, M.; Struzynska, L. Astroglial contribution to tau-dependent neurodegeneration. *Biochem. J.* **2019**, *476*, 3493–3504. [CrossRef]
58. Maphis, N.; Xu, G.; Kokiko-Cochran, O.N.; Jiang, S.; Cardona, A.; Ransohoff, R.M.; Lamb, B.T.; Bhaskar, K. Reactive microglia drive tau pathology and contribute to the spreading of pathological tau in the brain. *Brain* **2015**, *138*, 1738–1755. [CrossRef]
59. Ising, C.; Venegas, C.; Zhang, S.; Scheiblich, H.; Schmidt, S.V.; Vieira-Saecker, A.; Schwartz, S.; Albasset, R.; McManus, R.M.; Tejera, D.; et al. NLRP3 inflammasome activation drives tau pathology. *Nature* **2019**, *575*, 669–673. [CrossRef] [PubMed]
60. Asai, H.; Ikezu, S.; Tsunoda, S.; Medalla, M.; Luebke, J.; Haydar, T.; Wolozin, B.; Butovsky, O.; Kugler, S.; Ikezu, T. Depletion of microglia and inhibition of exosome synthesis halt tau propagation. *Nat. Neurosci.* **2015**, *18*, 1584–1593. [CrossRef]
61. Iwata, M.; Watanabe, S.; Yamane, A.; Miyasaka, T.; Misonou, H. Regulatory mechanisms for the axonal localization of tau protein in neurons. *Mol. Biol. Cell* **2019**, *30*, 2441–2457. [CrossRef]

62. Zempel, H.; Mandelkow, E. Lost after translation: Missorting of Tau protein and consequences for Alzheimer disease. *Trends Neurosci.* **2014**, *37*, 721–732. [CrossRef]
63. de Calignon, A.; Polydoro, M.; Suarez-Calvet, M.; William, C.; Adamowicz, D.H.; Kopeikina, K.J.; Pitstick, R.; Sahara, N.; Ashe, K.H.; Carlson, G.A.; et al. Propagation of tau pathology in a model of early Alzheimer's disease. *Neuron* **2012**, *73*, 685–697. [CrossRef]
64. Maia, L.F.; Kaeser, S.A.; Reichwald, J.; Hruscha, M.; Martus, P.; Staufenbiel, M.; Jucker, M. Changes in amyloid-beta and Tau in the cerebrospinal fluid of transgenic mice overexpressing amyloid precursor protein. *Sci. Transl. Med.* **2013**, *5*, 194re192. [CrossRef]
65. Siskova, Z.; Justus, D.; Kaneko, H.; Friedrichs, D.; Henneberg, N.; Beutel, T.; Pitsch, J.; Schoch, S.; Becker, A.; von der Kammer, H.; et al. Dendritic structural degeneration is functionally linked to cellular hyperexcitability in a mouse model of Alzheimer's disease. *Neuron* **2014**, *84*, 1023–1033. [CrossRef] [PubMed]
66. Wu, J.W.; Hussaini, S.A.; Bastille, I.M.; Rodriguez, G.A.; Mrejeru, A.; Rilett, K.; Sanders, D.W.; Cook, C.; Fu, H.; Boonen, R.A.; et al. Neuronal activity enhances tau propagation and tau pathology in vivo. *Nat. Neurosci.* **2016**, *19*, 1085–1092. [CrossRef] [PubMed]
67. Assefa, B.T.; Gebre, A.K.; Altaye, B.M. Reactive Astrocytes as Drug Target in Alzheimer's Disease. *Biomed. Res. Int.* **2018**, *2018*, 4160247. [CrossRef]
68. Amadoro, G.; Ciotti, M.T.; Costanzi, M.; Cestari, V.; Calissano, P.; Canu, N. NMDA receptor mediates tau-induced neurotoxicity by calpain and ERK/MAPK activation. *Proc. Natl. Acad. Sci. USA* **2006**, *103*, 2892–2897. [CrossRef] [PubMed]
69. Hynd, M.R.; Scott, H.L.; Dodd, P.R. Glutamate-mediated excitotoxicity and neurodegeneration in Alzheimer's disease. *Neurochem. Int.* **2004**, *45*, 583–595. [CrossRef] [PubMed]
70. Greenhalgh, A.D.; David, S.; Bennett, F.C. Immune cell regulation of glia during CNS injury and disease. *Nat. Rev. Neurosci.* **2020**, *21*, 139–152. [CrossRef] [PubMed]
71. Hopp, S.C.; Lin, Y.; Oakley, D.; Roe, A.D.; DeVos, S.L.; Hanlon, D.; Hyman, B.T. The role of microglia in processing and spreading of bioactive tau seeds in Alzheimer's disease. *J. Neuroinflam.* **2018**, *15*, 269. [CrossRef]
72. Lloyd, A.F.; Davies, C.L.; Miron, V.E. Microglia: Origins, homeostasis, and roles in myelin repair. *Curr. Opin. Neurobiol.* **2017**, *47*, 113–120. [CrossRef]
73. Song, L.; Yuan, X.; Jones, Z.; Vied, C.; Miao, Y.; Marzano, M.; Hua, T.; Sang, Q.A.; Guan, J.; Ma, T.; et al. Functionalization of Brain Region-specific Spheroids with Isogenic Microglia-like Cells. *Sci. Rep.* **2019**, *9*, 11895. [CrossRef]
74. Perea, J.R.; Llorens-Martin, M.; Avila, J.; Bolos, M. The Role of Microglia in the Spread of Tau: Relevance for Tauopathies. *Front. Cell Neurosci.* **2018**, *12*, 172. [CrossRef]
75. Wolf, S.A.; Boddeke, H.W.; Kettenmann, H. Microglia in Physiology and Disease. *Annu. Rev. Physiol.* **2017**, *79*, 619–643. [CrossRef] [PubMed]
76. Limatola, C.; Ransohoff, R.M. Modulating neurotoxicity through CX3CL1/CX3CR1 signaling. *Front. Cell Neurosci.* **2014**, *8*, 229. [CrossRef]
77. Graeber, M.B. Changing face of microglia. *Science* **2010**, *330*, 783–788. [CrossRef]
78. Cho, S.H.; Sun, B.; Zhou, Y.; Kauppinen, T.M.; Halabisky, B.; Wes, P.; Ransohoff, R.M.; Gan, L. CX3CR1 protein signaling modulates microglial activation and protects against plaque-independent cognitive deficits in a mouse model of Alzheimer disease. *J. Biol. Chem.* **2011**, *286*, 32713–32722. [CrossRef]
79. Kim, T.S.; Lim, H.K.; Lee, J.Y.; Kim, D.J.; Park, S.; Lee, C.; Lee, C.U. Changes in the levels of plasma soluble fractalkine in patients with mild cognitive impairment and Alzheimer's disease. *Neurosci. Lett.* **2008**, *436*, 196–200. [CrossRef]
80. Keren-Shaul, H.; Spinrad, A.; Weiner, A.; Matcovitch-Natan, O.; Dvir-Szternfeld, R.; Ulland, T.K.; David, E.; Baruch, K.; Lara-Astaiso, D.; Toth, B.; et al. A Unique Microglia Type Associated with Restricting Development of Alzheimer's Disease. *Cell* **2017**, *169*, 1276–1290.e1217. [CrossRef]
81. Bhaskar, K.; Konerth, M.; Kokiko-Cochran, O.N.; Cardona, A.; Ransohoff, R.M.; Lamb, B.T. Regulation of tau pathology by the microglial fractalkine receptor. *Neuron* **2010**, *68*, 19–31. [CrossRef]
82. Chidambaram, H.; Das, R.; Chinnathambi, S. Interaction of Tau with the chemokine receptor, CX3CR1 and its effect on microglial activation, migration and proliferation. *Cell Biosci.* **2020**, *10*, 1–9. [CrossRef]
83. Nash, K.R.; Lee, D.C.; Hunt, J.B., Jr.; Morganti, J.M.; Selenica, M.L.; Moran, P.; Reid, P.; Brownlow, M.; Guang-Yu Yang, C.; Savalia, M.; et al. Fractalkine overexpression suppresses tau pathology in a mouse model of tauopathy. *Neurobiol. Aging* **2013**, *34*, 1540–1548. [CrossRef]
84. Halle, A.; Hornung, V.; Petzold, G.C.; Stewart, C.R.; Monks, B.G.; Reinheckel, T.; Fitzgerald, K.A.; Latz, E.; Moore, K.J.; Golenbock, D.T. The NALP3 inflammasome is involved in the innate immune response to amyloid-beta. *Nat. Immunol.* **2008**, *9*, 857–865. [CrossRef]
85. Swanson, K.V.; Deng, M.; Ting, J.P. The NLRP3 inflammasome: Molecular activation and regulation to therapeutics. *Nat. Rev. Immunol.* **2019**, *19*, 477–489. [CrossRef] [PubMed]
86. Stancu, I.C.; Cremers, N.; Vanrusselt, H.; Couturier, J.; Vanoosthuyse, A.; Kessels, S.; Lodder, C.; Brone, B.; Huaux, F.; Octave, J.N.; et al. Aggregated Tau activates NLRP3-ASC inflammasome exacerbating exogenously seeded and non-exogenously seeded Tau pathology in vivo. *Acta Neuropathol.* **2019**, *137*, 599–617. [CrossRef] [PubMed]
87. Zhang, Y.; Dong, Z.; Song, W. NLRP3 inflammasome as a novel therapeutic target for Alzheimer's disease. *Signal Transduct. Target Ther.* **2020**, *5*, 37. [CrossRef]

88. Bahrini, I.; Song, J.H.; Diez, D.; Hanayama, R. Neuronal exosomes facilitate synaptic pruning by up-regulating complement factors in microglia. *Sci. Rep.* **2015**, *5*, 7989. [CrossRef] [PubMed]
89. Pascual, M.; Ibanez, F.; Guerri, C. Exosomes as mediators of neuron-glia communication in neuroinflammation. *Neural Regen. Res.* **2020**, *15*, 796–801. [CrossRef]
90. Calafate, S.; Buist, A.; Miskiewicz, K.; Vijayan, V.; Daneels, G.; de Strooper, B.; de Wit, J.; Verstreken, P.; Moechars, D. Synaptic Contacts Enhance Cell-to-Cell Tau Pathology Propagation. *Cell Rep.* **2015**, *11*, 1176–1183. [CrossRef]
91. Kalus, P.; Slotboom, J.; Gallinat, J.; Mahlberg, R.; Cattapan-Ludewig, K.; Wiest, R.; Nyffeler, T.; Buri, C.; Federspiel, A.; Kunz, D.; et al. Examining the gateway to the limbic system with diffusion tensor imaging: The perforant pathway in dementia. *Neuroimage* **2006**, *30*, 713–720. [CrossRef]
92. Perea, G.; Navarrete, M.; Araque, A. Tripartite synapses: Astrocytes process and control synaptic information. *Trends Neurosci.* **2009**, *32*, 421–431. [CrossRef]
93. Cahoy, J.D.; Emery, B.; Kaushal, A.; Foo, L.C.; Zamanian, J.L.; Christopherson, K.S.; Xing, Y.; Lubischer, J.L.; Krieg, P.A.; Krupenko, S.A.; et al. A transcriptome database for astrocytes, neurons, and oligodendrocytes: A new resource for understanding brain development and function. *J. Neurosci.* **2008**, *28*, 264–278. [CrossRef] [PubMed]
94. Kim, Y.; Park, J.; Choi, Y.K. The Role of Astrocytes in the Central Nervous System Focused on BK Channel and Heme Oxygenase Metabolites: A Review. *Antioxidants* **2019**, *8*, 121. [CrossRef] [PubMed]
95. Li, Y.; Cheng, D.; Cheng, R.; Zhu, X.; Wan, T.; Liu, J.; Zhang, R. Mechanisms of U87 astrocytoma cell uptake and trafficking of monomeric versus protofibril Alzheimer's disease amyloid-beta proteins. *PLoS ONE* **2014**, *9*, e99939. [CrossRef]
96. Martini-Stoica, H.; Cole, A.L.; Swartzlander, D.B.; Chen, F.; Wan, Y.W.; Bajaj, L.; Bader, D.A.; Lee, V.M.Y.; Trojanowski, J.Q.; Liu, Z.; et al. TFEB enhances astroglial uptake of extracellular tau species and reduces tau spreading. *J. Exp. Med.* **2018**, *215*, 2355–2377. [CrossRef]
97. Piacentini, R.; Li Puma, D.D.; Mainardi, M.; Lazzarino, G.; Tavazzi, B.; Arancio, O.; Grassi, C. Reduced gliotransmitter release from astrocytes mediates tau-induced synaptic dysfunction in cultured hippocampal neurons. *Glia* **2017**, *65*, 1302–1316. [CrossRef] [PubMed]
98. Scuderi, C.; Facchinetti, R.; Steardo, L.; Valenza, M. Neuroinflammation in Alzheimer's Disease: Friend or Foe? *FASEB J.* **2020**, *34*. [CrossRef]
99. Nilsen, L.H.; Rae, C.; Ittner, L.M.; Gotz, J.; Sonnewald, U. Glutamate metabolism is impaired in transgenic mice with tau hyperphosphorylation. *J. Cereb. Blood Flow Metab.* **2013**, *33*, 684–691. [CrossRef]
100. Sidoryk-Wegrzynowicz, M.; Gerber, Y.N.; Ries, M.; Sastre, M.; Tolkovsky, A.M.; Spillantini, M.G. Astrocytes in mouse models of tauopathies acquire early deficits and lose neurosupportive functions. *Acta Neuropathol. Commun.* **2017**, *5*, 89. [CrossRef] [PubMed]
101. Sonnewald, U.; Westergaard, N.; Schousboe, A. Glutamate transport and metabolism in astrocytes. *Glia* **1997**, *21*, 56–63. [CrossRef]
102. Corrêa, S.A.; Eales, K.L. The role of p38 MAPK and its substrates in neuronal plasticity and neurodegenerative disease. *J. Signal Transduct.* **2012**, *2012*. [CrossRef]
103. Tesseur, I.; Van Dorpe, J.; Spittaels, K.; Van den Haute, C.; Moechars, D.; Van Leuven, F. Expression of human apolipoprotein E4 in neurons causes hyperphosphorylation of protein tau in the brains of transgenic mice. *Am. J. Pathol.* **2000**, *156*, 951–964. [CrossRef]
104. Shi, Y.; Yamada, K.; Liddelow, S.A.; Smith, S.T.; Zhao, L.; Luo, W.; Tsai, R.M.; Spina, S.; Grinberg, L.T.; Rojas, J.C.; et al. ApoE4 markedly exacerbates tau-mediated neurodegeneration in a mouse model of tauopathy. *Nature* **2017**, *549*, 523–527. [CrossRef]
105. Lin, Y.T.; Seo, J.; Gao, F.; Feldman, H.M.; Wen, H.L.; Penney, J.; Cam, H.P.; Gjoneska, E.; Raja, W.K.; Cheng, J.; et al. APOE4 Causes Widespread Molecular and Cellular Alterations Associated with Alzheimer's Disease Phenotypes in Human iPSC-Derived Brain Cell Types. *Neuron* **2018**, *98*, 1294. [CrossRef]
106. Wang, C.; Najm, R.; Xu, Q.; Jeong, D.E.; Walker, D.; Balestra, M.E.; Yoon, S.Y.; Yuan, H.; Li, G.; Miller, Z.A.; et al. Gain of toxic apolipoprotein E4 effects in human iPSC-derived neurons is ameliorated by a small-molecule structure corrector. *Nat. Med.* **2018**, *24*, 647–657. [CrossRef]
107. Friedberg, J.S.; Aytan, N.; Cherry, J.D.; Xia, W.; Standring, O.J.; Alvarez, V.E.; Nicks, R.; Svirsky, S.; Meng, G.; Jun, G.; et al. Associations between brain inflammatory profiles and human neuropathology are altered based on apolipoprotein E epsilon4 genotype. *Sci. Rep.* **2020**, *10*, 2924. [CrossRef]
108. Alavi Naini, S.M.; Soussi-Yanicostas, N. Heparan Sulfate as a Therapeutic Target in Tauopathies: Insights from Zebrafish. *Front. Cell Dev. Biol.* **2018**, *6*, 163. [CrossRef]
109. Zahid, A.; Li, B.; Kombe, A.J.K.; Jin, T.; Tao, J. Pharmacological Inhibitors of the NLRP3 Inflammasome. *Front. Immunol.* **2019**, *10*, 2538. [CrossRef]
110. Thawkar, B.S.; Kaur, G. Inhibitors of NF-kappaB and P2X7/NLRP3/Caspase 1 pathway in microglia: Novel therapeutic opportunities in neuroinflammation induced early-stage Alzheimer's disease. *J. Neuroimmunol.* **2019**, *326*, 62–74. [CrossRef] [PubMed]
111. Shelton, L.B.; Baker, J.D.; Zheng, D.; Sullivan, L.E.; Solanki, P.K.; Webster, J.M.; Sun, Z.; Sabbagh, J.J.; Nordhues, B.A.; Koren, J., 3rd; et al. Hsp90 activator Aha1 drives production of pathological tau aggregates. *Proc. Natl. Acad. Sci. USA* **2017**, *114*, 9707–9712. [CrossRef]
112. Fan, Q.; He, W.; Gayen, M.; Benoit, M.R.; Luo, X.; Hu, X.; Yan, R. Activated CX3CL1/Smad2 Signals Prevent Neuronal Loss and Alzheimer's Tau Pathology-Mediated Cognitive Dysfunction. *J. Neurosci.* **2020**, *40*, 1133–1144. [CrossRef]

113. Vizi, E.S.; Kisfali, M.; Lorincz, T. Role of nonsynaptic GluN2B-containing NMDA receptors in excitotoxicity: Evidence that fluoxetine selectively inhibits these receptors and may have neuroprotective effects. *Brain Res. Bull.* **2013**, *93*, 32–38. [CrossRef] [PubMed]
114. Companys-Alemany, J.; Turcu, A.L.; Bellver-Sanchis, A.; Loza, M.I.; Brea, J.M.; Canudas, A.M.; Leiva, R.; Vazquez, S.; Pallas, M.; Grinan-Ferre, C. A Novel NMDA Receptor Antagonist Protects against Cognitive Decline Presented by Senescent Mice. *Pharmaceutics* **2020**, *12*, 284. [CrossRef]
115. Perez-Nievas, B.G.; Serrano-Pozo, A. Deciphering the Astrocyte Reaction in Alzheimer's Disease. *Front. Aging Neurosci.* **2018**, *10*, 114. [CrossRef] [PubMed]
116. Kong, Q.; Chang, L.C.; Takahashi, K.; Liu, Q.; Schulte, D.A.; Lai, L.; Ibabao, B.; Lin, Y.; Stouffer, N.; Das Mukhopadhyay, C.; et al. Small-molecule activator of glutamate transporter EAAT2 translation provides neuroprotection. *J. Clin. Invest.* **2014**, *124*, 1255–1267. [CrossRef] [PubMed]
117. Rosenberg, J.B.; Kaplitt, M.G.; De, B.P.; Chen, A.; Flagiello, T.; Salami, C.; Pey, E.; Zhao, L.; Ricart Arbona, R.J.; Monette, S.; et al. AAVrh.10-Mediated APOE2 Central Nervous System Gene Therapy for APOE4-Associated Alzheimer's Disease. *Hum. Gene Ther. Clin. Dev.* **2018**, *29*, 24–47. [CrossRef]

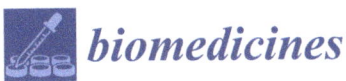 

Article

# SIRT1-Dependent Upregulation of BDNF in Human Microglia Challenged with Aβ: An Early but Transient Response Rescued by Melatonin

Grazia Ilaria Caruso [†], Simona Federica Spampinato, Giuseppe Costantino [‡], Sara Merlo [*,§] and Maria Angela Sortino [*,§]

Department of Biomedical and Biotechnological Sciences, Section of Pharmacology, University of Catania, Via Santa Sofia 97, 95123 Catania, Italy; grazia.caruso@outlook.it (G.I.C.); simona_spampinato@hotmail.com (S.F.S.); giuseppe.costantino@unifg.it (G.C.)
* Correspondence: sara_merlo@hotmail.com (S.M.); msortino@unict.it (M.A.S.)
† Ph.D. Program in Biotechnologies, Department of Biomedical and Biotechnological Sciences, University of Catania, 95123 Catania, Italy.
‡ Ph.D. Program in Neuroscience and Education, DISCUM, University of Foggia, 71121 Foggia, Italy.
§ Co-last authors that contributed equally to the supervision of this work.

**Citation:** Caruso, G.I.; Spampinato, S.F.; Costantino, G.; Merlo, S.; Sortino, M.A. SIRT1-Dependent Upregulation of BDNF in Human Microglia Challenged with Aβ: An Early but Transient Response Rescued by Melatonin. *Biomedicines* **2021**, *9*, 466. https://doi.org/10.3390/biomedicines9050466

Academic Editor: Lorenzo Falsetti

Received: 26 March 2021
Accepted: 21 April 2021
Published: 24 April 2021

**Publisher's Note:** MDPI stays neutral with regard to jurisdictional claims in published maps and institutional affiliations.

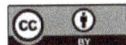

**Copyright:** © 2021 by the authors. Licensee MDPI, Basel, Switzerland. This article is an open access article distributed under the terms and conditions of the Creative Commons Attribution (CC BY) license (https://creativecommons.org/licenses/by/4.0/).

**Abstract:** Microglia represent a first-line defense in the brain. However, in pathological conditions such as Alzheimer's disease (AD), a pro-inflammatory switch may occur, leading to loss of protective functions. Using the human microglial cell line HMC3, we showed that exposure to low concentrations of β-amyloid peptide 1-42 (Aβ42; 0.2 μM) initially (6 h) upregulated anti-inflammatory markers interleukin (IL)-4, IL-13, and brain-derived neurotrophic factor (BDNF). BDNF increase was prevented by selective inhibition of SIRT1 with EX527 (2 μM). Accordingly, these early effects were accompanied by a significant Aβ42-induced increase of SIRT1 expression, nuclear localization, and activity. SIRT1 modulation involved adenosine monophosphate-regulated kinase (AMPK), which was promptly (30 min) phosphorylated by Aβ42, while the AMPK inhibitor BML-275 (2 μM) attenuated Aβ42-induced SIRT1 increase. Initially observed microglial responses appeared transient, as microglial features changed when exposure to Aβ42 was prolonged (0.2 μM for 72 h). While SIRT1 and BDNF levels were reduced, the expression of inflammatory markers IL-1β and tumor necrosis factor (TNF)-α increased. This coincided with a rise in NF-kB nuclear localization. The effects of melatonin (1 μM) on prolonged microglial exposure to Aβ42 were analyzed for their protective potential. Melatonin was able to prolong SIRT1 and BDNF upregulation, as well as to prevent NF-kB nuclear translocation and acetylation. These effects were sensitive to the melatonin receptor antagonist, luzindole (25 μM). In conclusion, our data define an early microglial defensive response to Aβ42, featuring SIRT1-mediated BDNF upregulation that can be exogenously modulated by melatonin, thus identifying an important target for neuroprotection.

**Keywords:** Alzheimer's disease; HMC3 human microglia; inflammation; microglial switch; NF-kB; Silent Information Regulator 2 homolog 1; brain-derived neurotrophic factor

## 1. Introduction

Alzheimer's disease (AD) is a progressive neurodegenerative disorder affecting primarily the elderly. A salient feature of AD is that it develops slowly over the years, remaining asymptomatic for up to two decades before diagnosis is possible [1,2]. By this time, neurodegeneration is so advanced that chances for treatment are reduced, accounting at least in part for current failure to develop effective disease-modifying therapies [1,3].

From a molecular point of view, hallmarks of AD are the increased brain levels of the beta amyloid peptide (Aβ) and phosphorylated tau protein, which respectively aggregate into extracellular plaques and intracellular tangles [4–7]. According to the amyloid cascade hypothesis, initial accumulation of the aggregation-prone 42 amino acid-long isoform of Aβ (Aβ42) is the result of an imbalance between its production and/or clearance, leading to abnormally high concentrations of oligomers that hold potential for neurotoxicity upon chronic exposure [5]. Aβ can directly interact with neuronal surface molecules, damage the cell membrane, and be internalized with ensuing oxidative stress [8]. Interestingly, however, glial cells can respond to rising concentrations of Aβ oligomers activating to oppose its buildup and its neurotoxicity. Microglia, in particular, interact with Aβ through a variety of receptors and are the main effectors of its clearance, exerting an initial anti-inflammatory response [9–12]. However, the clearing and neuroprotective functions of microglia may become insufficient upon excessive Aβ buildup, triggering a pro-inflammatory phenotypic switch [13]. In agreement, data from both AD patients and animal studies reported an increased expression of neuroinflammatory cytokines with disease progression, which coincided with a significant reduction of BDNF levels in cognition-related brain structures and in serum [14]. On these bases, targeting microglia to enhance/prolong their beneficial functions and halt/delay pro-inflammatory polarization has been proposed to represent a successful strategy [15,16].

Among candidate effectors for neuroprotection against neurodegenerative diseases, including AD, is Silent Information Regulator 2 homolog 1 (SIRT1) [17–20]. SIRT1 is an NAD$^+$-dependent deacetylase that modulates gene expression by deacetylation of histones and transcription factors. Among its targets is NF-kB, accounting for the anti-inflammatory actions of the enzyme [21,22]. In particular, SIRT1 has been shown to affect several processes in the pathogenesis of AD, from Aβ synthesis to tau toxicity, and declines in its levels have been suggested to mirror disease progression [23–25].

An interesting candidate activator of SIRT1 is melatonin, an endogenous neurohormone shown to be pleiotropic and neuroprotective in neurodegenerative conditions [26] including AD [27], Parkinson's disease [28], hypoxia/ischemia [29], and spinal cord injury [30]. Animal and human studies showed that the use of melatonin is safe in short- and long-term treatments. Only mild and no serious adverse effects have in fact been reported so far [31]. Melatonin is able to exert neuroprotection through different cellular mechanisms, including activation of antiapoptotic pathways, upregulation of anti-oxidant enzymes, and inhibition of pro-inflammatory signaling [26,32]. The hormone mainly acts through cell membrane G protein-coupled receptors, MT1 and MT2 [33,34], both widely distributed in different brain areas and expressed by both neuronal and glial cells [35]. In addition, intracellular binding sites have been reported, namely the quinone reductase enzyme MT3 [36] and the retinoic acid-related orphan receptors RORs [37]. Non-receptor-mediated actions reported for melatonin include the direct detoxification of reactive oxygen and nitrogen species [38]. In AD, melatonin-mediated neuroprotective mechanisms include anti-amyloidogenic actions [39,40], synaptic stabilization [41], and promotion of neurogenesis [42]. Clinical studies are currently underway to determine the potential of melatonin administration against sleep alterations and related decline in cognitive functions in AD, with so far positive results [43].

Based on these premises, and moving from our previous work showing the early contribution of microglia to neuroprotection [11], we here aimed to characterize the time course of beneficial microglial responses to low concentrations of Aβ, using an in vitro system to mimic the very initial events in AD development. For this purpose, we used the human microglial cell line HMC3. Furthermore, we evaluated the involvement of SIRT1 and the ability of melatonin to target SIRT1 in order to enhance microglial anti-inflammatory functions, hindering the pro-inflammatory switch.

## 2. Materials and Methods

### 2.1. Drugs and Reagents

Amyloid β peptide 1-42 (Aβ42) from Innovagen (Lund, Sweden) was prepared according to the protocol previously used in our lab [44]. Briefly, Aβ was dissolved in dimethylsulfoxide (DMSO; Sigma-Merck, Darmstadt, Germany) as a 5 mM stock, subsequently diluted to 100 μM in a culture medium, and enriched in oligomers by aggregation at RT for 24 h, followed by at least two freeze–thaw cycles prior to use. Melatonin, EX527 (Santa Cruz Biotechnologies, Santa Cruz, CA, USA), and BML-275 (Enzo Life Sciences Inc., Farmingdale, NY, USA) were dissolved in DMSO as 10 mM stocks and further diluted in a culture medium for experiments. Both EX527 and BML-275 were always added 15 min before other drugs. Luzindole (Tocris, Bristol, UK) was dissolved in DMSO as 50 mM stock and further diluted in culture medium for experiments, where it was always added 30 min before other drugs. Golgi inhibitor brefeldin-A (Thermofisher Scientific, Waltham, MA, USA) was dissolved in DMSO as a 10 mg/mL stock and added during the last 3 h of treatment.

*2.2. Cell Cultures*

The HMC3 human microglial cell line (ATTC, LGC Standards, Manassas, VA, USA) was grown in Eagle's Minimum Essential Medium (EMEM; Thermofisher Scientific, Waltham, MA, USA) supplemented with 10% fetal bovine serum (FBS; Thermofisher Scientific,Waltham, MA, USA) and penicillin (100 U/mL)/streptomycin (100 μg/mL) at 37 °C and in a 5% $CO_2$ atmosphere. Based on experimental needs, cells were plated with the following densities: 800 k cells/well in six-well plates, 15 k cells/well in 96-well plates (all plastic from Falcon, Milan, Italy), or 8 k cells/well in eight-well microslides (Ibidi, Gräfelfing, Germany). For morphological observation, cells were stained with the fluorescent dye FM® 1–43 (5 μM for 15 min; Thermofisher Scientific, Waltham, MA, USA).

*2.3. Quantitative Real-Time Polymerase Chain Reaction*

Cells were collected and total RNA extracted using the RNeasy Plus Mini Kit (Qiagen, Milan, Italy). RNA concentration was determined using Nanodrop spectrophotometer ND-1000 (Thermofisher Scientific, Waltham, MA, USA), and 2 μg of RNA were reverse transcribed using Superscript-VILO kit (Thermofisher Scientific, Waltham, MA, USA) according to the manufacturer's instructions. Quantitative real-time PCR (qRT-PCR) was performed on a 1:300 dilution of the reverse transcription reaction per sample, using the Rotor-Gene Q and Qiagen QuantiNova SYBR Green Real Time-PCR Kit. Primers are listed in Table 1 and were all from Qiagen. RPLP0 was used as the endogenous control. Melting curve analysis confirmed the specificity of the amplified products. Data were analyzed applying the $\Delta\Delta Ct$ method and expressed as fold change vs. control.

**Table 1.** Primers used for qRT-PCR.

| Gene | Primer | Cat. No. |
| --- | --- | --- |
| BDNF | Hs_BDNF_1_SG QuantiTect Primer Assay | QT00235368 |
| IL-13 | Hs_IL13_1_SG QuantiTect Primer Assay | QT00000511 |
| IL-4 | Hs_IL4_1_SG QuantiTect Primer Assay | QT00012565 |
| TNFα | Hs_TNF_1_SG QuantiTect Primer Assay | QT00029162 |
| IL-1β | Hs_IL1B_1_SG QuantiTect Primer Assay | QT00021385 |
| RPLP0 | Hs_RPLP0_1_SG QuantiTect Primer Assay | QT00075012 |

*2.4. Enzyme-Linked Immunosorbent Assay (ELISA)*

Levels of BDNF in medium from HMC3 cells plated in 96-well microplates were determined using the Biosensis® BDNF RapidTM ELISA kit (Biosensis Pty Ltd., Thebarton, SA, Australia), strictly following the manufacturer's instructions. Absorbance at 450 nm was measured with a VarioskanTM Flash Multimode Reader.

*2.5. Western Blot*

Cells were collected and lysed in M-PER® Mammalian Protein Extraction Reagent (Thermofisher Scientific, Waltham, MA, USA) supplemented with anti-protease and anti-phosphatase cocktails (Sigma-Merck, Darmstadt, Germany). Samples were sonicated, and centrifuged at high speed for 5 min at 4 °C, and protein concentration was determined by a Bradford reagent (Sigma-Merck, Darmstadt, Germany), according to the manufacturer's instructions. Absorbance was measured with a VarioskanTM Flash Multimode Reader. Nuclear and cytoplasmic fractions were extracted using the Subcellular Protein Fractionation Kit for Cultured Cells (Thermofisher Scientific, Waltham, MA, USA), according to the manufacturer's instructions. Sodium dodecyl sulfate-poly-acrylamide gel electrophoresis (SDS-PAGE) was performed by loading equal amounts of protein extracts per experiment on pre-cast "any-kDa" or 4–20% gradient gels (Bio-Rad, Hercules, CA, USA) followed by transfer to nitrocellulose membrane (Hybond ECL, Amersham Biosciences Europe GmbH, Milan, Italy) using a Transblot semidry transfer cell (Bio-Rad, Hercules, CA, USA). Membranes were blocked with a Blocker FL Fluorescent Blocking buffer (Thermofisher Scientific, Waltham, MA, USA) and incubated with primary antibodies overnight at 4 °C. The primary antibodies used were mouse anti-BDNF (1:900; Thermofisher Scientific, Waltham, MA, USA, Cat. No. MA5-34960), rabbit anti-SIRT1(H300) (1:400; Santa Cruz Biotechnologies, Santa Cruz, CA, USA, Cat. No. sc-15404), rabbit anti-NF-kBp65 (1:400; Thermofisher Scientific, Waltham, MA, USA, Cat. No. PA1-186), rabbit anti-β-actin (1:5000; Sigma-Merck, Darmstadt, Germany, Cat. No. A2066), mouse anti-glyceraldehyde 3-phosphate dehydrogenase (GAPDH) (1:5000; Millipore, Billerica, MA, USA, Cat. No. MAB374), and mouse anti-lamin B1 (1:1000; Santa Cruz Biotechnologies, Santa Cruz, CA, USA, Cat. No. sc-365214). Membranes were then washed and exposed to appropriate secondary antibodies for 45 min at RT as follows: AlexaFluor (AF) 647-conjugated anti-rabbit (1:2000; Thermofisher Scientific, Waltham, MA, USA), AF488 Plus-conjugated anti-rabbit (1:2000; Thermofisher Scientific, Waltham, MA, USA), and AF488 Plus-conjugated anti-mouse (1:5000; Thermofisher Scientific, Waltham, MA, USA). The detection of specific bands was carried out using the iBright FL1500 Imaging System (Thermofisher Scientific, Waltham, MA, USA). Band intensity was analyzed using the ImageJ software, developed by the National Institutes of Health (NIH) and in the public domain.

*2.6. Immunoprecipitation (IP) & SIRT1 Activity Assay*

Cell lysates were obtained as described in the Western blot section above. An amount of 350 μg of extracted proteins was diluted in a final volume of 500 μL with M-PER lysis buffer and incubated with 2 μg of rabbit anti-SIRT1(H300) primary antibody (1:400; Santa Cruz Biotechnologies, Santa Cruz, CA, USA, Cat. No. sc-15404) for 24 h at 4 °C. Next, 20 μL of Protein A/G PLUS-Agarose beads (Santa Cruz Biotechnologies, Santa Cruz, CA, USA, Sc-2002) were added, followed by incubation at 4 °C overnight. The mixture was centrifuged at 2500 rpm for 5 min at 4 °C. The supernatant was discarded, and the co-IP products were washed five times with PBS. After the final wash, the precipitates were resuspended in 30 μL of assay buffer from the SIRT1 activity assay kit. Enzyme activity was assayed with SIRT1 Fluorometric Drug Discovery Kit (Enzo Life Sciences Inc., Farmingdale, NY, USA) according to the manufacturer's instructions.

*2.7. Immunocytochemistry*

Cells were fixed using InsideFix Solution (Miltenyi Biotec, Bologna, Italy) and incubated overnight at 4 °C with primary antibodies diluted in InsidePerm solution (Miltenyi, Bologna, Italy). The antibodies used were rabbit anti-SIRT1(H300) (1:400; Santa Cruz Biotechnologies, Santa Cruz, CA, USA, Cat. No. sc-15404) and rabbit anti-acetyl-NF-kB p65 (Lys310) (1:30; Cell Signaling, Danvers, MA, USA, Cat. No. 3045). After washing, cells were incubated with secondary antibodies, diluted in InsidePerm solution, for 45 min RT. The secondary antibodies used were AF488-anti-mouse (1:300; Thermofisher Scientific, Waltham, MA, USA) and AF488-anti-rabbit (1:300; Thermofisher Scientific, Waltham, MA, USA). After washing, slides were mounted with 4′,6-diamidino-2-phenylindole (DAPI)-containing mounting solution (Sigma-Merck, Darmstadt, Germany). Digital images were captured with a Zeiss Observer.Z1 microscope equipped with the Apotome.2 acquisition system (Zeiss, Oberkochen, Germany). The number of immunopositive cells with nuclear SIRT1 was determined by cell counting in at least five randomly selected fields/well.

## 2.8. Statistical Analysis

All data were from three or more independent experiments run at least in triplicate. All experimental values are presented as the mean ± SEM. Statistical analyses were performed, as appropriate, by Student's t-test and one- or two-way ANOVA followed by Newman–Keuls post-hoc test using GraphPad Prism Software (GraphPad Software, San Diego, CA, USA). $p < 0.05$ was the criterion for statistical significance.

## 3. Results

### 3.1. Microglia Respond to Aβ42 with Transient SIRT1-Mediated BDNF Upregulation That Is Prolonged by Melatonin

The ability of HMC3 microglia to upregulate BDNF in response to a short exposure to Aβ42 was initially analyzed at the mRNA level by qRT-PCR. To this end, a low concentration of 0.2 µM and a higher one of 2 µM were initially tested. Results confirmed that only the lowest concentration (0.2 µM) induced a significant short-term increase of BDNF mRNA at 6 h (fold change of 1.42 ± 0.06 vs. C). In contrast, at the higher concentration of 2 µM, this effect was not present (fold change of 0.96 ± 0.12 vs. C). Based on this preliminary evidence, subsequent experiments were carried out using 0.2 µM of Aβ42.

Western blot analysis was then performed to determine protein levels of BDNF shortly after Aβ42 exposure. In these experiments, brefeldin A (5 µg/mL) was added during the last 3 h of treatment, in order to prevent BDNF release and maximize its detection. Because of brefeldin A interference with the protein maturation pathway, a pre-pro isoform of BDNF of about 35 kDa was detected. Microglia responded to Aβ42 with a significant increase in BDNF protein expression (Figure 1A). To examine the involvement of SIRT1 as a mediator of this effect, selective SIRT1 inhibitor EX527 (5 µM) was added in combination with Aβ42. Results show that in these conditions, the BDNF increase was prevented (Figure 1A). Released BDNF levels were then assayed by ELISA in a conditioned medium at 6 and 24 h and after a prolonged exposure to Aβ42 for 72 h. While no effect was detected at 6 h (not shown), released BDNF levels were significantly augmented compared to control at 24 h, an effect sensitive to EX527 (5 µM; Figure 1B). When treatments were prolonged to 72 h, microglia lost their ability to upregulate BDNF release in response to Aβ42 (Figure 1C). Melatonin was thus tested in these conditions for its ability to contrast BDNF reduction. As shown in Figure 1C, in the presence of 1 µM of melatonin, BDNF levels were still significantly higher than in control or Aβ42-treated cells. Notably, melatonin's effect was prevented by the addition of EX527 (5 µM) and of the mixed MT1/MT2 melatonin receptor antagonist luzindole (25 µM), indicating a SIRT1-mediated and receptor-dependent action.

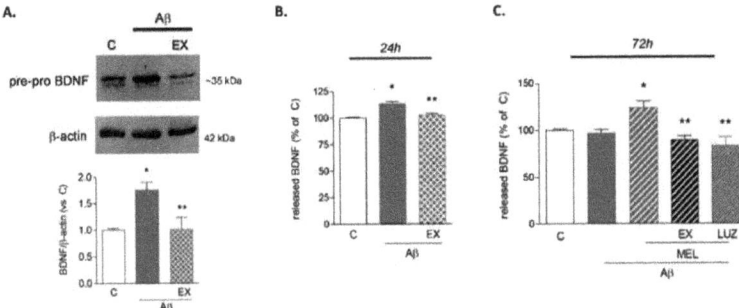

**Figure 1.** BDNF expression in HMC3 cells upon Aβ42 exposure. In (**A**,**B**), cells were treated with Aβ42 (0.2 µM) alone or in combination with SIRT1-selective inhibitor EX527 (EX, 5 µM). In (**A**), Western blot analysis of the intracellular content of BDNF at 6 h in the presence of brefeldin A (5 µg/mL). A representative blot is shown. ELISA determinations of released BDNF are reported at 24 h (**B**) and 72 h (**C**). In panel (**C**), melatonin (MEL, 1 µM) was added to Aβ42, alone or in combination with EX or luzindole (LUZ, 25 µM). Results are the mean ± SEM of 3–5 independent experiments. * $p < 0.05$ vs. C and ** $p < 0.05$ vs. Aβ (**B**) or vs. Aβ+MEL (**C**) by one-way ANOVA followed by Newman Keuls test for significance.

### 3.2. Microglia Undergo a Pro-Inflammatory Switch Following Prolonged Aβ42 Exposure

To correlate transient BDNF induction after exposure to Aβ42 with the state of polarization of human HMC3 microglial cells, gene expression of anti- and pro-inflammatory markers was evaluated by qRT-PCR at 3 and 72 h. The anti-inflammatory markers interleukin (IL) 13 and IL4 were significantly induced shortly after exposure to Aβ42 (Figure 2A), but were downregulated after prolonged treatment (Figure 2B). On the contrary, pro-inflammatory markers TNFα and IL1β were not modified after short exposure to Aβ42 (Figure 2A), but were increased after prolonged exposure (Figure 2B). This is indicative of a microglial switch towards a pro-inflammatory phenotype after prolonged Aβ42 exposure.

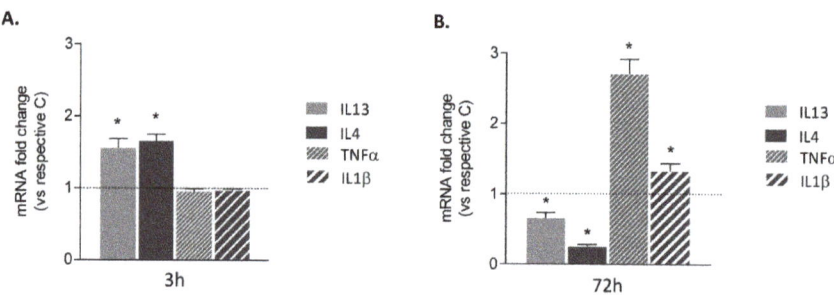

**Figure 2.** Time course of HMC3 microglial polarization. Cells were treated with 0.2 µM of Aβ42. 3 h (**A**) or 72 h (**B**). Expression of anti-inflammatory (IL4 and IL13) and pro-inflammatory (TNFα and IL1β) markers was investigated by qRT-PCR. Dotted lines indicate control values. Results are the mean ± SEM of three independent experiments. * $p < 0.05$ vs. respective control by Student's *t*-test for significance.

### 3.3. Melatonin Prolongs Transient Aβ42-Induced Upregulation of SIRT1 Activity and Expression

Given the involvement of SIRT1 in mediating Aβ42- and melatonin-induced effects on BDNF levels, the time course of its expression was characterized in more detail. Based on the well-established interdependence of SIRT1 with the activation of the AMP-regulated protein kinase (AMPK) pathway, we first analyzed phosphorylated AMPK (pAMPK) induction by Western blot. Thirty minutes after exposure to Aβ42, pAMPK was significantly upregulated (Figure 3A). Next, we examined the modulation of SIRT1 levels in response to Aβ42 and the effects of pharmacological AMPK blockade with BML-275. Western blot showed that within 6 h, SIRT1 content was increased, an effect slightly but significantly reduced by BML-275 (2 µM; Figure 3B). After 72 h, SIRT1 returned to control levels in microglia exposed to Aβ42 alone (Figure 3C). Again, we tested the effects of melatonin (1 µM) in combination with Aβ42. As shown in Figure 3C, in these conditions SIRT1 levels remained significantly higher than control or Aβ42-treated cells. This effect was sensitive to MT receptors antagonist luzindole (25 µM; Figure 3C).

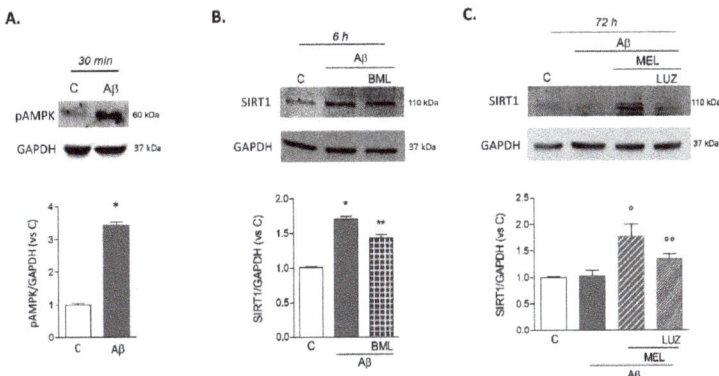

**Figure 3.** Involvement of pAMPK and time-course of SIRT1 expression in HMC3 cells upon Aβ42 exposure. Intracellular content of pAMPK (**A**) and SIRT1 (**B**,**C**) was evaluated by Western blot analysis at the time points indicated. Cells were exposed to either Aβ42 (0.2 μM) alone or in combination with AMPK inhibitor BML-275 (BML, 2 μM; **B**), with melatonin (MEL, 1 μM; **C**) or with MEL+luzindole (LUZ, 25 μM; **C**). Representative blots are shown. Results are the mean ± SEM of 3–5 independent experiments. * $p < 0.05$ vs. C by Student's t-test (**A**), * $p < 0.05$ vs. C, ** $p < 0.05$ vs. Aβ (**B**); ° $p < 0.05$ vs. C and Aβ, °° $p < 0.05$ vs. Aβ+MEL (**C**) by one-way ANOVA followed by Newman Keuls test for significance.

In order to analyze the activation of SIRT1, we carried out an enzymatic activity assay and Western analysis of its nuclear localization. The activity assay was selectively performed on SIRT1 immunoprecipitates in order to exclude contribution from other sirtuins. Results confirmed that after 6 h of exposure to Aβ42 (0.2 μM), SIRT1 activity was significantly increased compared to control (Figure 4A). In agreement, analysis of the subcellular localization of upregulated SIRT1 showed an increase in the nuclear fraction (Figure 4B) and a parallel reduction in the cytosolic fraction (Figure 4C).

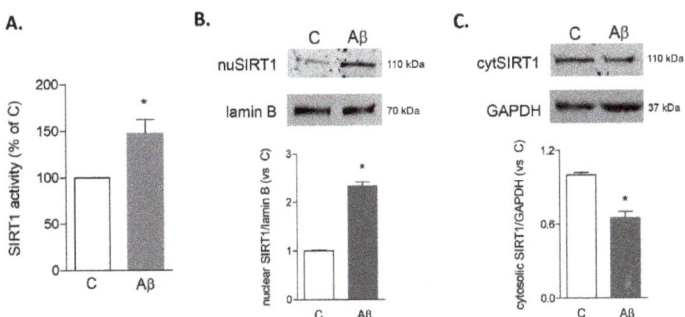

**Figure 4.** Activity and subcellular localization of SIRT1 in HMC3 cells upon Aβ42 exposure. Cells were treated for 6 h with Aβ42 (0.2 μM). SIRT1 enzymatic activity was evaluated in lysates immunoprecipitated for SIRT1 (**A**). Nuclear (**B**) and cytosolic (**C**) expression of SIRT1 were investigated by Western blot analysis on purified fractions. Representative blots are shown. Results are the mean ± SEM of three independent experiments. * $p < 0.05$ vs. C by Student's *t*-test for significance.

To further strengthen this result and monitor the sub-cellular localization of SIRT1 in time, cells were immunostained and counted for nuclear SIRT1 positivity. Representative images of SIRT1-labeled cells (green) counterstained with DAPI (blue) are reported in Figure 5A–C. After 6 h of exposure to Aβ42 alone, the population of nuclear SIRT1-positive cells was increased by 108% over the control (Figure 5D). When in combination with melatonin, Aβ induced a significantly more pronounced increase (165% over the control; Figure 5D). With Aβ42 alone, this effect was progressively reduced at 24 h (26.7% over the control; Figure 5D) and disappeared at 72 h (−5% vs. control; Figure 5D), but remained higher when in combination with melatonin (+128% vs. control at 24 h and +27% vs. control at 72 h; Figure 5D). Overall, these results confirm that SIRT1 is shortly but transiently upregulated by microglia in response to Aβ42 and that melatonin is able to potentiate and prolong this effect.

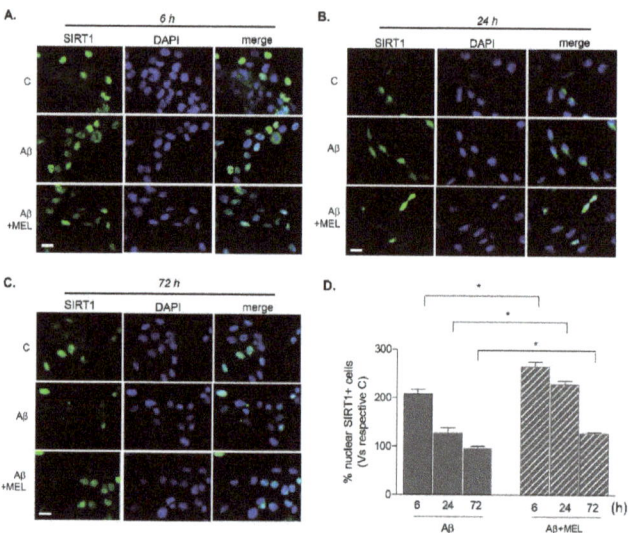

**Figure 5.** Time course of SIRT1 nuclear localization in HMC3 cells upon Aβ42 exposure. Cells were treated with 0.2 µM of Aβ42 alone or in combination with 1 µM melatonin (MEL) for 6, 24, or 72 h. In panels (**A–C**), representative images of immunostaining for SIRT1 (green) and nuclear counterstaining with DAPI (blue). Scale bar = 40 µm. In panel (**D**), graph reporting the percentage of nuclear SIRT1-positive cells over total SIRT1-positive cells, each vs. respective control, set as 100%. Results are the mean ± SEM of 3–5 independent experiments. * $p < 0.05$ vs. treatment with Aβ alone at corresponding time points (two-way ANOVA followed by Newman–Keuls test for significance; treatment vs. time).

*3.4. Melatonin Reduces Microglial NF-kB Expression Induced by Prolonged Aβ42 Exposure*

We next focused on NF-kB, a well-known target of SIRT1, with a crucial role in microglial pro-inflammatory activation. Western blot analysis on nuclear fractions confirmed an increase of NF-kB p65 after a 72 h-exposure to Aβ42 (Figure 6A). Addition of melatonin (1 µM) prevented this effect in an EX527- (5 µM) and luzindole- (25 µM) dependent fashion (Figure 6A). Since SIRT1 can directly inactivate NF-kB by deacetylation at lysine 310 (Lys310), immunostaining of acetylated NF-kB p65 was performed (green; Figure 6B). Results confirmed an increase of nuclear acetylated NF-kB-positive cells following Aβ42 exposure for 72 h. This effect was counteracted by melatonin but reappeared when cells were exposed to Aβ42+melatonin under a blockade of SIRT1 by EX527 (Figure 6B). The long-term effects of Aβ42 were also accompanied by slight morphological changes, as visualized by staining with fluorescent dye FM 1–43 (5 µM for 15 min). As shown in Figure 6C, HMC3 cells exhibited an elongated, bipolar phenotype upon exposure to Aβ42 (0.2 µM), which was partially reversed by treatment with melatonin.

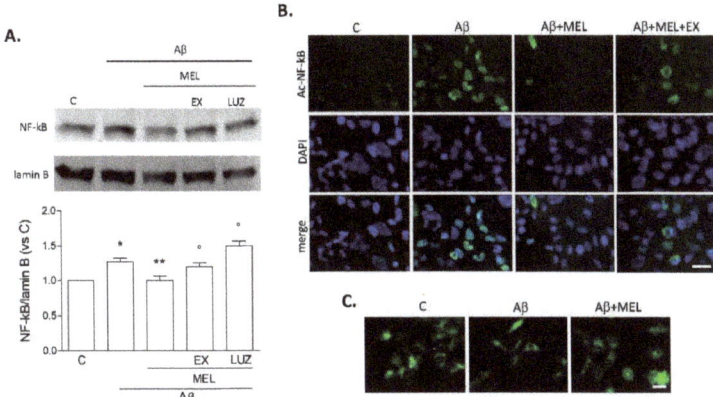

**Figure 6.** Pro-inflammatory switch of HMC3 cells upon prolonged Aβ42 exposure. Cells were treated for 72 h with Aβ42 alone (0.2 μM), in combination with melatonin (MEL, 1 μM), MEL+EX527 (EX; 5 μM), or MEL+luzindole (LUZ; 25 μM). In (**A**), Western blot of NF-kB p65 on nuclear fractions. Results are the mean ± SEM of three independent experiments, and a representative blot is shown. * $p < 0.05$ vs. C, ** $p < 0.05$ vs. Aβ, ° $p < 0.05$ vs. Aβ+MEL by one-way ANOVA followed by Newman–Keuls test for significance. In (**B**), representative images of immunostaining for acetyl-Lys310-NF-kB p65 (green) with DAPI counterstaining (blue; scale bar = 40 μm). In (**C**), morphological appearance of cells stained with fluorescent dye FM 1–43 (5 μM for 15 min; scale bar = 50 μm).

## 4. Discussion

Microglia are the resident immune cells in the brain and play a crucial role of surveillance against micro-environmental changes that could pose a threat to brain homeostasis. Microglial activation is finely balanced between pro- and anti-inflammatory phenotypes that act in concert to restore homeostasis through self-limited inflammatory events. However, this balance can be disrupted under chronic toxicity, leading to a switch from protective to detrimental [45–48]. This has been proposed to occur also in AD, where progressive accumulation of Aβ42 oligomers, over a time span of up to two decades, slowly but relentlessly leads to progressive cellular distress and chronic toxicity. This in time will push microglia towards an inflammation-sustaining phenotype [5,49–51].

The focus on microglial contribution in AD has been especially, though mainly unsuccessfully, aimed at contrasting inflammation [52,53]. However, targeting microglia to enhance their initial protective features, rather than entirely turning off their activation, appears as an appealing strategy. To this end, the very initial responses of microglia to Aβ still need to be fully characterized.

Our present study moves from our previous work, where we established in vitro models of slow-developing neuronal damage using low concentrations of oligomeric Aβ [11,54]. This allowed us to show that early Aβ-induced microglial BDNF was the mediator of an early compensatory and protective response against Aβ toxicity in neuronal cells [11,54]. On these bases, the next step was to study the time course and the mechanisms underlying Aβ-induced BDNF increase in microglia. For our purposes, we were now able to use microglia of human origin, the HMC3 cell line [55]. This appears relevant due to the different responses between murine and human microglia, as recently pointed out [56]. Notably, the early increase in BDNF and the time-dependent fluctuations in anti- and pro-inflammatory gene expression confirmed that our model, based on low Aβ42 as a light noxious stimulus, well recapitulated the dual microglial activation and the intrinsic decline of the initial neurotrophic response. In agreement, BDNF reduction has been largely linked to cognitive decline in AD patients [57–59] and preclinical in vivo models, where its administration proved to be neuro- and synapto-protective [60–62]. In vitro models provided concordant observations [63–65]. Notably, it was also shown that aging itself can cause a decline in microglial BDNF, which correlates with a pro-inflammatory switch [66].

Since the ability to support BDNF-producing, protective microglia entails the identification of an appropriate target, we here contemplated a role for SIRT1. In order to fully characterize the involvement of SIRT1 in our model and to exclude the contribution of other cellular sirtuins to the measured deacetylase activity, an in vitro activity assay was firstly carried out using SIRT1-immunoprecipitated lysates. Furthermore, SIRT1 nuclear localization was evaluated as an index of enzyme activation. Evidence from different cell types shows in fact that SIRT1 can shuttle between the nucleus and cytoplasm, exerting differential functions [67,68]. It has been pointed out that SIRT1 activity may be hampered depending on local $NAD^+$ availability [69]. However, this was not the case in our conditions, as shown by the inhibitory effects of EX527. Finally, because SIRT1 activity has been reported to be interconnected with the activation of the AMPK pathway [70,71], we confirmed AMPK involvement both by looking at its direct induction by Aβ42, and by evidencing the effects of its pharmacological blockade on SIRT1 expression. The choice to focus on SIRT1 was based on its established neuroprotective role, particularly relevant against aging and age-related diseases. SIRT1 has multiple beneficial actions in the central nervous system [72], including modulation of synaptic plasticity, learning, and memory [73,74], anti-apoptotic activity, and antioxidant and anti-inflammatory properties [75]. Deacetylation of key transcription factors such as forkhead box O3 (FOXO3), peroxisome proliferator-activated receptor γ (PPARγ), and NF-kB appear mainly involved in these effects [39,75–77]. Also in AD animal models, activation or overexpression of SIRT1 was linked to neuroprotection and improved cognitive function [78–80], whereas cognitive deficits in SIRT1 knockout mice were aggravated (Bonda et al., 2011). Interestingly, in AD patients, levels of SIRT1 appeared reduced in the serum [81], hippocampus [82], and cortex [24] and inversely correlated with neuropathological changes [23]. These data are supported by in vitro studies showing that SIRT1 directly affected Aβ production in neurons [83], promoted Aβ clearance in astrocytes [84], and inhibited inflammatory signaling in microglia [22].

Our results showed that in microglia, SIRT1 peaked early, but transiently, after Aβ42 exposure, mediating an initial BDNF-sustained neurotrophic response. In an attempt to prolong the beneficial microglial polarization, we considered as a potential candidate melatonin, a safe molecule that easily crosses the blood–brain barrier [31,85]. Indeed, melatonin in combination with Aβ prolonged the BDNF-producing state of human microglial cells, an effect majorly dependent on the induction of SIRT1 and on surface signaling through MT1/MT2 receptors. At the same time, melatonin prevented nuclear induction of pro-inflammatory transcription factor NF-kB and, importantly, attenuated its acetylation at Lys310. This is consistent with the reported ability of SIRT1 to inactivate NF-kB by the removal of the acetylic group in Lys 310 [86], which is required for NF-kB full transcriptional activity on target promoters [87]. Indeed, NF-kB inactivation prevents the microglia pro-inflammatory switch and appears relevant for neuroprotection in AD, as previously shown [21,22,88]. In our hands, the Aβ-induced microglial switch correlated with a slight trend towards a more elongated cell morphology, which melatonin was able to prevent. Data on morphological changes connected to pro-inflammatory activation of the HMC3 cell line are currently scarce and somewhat discordant. In one study, HMC3 cells appeared elongated and bipolar following stimulation with IFNγ+IL1β for 24 h [89]. In another report, activation with a high concentration of Aβ42 (5 μM) for 24 h corresponded to the acquisition of an amoeboid shape [90].

Overall, our results on melatonin's effects are in agreement with its reported multiple beneficial actions that go well beyond a mere regulation of circadian rhythms. The compound is in fact endowed with anti-inflammatory, antioxidant, and neuroprotective activity against a number of neurodegenerative conditions that share neuroinflammatory features [35,91], including Parkinson's disease [92], hypoxia [29,93], amyotrophic lateral sclerosis [94], traumatic brain injury, spinal cord injury [95], and neuropsychiatric disorders [96]. A role for melatonin has convincingly emerged also in AD, where an inverse correlation between melatonin levels and disease progression has been reported in patients, along with sleep–wake cycle disturbances [43,97]. This could be indicative of a potential loss of endogenous protection when melatonin levels are reduced. Preclinical studies on AD transgenic mice models confirmed the rescue of cognitive functions by melatonin administration, also in association with AD-approved symptomatic drug memantine [98–101]. However, molecular mechanisms involved in melatonin-mediated neuroprotection have been majorly investigated in neurons, whereas studies on glial cells are limited. Melatonin was reported to suppress the hippocampal glial activation induced by Aβ25-35 in rats [102], but, to our knowledge, there are no other detailed studies on glial cells as potential targets for melatonin in AD. We here showed for the first time that the addition of melatonin to Aβ was efficient in prolonging the peak in SIRT1 and related BDNF expression, maintaining human microglia in an anti-inflammatory state.

## 5. Conclusions

Long before AD patients enter the clinical phase, attempted protective responses take place at the cellular level that may be important in determining some degree of resilience to neurodegeneration [103,104]. Among these, microglial protective activation seems to play a key role. In the present study, we demonstrated that following a subtle challenge with Aβ, human microglial cells upregulate BDNF synthesis and release, via induction of deacetylase SIRT1. This effect is accompanied by anti-inflammatory features, but is only transient. We here show that the addition of melatonin can maintain high SIRT1/BDNF levels in the presence of Aβ for a prolonged time (Figure 7). Our study thus identifies microglial SIRT1 as a potential target in AD and highlights a therapeutic potential for melatonin as a SIRT1/BDNF inducer in microglial cells.

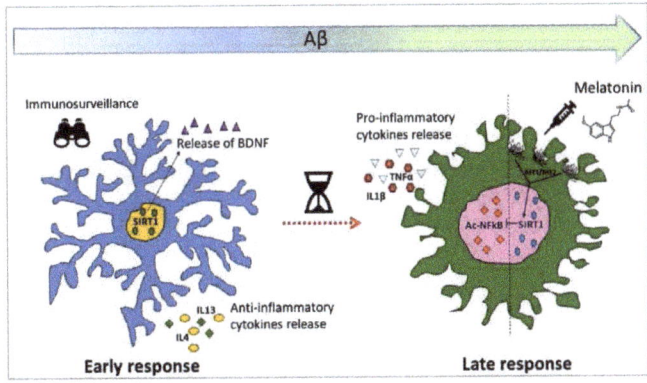

**Figure 7.** Dual response of microglia to Aβ challenge.

**Author Contributions:** Conceptualization: S.M. and M.A.S.; data curation: G.I.C., S.M., and M.A.S.; formal analysis, G.I.C., S.F.S., and S.M.; funding acquisition: M.A.S.; investigation: G.I.C., S.F.S., G.C., and S.M.; supervision: S.M. and M.A.S.; writing—original draft: G.I.C., S.M., and M.A.S. All authors have read and agreed to the published version of the manuscript.

**Funding:** This research was funded by PRIN2017 from the Italian Ministry of University and Research, grant number 2017XZ7A37_004.

**Acknowledgments:** The authors wish to acknowledge the support of Depofarma S.p.A., Italy.

**Conflicts of Interest:** The authors declare no conflict of interest.

## References

1. Holtzman, D.M.; Morris, J.C.; Goate, A.M. Alzheimer's disease: The challenge of the second century. *Sci. Transl. Med.* **2011**, *3*, 77sr71. [CrossRef]
2. Dubois, B.; Hampel, H.; Feldman, H.H.; Scheltens, P.; Aisen, P.; Andrieu, S.; Bakardjian, H.; Benali, H.; Bertram, L.; Blennow, K.; et al. Preclinical Alzheimer's disease: Definition, natural history, and diagnostic criteria. *Alzheimer's Dement. J. Alzheimer's Assoc.* **2016**, *12*, 292–323. [CrossRef]
3. Cummings, J.; Lee, G.; Ritter, A.; Sabbagh, M.; Zhong, K. Alzheimer's disease drug development pipeline: 2020. *Alzheimer's Dement.* **2020**, *6*, e12050. [CrossRef]
4. Polanco, J.C.; Li, C.; Bodea, L.G.; Martinez-Marmol, R.; Meunier, F.A.; Gotz, J. Amyloid-beta and tau complexity—Towards improved biomarkers and targeted therapies. *Nat. Rev. Neurol.* **2018**, *14*, 22–39. [CrossRef]
5. Selkoe, D.J.; Hardy, J. The amyloid hypothesis of Alzheimer's disease at 25 years. *EMBO Mol. Med.* **2016**, *8*, 595–608. [CrossRef] [PubMed]
6. Pereira, J.B.; Janelidze, S.; Ossenkoppele, R.; Kvartsberg, H.; Brinkmalm, A.; Mattsson-Carlgren, N.; Stomrud, E.; Smith, R.; Zetterberg, H.; Blennow, K.; et al. Untangling the association of amyloid-beta and tau with synaptic and axonal loss in Alzheimer's disease. *Brain J. Neurol.* **2020**. [CrossRef]
7. Gao, Y.; Tan, L.; Yu, J.T.; Tan, L. Tau in Alzheimer's disease: Mechanisms and therapeutic strategies. *Curr. Alzheimer Res.* **2018**, *15*, 283–300. [CrossRef]
8. Caruso, G.; Spampinato, S.F.; Cardaci, V.; Caraci, F.; Sortino, M.A.; Merlo, S. Beta-amyloid and oxidative stress: Perspectives in drug development. *Curr. Pharm. Des.* **2019**, *25*, 4771–4781. [CrossRef] [PubMed]
9. Zuroff, L.; Daley, D.; Black, K.L.; Koronyo-Hamaoui, M. Clearance of cerebral Abeta in Alzheimer's disease: Reassessing the role of microglia and monocytes. *Cell. Mol. Life Sci. CMLS* **2017**, *74*, 2167–2201. [CrossRef] [PubMed]
10. Merlo, S.; Spampinato, S.F.; Caruso, G.I.; Sortino, M.A. The ambiguous role of microglia in abeta toxicity: Chances for therapeutic intervention. *Curr. Neuropharmacol.* **2020**, *18*, 446–455. [CrossRef]
11. Merlo, S.; Spampinato, S.F.; Beneventano, M.; Sortino, M.A. The contribution of microglia to early synaptic compensatory responses that precede beta-amyloid-induced neuronal death. *Sci. Rep.* **2018**, *8*, 7297. [CrossRef] [PubMed]
12. Rivest, S. TREM2 enables amyloid beta clearance by microglia. *Cell Res.* **2015**, *25*, 535–536. [CrossRef] [PubMed]
13. Whittington, R.A.; Planel, E.; Terrando, N. Impaired resolution of inflammation in Alzheimer's disease: A review. *Front. Immunol.* **2017**, *8*, 1464. [CrossRef] [PubMed]
14. Lima Giacobbo, B.; Doorduin, J.; Klein, H.C.; Dierckx, R.; Bromberg, E.; de Vries, E.F.J. Brain-derived neurotrophic factor in brain disorders: Focus on neuroinflammation. *Mol. Neurobiol.* **2019**, *56*, 3295–3312. [CrossRef]
15. Deczkowska, A.; Keren-Shaul, H.; Weiner, A.; Colonna, M.; Schwartz, M.; Amit, I. Disease-associated microglia: A universal immune sensor of neurodegeneration. *Cell* **2018**, *173*, 1073–1081. [CrossRef] [PubMed]
16. Rangaraju, S.; Dammer, E.B.; Raza, S.A.; Rathakrishnan, P.; Xiao, H.; Gao, T.; Duong, D.M.; Pennington, M.W.; Lah, J.J.; Seyfried, N.T.; et al. Identification and therapeutic modulation of a pro-inflammatory subset of disease-associated-microglia in Alzheimer's disease. *Mol. Neurodegener.* **2018**, *13*, 24. [CrossRef] [PubMed]
17. Xu, J.; Jackson, C.W.; Khoury, N.; Escobar, I.; Perez-Pinzon, M.A. Brain SIRT1 mediates metabolic homeostasis and neuroprotection. *Front. Endocrinol.* **2018**, *9*, 702. [CrossRef]
18. Wong, S.Y.; Tang, B.L. SIRT1 as a therapeutic target for Alzheimer's disease. *Rev. Neurosci.* **2016**, *27*, 813–825. [CrossRef]
19. Herskovits, A.Z.; Guarente, L. Sirtuin deacetylases in neurodegenerative diseases of aging. *Cell Res.* **2013**, *23*, 746–758. [CrossRef]
20. Zhang, F.; Wang, S.; Gan, L.; Vosler, P.S.; Gao, Y.; Zigmond, M.J.; Chen, J. Protective effects and mechanisms of sirtuins in the nervous system. *Prog. Neurobiol.* **2011**, *95*, 373–395. [CrossRef]
21. Kauppinen, A.; Suuronen, T.; Ojala, J.; Kaarniranta, K.; Salminen, A. Antagonistic crosstalk between NF-kappaB and SIRT1 in the regulation of inflammation and metabolic disorders. *Cell. Signal.* **2013**, *25*, 1939–1948. [CrossRef]
22. Chen, J.; Zhou, Y.; Mueller-Steiner, S.; Chen, L.-F.; Kwon, H.; Yi, S.; Mucke, L.; Gan, L. SIRT1 Protects against microglia-dependent amyloid-β toxicity through inhibiting NF-κB signaling. *J. Biol. Chem.* **2005**, *280*, 40364–40374. [CrossRef]
23. Lutz, M.I.; Milenkovic, I.; Regelsberger, G.; Kovacs, G.G. Distinct patterns of sirtuin expression during progression of Alzheimer's disease. *Neuromolecular Med.* **2014**, *16*, 405–414. [CrossRef]
24. Julien, C.; Tremblay, C.; Emond, V.; Lebbadi, M.; Salem, N., Jr.; Bennett, D.A.; Calon, F. Sirtuin 1 reduction parallels the accumulation of tau in Alzheimer disease. *J. Neuropathol. Exp. Neurol.* **2009**, *68*, 48–58. [CrossRef] [PubMed]
25. Lee, H.R.; Shin, H.K.; Park, S.Y.; Kim, H.Y.; Lee, W.S.; Rhim, B.Y.; Hong, K.W.; Kim, C.D. Cilostazol suppresses beta-amyloid production by activating a disintegrin and metalloproteinase 10 via the upregulation of SIRT1-coupled retinoic acid receptor-beta. *J. Neurosci. Res.* **2014**, *92*, 1581–1590. [CrossRef]
26. Mahmood, D. Pleiotropic effects of melatonin. *Drug Res.* **2019**, *69*, 65–74. [CrossRef] [PubMed]
27. Vincent, B. Protective roles of melatonin against the amyloid-dependent development of Alzheimer's disease: A critical review. *Pharmacol. Res.* **2018**, *134*, 223–237. [CrossRef] [PubMed]
28. Mack, J.M.; Schamne, M.G.; Sampaio, T.B.; Pertile, R.A.; Fernandes, P.A.; Markus, R.P.; Prediger, R.D. Melatoninergic system in Parkinson's disease: From neuroprotection to the management of motor and nonmotor symptoms. *Oxidative Med. Cell. Longev.* **2016**, *2016*, 3472032. [CrossRef]

29. Paprocka, J.; Kijonka, M.; Rzepka, B.; Sokol, M. Melatonin in hypoxic-ischemic brain injury in term and preterm babies. *Int. J. Endocrinol.* **2019**, *2019*, 9626715. [CrossRef] [PubMed]
30. Shen, Z.; Zhou, Z.; Gao, S.; Guo, Y.; Gao, K.; Wang, H.; Dang, X. melatonin inhibits neural cell apoptosis and promotes locomotor recovery via activation of the Wnt/beta-catenin signaling pathway after spinal cord injury. *Neurochem. Res.* **2017**, *42*, 2336–2343. [CrossRef] [PubMed]
31. Andersen, L.P.; Gogenur, I.; Rosenberg, J.; Reiter, R.J. The safety of melatonin in humans. *Clin. Drug Investig.* **2016**, *36*, 169–175. [CrossRef] [PubMed]
32. Shukla, M.; Chinchalongporn, V.; Govitrapong, P.; Reiter, R.J. The role of melatonin in targeting cell signaling pathways in neurodegeneration. *Ann. N. Y. Acad. Sci.* **2019**, *1443*, 75–96. [CrossRef]
33. Emet, M.; Ozcan, H.; Ozel, L.; Yayla, M.; Halici, Z.; Hacimuftuoglu, A. A review of melatonin, its receptors and drugs. *Eurasian J. Med.* **2016**, *48*, 135–141. [CrossRef]
34. Ng, K.Y.; Leong, M.K.; Liang, H.; Paxinos, G. Melatonin receptors: Distribution in mammalian brain and their respective putative functions. *Brain Struct. Funct.* **2017**, *222*, 2921–2939. [CrossRef]
35. Alghamdi, B.S. The neuroprotective role of melatonin in neurological disorders. *J. Neurosci. Res.* **2018**, *96*, 1136–1149. [CrossRef]
36. Boutin, J.A.; Ferry, G. Is there sufficient evidence that the melatonin binding site MT3 Is quinone reductase 2? *J. Pharmacol. Exp. Ther.* **2019**, *368*, 59–65. [CrossRef] [PubMed]
37. Smirnov, A.N. Nuclear melatonin receptors. *Biochemistry* **2001**, *66*, 19–26. [CrossRef]
38. Reiter, R.J.; Paredes, S.D.; Manchester, L.C.; Tan, D.X. Reducing oxidative/nitrosative stress: A newly-discovered genre for melatonin. *Crit. Rev. Biochem. Mol. Biol.* **2009**, *44*, 175–200. [CrossRef]
39. Chen, C.; Zhou, M.; Ge, Y.; Wang, X. SIRT1 and aging related signaling pathways. *Mech. Ageing Dev.* **2020**, *187*, 111215. [CrossRef]
40. Li, Y.; Zhang, J.; Wan, J.; Liu, A.; Sun, J. Melatonin regulates Abeta production/clearance balance and Abeta neurotoxicity: A potential therapeutic molecule for Alzheimer's disease. *Biomed. Pharmacother.* **2020**, *132*, 110887. [CrossRef]
41. Shi, Y.; Fang, Y.Y.; Wei, Y.P.; Jiang, Q.; Zeng, P.; Tang, N.; Lu, Y.; Tian, Q. Melatonin in synaptic impairments of Alzheimer's Disease. *J. Alzheimer's Dis.* **2018**, *63*, 911–926. [CrossRef]
42. Mihardja, M.; Roy, J.; Wong, K.Y.; Aquili, L.; Heng, B.C.; Chan, Y.S.; Fung, M.L.; Lim, L.W. Therapeutic potential of neurogenesis and melatonin regulation in Alzheimer's disease. *Ann. N. Y. Acad. Sci.* **2020**, *1478*, 43–62. [CrossRef]
43. Wade, A.G.; Farmer, M.; Harari, G.; Fund, N.; Laudon, M.; Nir, T.; Frydman-Marom, A.; Zisapel, N. Add-on prolonged-release melatonin for cognitive function and sleep in mild to moderate Alzheimer's disease: A 6-month, randomized, placebo-controlled, multicenter trial. *Clin. Interv. Aging* **2014**, *9*, 947–961. [CrossRef]
44. Merlo, S.; Sortino, M.A. Estrogen activates matrix metalloproteinases-2 and -9 to increase beta amyloid degradation. *Mol. Cell. Neurosci.* **2012**, *49*, 423–429. [CrossRef]
45. Cianciulli, A.; Porro, C.; Calvello, R.; Trotta, T.; Lofrumento, D.D.; Panaro, M.A. Microglia mediated neuroinflammation: Focus on PI3K modulation. *Biomolecules* **2020**, *10*, 135. [CrossRef]
46. Du, L.; Zhang, Y.; Chen, Y.; Zhu, J.; Yang, Y.; Zhang, H.L. role of microglia in neurological disorders and their potentials as a therapeutic target. *Mol. Neurobiol.* **2017**, *54*, 7567–7584. [CrossRef]
47. Gupta, N.; Shyamasundar, S.; Patnala, R.; Karthikeyan, A.; Arumugam, T.V.; Ling, E.A.; Dheen, S.T. Recent progress in therapeutic strategies for microglia-mediated neuroinflammation in neuropathologies. *Expert Opin. Ther. Targets* **2018**, *22*, 765–781. [CrossRef] [PubMed]
48. Hu, X.; Leak, R.K.; Shi, Y.; Suenaga, J.; Gao, Y.; Zheng, P.; Chen, J. Microglial and macrophage polarization-new prospects for brain repair. *Nat. Rev. Neurol.* **2015**, *11*, 56–64. [CrossRef]
49. Hamelin, L.; Lagarde, J.; Dorothee, G.; Leroy, C.; Labit, M.; Comley, R.A.; de Souza, L.C.; Corne, H.; Dauphinot, L.; Bertoux, M.; et al. Early and protective microglial activation in Alzheimer's disease: A prospective study using 18F-DPA-714 PET imaging. *Brain J. Neurol.* **2016**, *139*, 1252–1264. [CrossRef] [PubMed]
50. Fan, Z.; Brooks, D.J.; Okello, A.; Edison, P. An early and late peak in microglial activation in Alzheimer's disease trajectory. *Brain J. Neurol.* **2017**, *140*, 792–803. [CrossRef]
51. Shen, Z.; Bao, X.; Wang, R. Clinical PET imaging of microglial activation: Implications for microglial therapeutics in Alzheimer's disease. *Front. Aging Neurosci.* **2018**, *10*, 314. [CrossRef]
52. Ozben, T.; Ozben, S. Neuro-inflammation and anti-inflammatory treatment options for Alzheimer's disease. *Clin. Biochem.* **2019**, *72*, 87–89. [CrossRef] [PubMed]
53. Gyengesi, E.; Munch, G. In search of an anti-inflammatory drug for Alzheimer disease. *Nat. Rev. Neurol.* **2020**, *16*, 131–132. [CrossRef]
54. Merlo, S.; Spampinato, S.F.; Capani, F.; Sortino, M.A. Early beta-Amyloid-induced synaptic dysfunction is counteracted by estrogen in organotypic hippocampal cultures. *Curr. Alzheimer Res.* **2016**, *13*, 631–640. [CrossRef]
55. Dello Russo, C.; Cappoli, N.; Coletta, I.; Mezzogori, D.; Paciello, F.; Pozzoli, G.; Navarra, P.; Battaglia, A. The human microglial HMC3 cell line: Where do we stand? A systematic literature review. *J. Neuroinflammation* **2018**, *15*, 259. [CrossRef]
56. Smith, A.M.; Dragunow, M. The human side of microglia. *Trends Neurosci.* **2014**, *37*, 125–135. [CrossRef] [PubMed]
57. Ng, T.K.S.; Ho, C.S.H.; Tam, W.W.S.; Kua, E.H.; Ho, R.C. decreased serum brain-derived neurotrophic factor (BDNF) levels in patients with Alzheimer's disease (AD): A systematic review and meta-analysis. *Int. J. Mol. Sci.* **2019**, *20*, 257. [CrossRef]

58. Laske, C.; Stellos, K.; Hoffmann, N.; Stransky, E.; Straten, G.; Eschweiler, G.W.; Leyhe, T. Higher BDNF serum levels predict slower cognitive decline in Alzheimer's disease patients. *Int. J. Neuropsychopharmacol.* **2011**, *14*, 399–404. [CrossRef]
59. Laske, C.; Stransky, E.; Leyhe, T.; Eschweiler, G.W.; Wittorf, A.; Richartz, E.; Bartels, M.; Buchkremer, G.; Schott, K. Stage-dependent BDNF serum concentrations in Alzheimer's disease. *J. Neural Transm.* **2006**, *113*, 1217–1224. [CrossRef]
60. Lee, S.T.; Chu, K.; Jung, K.H.; Kim, J.H.; Huh, J.Y.; Yoon, H.; Park, D.K.; Lim, J.Y.; Kim, J.M.; Jeon, D.; et al. miR-206 regulates brain-derived neurotrophic factor in Alzheimer disease model. *Ann. Neurol.* **2012**, *72*, 269–277. [CrossRef]
61. Iwasaki, Y.; Negishi, T.; Inoue, M.; Tashiro, T.; Tabira, T.; Kimura, N. Sendai virus vector-mediated brain-derived neurotrophic factor expression ameliorates memory deficits and synaptic degeneration in a transgenic mouse model of Alzheimer's disease. *J. Neurosci. Res.* **2012**, *90*, 981–989. [CrossRef]
62. Nagahara, A.H.; Merrill, D.A.; Coppola, G.; Tsukada, S.; Schroeder, B.E.; Shaked, G.M.; Wang, L.; Blesch, A.; Kim, A.; Conner, J.M.; et al. Neuroprotective effects of brain-derived neurotrophic factor in rodent and primate models of Alzheimer's disease. *Nat. Med.* **2009**, *15*, 331–337. [CrossRef] [PubMed]
63. Tagai, N.; Tanaka, A.; Sato, A.; Uchiumi, F.; Tanuma, S.I. low levels of brain-derived neurotrophic factor trigger self-aggregated amyloid beta-induced neuronal cell death in an alzheimer's cell model. *Biol. Pharm. Bull.* **2020**, *43*, 1073–1080. [CrossRef]
64. Mitroshina, E.V.; Yarkov, R.S.; Mishchenko, T.A.; Krut, V.G.; Gavrish, M.S.; Epifanova, E.A.; Babaev, A.A.; Vedunova, M.V. Brain-Derived Neurotrophic Factor (BDNF) preserves the functional integrity of neural networks in the beta-amyloidopathy model in vitro. *Front. Cell Dev. Biol.* **2020**, *8*, 582. [CrossRef]
65. Arancibia, S.; Silhol, M.; Mouliere, F.; Meffre, J.; Hollinger, I.; Maurice, T.; Tapia-Arancibia, L. Protective effect of BDNF against beta-amyloid induced neurotoxicity in vitro and in vivo in rats. *Neurobiol. Dis.* **2008**, *31*, 316–326. [CrossRef] [PubMed]
66. Wu, S.Y.; Pan, B.S.; Tsai, S.F.; Chiang, Y.T.; Huang, B.M.; Mo, F.E.; Kuo, Y.M. BDNF reverses aging-related microglial activation. *J. Neuroinflammation* **2020**, *17*, 210. [CrossRef]
67. Hisahara, S.; Chiba, S.; Matsumoto, H.; Tanno, M.; Yagi, H.; Shimohama, S.; Sato, M.; Horio, Y. Histone deacetylase SIRT1 modulates neuronal differentiation by its nuclear translocation. *Proc. Natl. Acad. Sci. USA* **2008**, *105*, 15599–15604. [CrossRef] [PubMed]
68. Tanno, M.; Sakamoto, J.; Miura, T.; Shimamoto, K.; Horio, Y. Nucleocytoplasmic shuttling of the NAD+-dependent histone deacetylase SIRT1. *J. Biol. Chem.* **2007**, *282*, 6823–6832. [CrossRef]
69. Hardeland, R. Aging, melatonin, and the pro- and anti-inflammatory networks. *Int. J. Mol. Sci.* **2019**, *20*, 1223. [CrossRef]
70. Canto, C.; Gerhart-Hines, Z.; Feige, J.N.; Lagouge, M.; Noriega, L.; Milne, J.C.; Elliott, P.J.; Puigserver, P.; Auwerx, J. AMPK regulates energy expenditure by modulating NAD+ metabolism and SIRT1 activity. *Nature* **2009**, *458*, 1056–1060. [CrossRef]
71. Ruderman, N.B.; Xu, X.J.; Nelson, L.; Cacicedo, J.M.; Saha, A.K.; Lan, F.; Ido, Y. AMPK and SIRT1: A long-standing partnership? *Am. J. Physiol. Endocrinol. Metab.* **2010**, *298*, E751–E760. [CrossRef] [PubMed]
72. Lee, S.H.; Lee, J.H.; Lee, H.Y.; Min, K.J. Sirtuin signaling in cellular senescence and aging. *BMB Rep.* **2019**, *52*, 24–34. [CrossRef]
73. Michan, S.; Li, Y.; Chou, M.M.; Parrella, E.; Ge, H.; Long, J.M.; Allard, J.S.; Lewis, K.; Miller, M.; Xu, W.; et al. SIRT1 is essential for normal cognitive function and synaptic plasticity. *J. Neurosci.* **2010**, *30*, 9695–9707. [CrossRef]
74. Gao, J.; Wang, W.Y.; Mao, Y.W.; Graff, J.; Guan, J.S.; Pan, L.; Mak, G.; Kim, D.; Su, S.C.; Tsai, L.H. A novel pathway regulates memory and plasticity via SIRT1 and miR-134. *Nature* **2010**, *466*, 1105–1109. [CrossRef] [PubMed]
75. Bonda, D.J.; Lee, H.G.; Camins, A.; Pallas, M.; Casadesus, G.; Smith, M.A.; Zhu, X. The sirtuin pathway in ageing and Alzheimer disease: Mechanistic and therapeutic considerations. *Lancet Neurol.* **2011**, *10*, 275–279. [CrossRef]
76. Brunet, A.; Sweeney, L.B.; Sturgill, J.F.; Chua, K.F.; Greer, P.L.; Lin, Y.; Tran, H.; Ross, S.E.; Mostoslavsky, R.; Cohen, H.Y.; et al. Stress-dependent regulation of FOXO transcription factors by the SIRT1 deacetylase. *Science* **2004**, *303*, 2011–2015. [CrossRef]
77. Elibol, B.; Kilic, U. High Levels of SIRT1 expression as a protective mechanism against disease-related conditions. *Front. Endocrinol.* **2018**, *9*, 614. [CrossRef]
78. Ng, F.; Wijaya, L.; Tang, B.L. SIRT1 in the brain—Connections with aging-associated disorders and lifespan. *Front. Cell. Neurosci.* **2015**, *9*, 64. [CrossRef] [PubMed]
79. Kim, D.; Nguyen, M.D.; Dobbin, M.M.; Fischer, A.; Sananbenesi, F.; Rodgers, J.T.; Delalle, I.; Baur, J.A.; Sui, G.; Armour, S.M.; et al. SIRT1 deacetylase protects against neurodegeneration in models for Alzheimer's disease and amyotrophic lateral sclerosis. *EMBO J.* **2007**, *26*, 3169–3179. [CrossRef] [PubMed]
80. Corpas, R.; Revilla, S.; Ursulet, S.; Castro-Freire, M.; Kaliman, P.; Petegnief, V.; Gimenez-Llort, L.; Sarkis, C.; Pallas, M.; Sanfeliu, C. SIRT1 Overexpression in mouse hippocampus induces cognitive enhancement through proteostatic and neurotrophic mechanisms. *Mol. Neurobiol.* **2017**, *54*, 5604–5619. [CrossRef]
81. Kumar, R.; Chaterjee, P.; Sharma, P.K.; Singh, A.K.; Gupta, A.; Gill, K.; Tripathi, M.; Dey, A.B.; Dey, S. Sirtuin1: A promising serum protein marker for early detection of Alzheimer's disease. *PLoS ONE* **2013**, *8*, e61560. [CrossRef]
82. Pukhalskaia, A.E.; Dyatlova, A.S.; Linkova, N.S.; Kozlov, K.L.; Kvetnaia, T.V.; Koroleva, M.V.; Kvetnoy, I.M. Sirtuins as possible predictors of aging and Alzheimer's disease development: Verification in the hippocampus and saliva. *Bull. Exp. Biol. Med.* **2020**, *169*, 821–824. [CrossRef]
83. Marwarha, G.; Raza, S.; Meiers, C.; Ghribi, O. Leptin attenuates BACE1 expression and amyloid-beta genesis via the activation of SIRT1 signaling pathway. *Biochim. Biophys. Acta* **2014**, *1842*, 1587–1595. [CrossRef] [PubMed]
84. Li, M.Z.; Zheng, L.J.; Shen, J.; Li, X.Y.; Zhang, Q.; Bai, X.; Wang, Q.S.; Ji, J.G. SIRT1 facilitates amyloid beta peptide degradation by upregulating lysosome number in primary astrocytes. *Neural. Regen. Res.* **2018**, *13*, 2005–2013. [CrossRef] [PubMed]

85. Ferlazzo, N.; Andolina, G.; Cannata, A.; Costanzo, M.G.; Rizzo, V.; Curro, M.; Ientile, R.; Caccamo, D. Is melatonin the cornucopia of the 21st century? *Antioxidants* **2020**, *9*, 1088. [CrossRef]
86. Yang, H.; Zhang, W.; Pan, H.; Feldser, H.G.; Lainez, E.; Miller, C.; Leung, S.; Zhong, Z.; Zhao, H.; Sweitzer, S.; et al. SIRT1 activators suppress inflammatory responses through promotion of p65 deacetylation and inhibition of NF-kappaB activity. *PLoS ONE* **2012**, *7*, e46364. [CrossRef]
87. Chen, L.F.; Mu, Y.; Greene, W.C. Acetylation of RelA at discrete sites regulates distinct nuclear functions of NF-kappaB. *EMBO J.* **2002**, *21*, 6539–6548. [CrossRef] [PubMed]
88. Thawkar, B.S.; Kaur, G. Inhibitors of NF-kappaB and P2X7/NLRP3/Caspase 1 pathway in microglia: Novel therapeutic opportunities in neuroinflammation induced early-stage Alzheimer's disease. *J. Neuroimmunol.* **2019**, *326*, 62–74. [CrossRef] [PubMed]
89. Cappoli, N.; Mezzogori, D.; Tabolacci, E.; Coletta, I.; Navarra, P.; Pani, G.; Dello Russo, C. The mTOR kinase inhibitor rapamycin enhances the expression and release of pro-inflammatory cytokine interleukin 6 modulating the activation of human microglial cells. *EXCLI J.* **2019**, *18*, 779–798. [CrossRef]
90. Akhter, R.; Shao, Y.; Formica, S.; Khrestian, M.; Bekris, L.M. TREM2 alters the phagocytic, apoptotic and inflammatory response to Abeta42 in HMC3 cells. *Mol. Immunol.* **2021**, *131*, 171–179. [CrossRef]
91. Tan, H.Y.; Ng, K.Y.; Koh, R.Y.; Chye, S.M. Pharmacological effects of melatonin as neuroprotectant in rodent model: A review on the current biological evidence. *Cell. Mol. Neurobiol.* **2020**, *40*, 25–51. [CrossRef] [PubMed]
92. Singhal, N.K.; Srivastava, G.; Agrawal, S.; Jain, S.K.; Singh, M.P. Melatonin as a neuroprotective agent in the rodent models of Parkinson's disease: Is it all set to irrefutable clinical translation? *Mol. Neurobiol.* **2012**, *45*, 186–199. [CrossRef]
93. Merlo, S.; Luaces, J.P.; Spampinato, S.F.; Toro-Urrego, N.; Caruso, G.I.; D'Amico, F.; Capani, F.; Sortino, M.A. SIRT1 mediates melatonin's effects on microglial activation in hypoxia: In vitro and in vivo evidence. *Biomolecules* **2020**, *10*, 364. [CrossRef] [PubMed]
94. Bald, E.M.; Nance, C.S.; Schultz, J.L. Melatonin may slow disease progression in amyotrophic lateral sclerosis: Findings from the pooled resource open-access ALS clinic trials database. *Muscle Nerve* **2021**. [CrossRef]
95. Naseem, M.; Parvez, S. Role of melatonin in traumatic brain injury and spinal cord injury. *Sci. World J.* **2014**, *2014*, 586270. [CrossRef]
96. Lee, J.G.; Woo, Y.S.; Park, S.W.; Seog, D.H.; Seo, M.K.; Bahk, W.M. The neuroprotective effects of melatonin: Possible role in the pathophysiology of neuropsychiatric disease. *Brain Sci.* **2019**, *9*, 285. [CrossRef]
97. Nous, A.; Engelborghs, S.; Smolders, I. Melatonin levels in the Alzheimer's disease continuum: A systematic review. *Alzheimer's Res. Ther.* **2021**, *13*, 52. [CrossRef]
98. Labban, S.; Alghamdi, B.S.; Alshehri, F.S.; Kurdi, M. Effects of melatonin and resveratrol on recognition memory and passive avoidance performance in a mouse model of Alzheimer's disease. *Behav. Brain. Res.* **2021**, *402*, 113100. [CrossRef] [PubMed]
99. Liu, Y.C.; Hsu, W.L.; Ma, Y.L.; Lee, E.H.Y. Melatonin induction of APP intracellular domain 50 SUMOylation alleviates AD through enhanced transcriptional activation and abeta degradation. *Mol. Ther.* **2021**, *29*, 376–395. [CrossRef] [PubMed]
100. Sun, C.; Qiu, X.; Wang, Y.; Liu, J.; Li, Q.; Jiang, H.; Li, S.; Song, C. Long-term oral melatonin alleviates memory deficits, reduces amyloid-beta deposition associated with downregulation of BACE1 and mitophagy in APP/PS1 transgenic mice. *Neurosci. Lett.* **2020**, *735*, 135192. [CrossRef]
101. Jurgenson, M.; Zharkovskaja, T.; Noortoots, A.; Morozova, M.; Beniashvili, A.; Zapolski, M.; Zharkovsky, A. Effects of the drug combination memantine and melatonin on impaired memory and brain neuronal deficits in an amyloid-predominant mouse model of Alzheimer's disease. *J. Pharm. Pharmacol.* **2019**, *71*, 1695–1705. [CrossRef]
102. Shen, Y.; Zhang, G.; Liu, L.; Xu, S. Suppressive effects of melatonin on amyloid-beta-induced glial activation in rat hippocampus. *Arch. Med Res.* **2007**, *38*, 284–290. [CrossRef] [PubMed]
103. De Strooper, B.; Karran, E. The cellular phase of Alzheimer's disease. *Cell* **2016**, *164*, 603–615. [CrossRef]
104. Merlo, S.; Spampinato, S.F.; Sortino, M.A. Early compensatory responses against neuronal injury: A new therapeutic window of opportunity for Alzheimer's Disease? *CNS Neurosci. Ther.* **2019**, *25*, 5–13. [CrossRef]

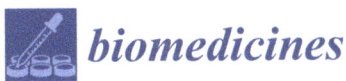 

*Review*

# Systemic Actions of SGLT2 Inhibition on Chronic mTOR Activation as a Shared Pathogenic Mechanism between Alzheimer's Disease and Diabetes

Gabriela Dumitrita Stanciu [1], Razvan Nicolae Rusu [2], Veronica Bild [1,2], Leontina Elena Filipiuc [1,3], Bogdan-Ionel Tamba [1,3,*] and Daniela Carmen Ababei [2]

[1] Center for Advanced Research and Development in Experimental Medicine (CEMEX), Grigore T. Popa University of Medicine and Pharmacy, 16 Universitatii Street, 700115 Iasi, Romania; gabriela-dumitrita.s@umfiasi.ro (G.D.S.); veronica.bild@gmail.com (V.B.); leontina.filipiuc@umfiasi.ro (L.E.F.)

[2] Pharmacodynamics and Clinical Pharmacy Department, Grigore T. Popa University of Medicine and Pharmacy, 16 Universitatii Street, 700115 Iasi, Romania; razvan.nicolae.rusu@gmail.com (R.N.R.); dana.ababei@gmail.com (D.C.A.)

[3] Department of Pharmacology, Clinical Pharmacology and Algesiology, Grigore T. Popa University of Medicine and Pharmacy, 16 Universitatii Street, 700115 Iasi, Romania

* Correspondence: bogdan.tamba@umfiasi.ro

**Abstract:** Alzheimer's disease (AD) affects tens of millions of people worldwide. Despite the advances in understanding the disease, there is an increased urgency for pharmacological approaches able of impacting its onset and progression. With a multifactorial nature, high incidence and prevalence in later years of life, there is growing evidence highlighting a relationship between metabolic dysfunction related to diabetes and subject's susceptibility to develop AD. The link seems so solid that sometimes AD and type 3 diabetes are used interchangeably. A candidate for a shared pathogenic mechanism linking these conditions is chronically-activated mechanistic target of rapamycin (mTOR). Chronic activation of unrestrained mTOR could be responsible for sustaining metabolic dysfunction that causes the breakdown of the blood-brain barrier, tau hyperphosphorylation and senile plaques formation in AD. It has been suggested that inhibition of sodium glucose cotransporter 2 (SGLT2) mediated by constant glucose loss, may restore mTOR cycle via nutrient-driven, preventing or even decreasing the AD progression. Currently, there is an unmet need for further research insight into molecular mechanisms that drive the onset and AD advancement as well as an increase in efforts to expand the testing of potential therapeutic strategies aimed to counteract disease progression in order to structure effective therapies.

**Keywords:** Alzheimer's disease; sodium glucose cotransporter 2 inhibition; mechanistic target of rapamycin; metabolic dysfunction hypothesis; diabetes

## 1. Introduction

Alzheimer's disease (AD), the leading cause of dementia in aging people, is characterized by a cognitive decline that involves memory, orientation, judgment, communication and reasoning, and is a major threat to people's health and quality of life worldwide [1,2]. According to the World Health Organization, over 47 million people are afflicted by AD globally, and this number is expected to reach almost 76 million by 2030 and about 115 million by 2050 [3]. The incidence of AD continues to rise steadily; as aging demographics of the global human population and life expectancy are increasing, leading to a heavy economic and societal burden. Undoubtedly, extensive research into the pathogenesis and AD therapies continues to stimulate in-depth efforts by academia, pharmaceutical companies and government attention to finding curative compounds or at least slow the disease progression.

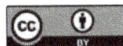

To date, with a multifactorial nature, the ultimate cause of AD remains elusive, and is generally considered to be related to genetic, neuroendocrine, biochemical, environmental, and immune factors based on aging [4,5]. In recent decades, several hypotheses have been designed to explain the AD pathogenesis mechanisms, such as amyloid-β (Aβ) deposition as the core of neuritic plaques, tau protein hyperphosphorylation as the key constituent of neurofibrillary tangles, degeneration of cholinergic neurons, or death [2,6–9]. Figure 1 highlights some of the most studied hypotheses for AD, including Aβ aggregation [10–12], cholinergic dysfunction [13,14], tau aggregation [15,16], oxidative stress [17,18], inflammation [19–21]. Challenges and future prospects include extensive testing of new hypotheses such as endo-lysosomal [22–24], mitochondrial [25–28] and metabolic dysfunctions [29,30]. It remains to be determined whether the root cause of AD is the Aβ aggregates formation and accretion between neurons or tau neurofibrillary tangle developments within neurons or the cumulative end-effects of other causal epigenetic and/or genetic processes, or a fusion of both [10,31–33]. In addition, growing evidence suggests that endo-lysosomal, mitochondrial and metabolic dysfunction display a critical role in the multiple memory and attention processes of the elderly and are viable early drivers in the onset and progression of AD [34–36]. Thus, it is more and more evident that there is a solid interplay between metabolic dysfunction related to metabolic syndrome, diabetes, obesity and patient's susceptibility to AD development [37,38]. From the strong relationship between AD and the pathological conditions of diabetes mellitus, AD can be referred to as "diabetes type 3" or "brain diabetes" [39,40].

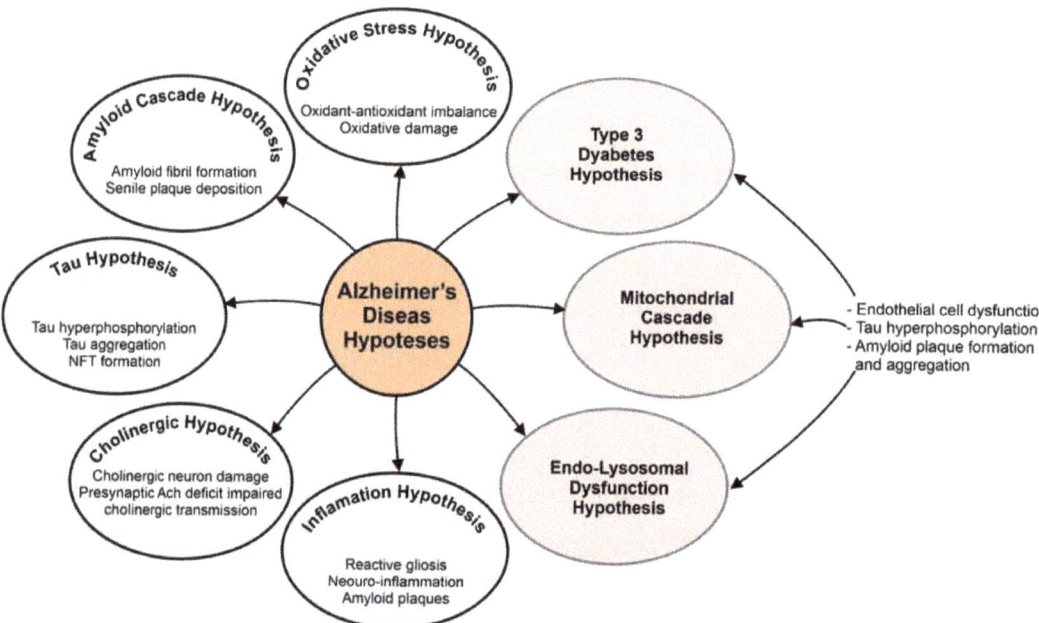

**Figure 1.** Alzheimer's disease is a neurodegenerative disease that involves a multitude of factors. Given the complexity of the human brain, the lack of effective research tools and reasonable animal models, the detailed pathophysiology of the disease remains unclear. Based on multifaceted nature of AD, there have been proposed various hypotheses, including Aβ aggregation, cholinergic dysfunction, tau aggregation, oxidative stress, inflammation, etc. Challenges and future prospects include extensive testing of new hypotheses such as endo-lysosomal, mitochondrial and metabolic dysfunctions to attack the disease from different angles for the effective development of an early diagnosis and successful drugs for therapies. NTF, neurofibrillary tangle; Ach, acetylcholine.

Overwhelming results suggest that there are early abnormalities in cerebral glucose metabolism in people with AD [41,42], involving deficiencies in glycolysis and glucose transporters [43,44]. A candidate for a shared pathogenic mechanism linking these metabolically-driven conditions is represented by a chronic mechanistic target of rapamycin (mTOR) signaling activation [45]. Chronic unrestrained mTOR activation may be behind AD lysosomal, mitochondrial and metabolic alteration, causing the failure of the blood-brain barrier (BBB) through endothelial cell dysfunction; as well as leading to tau hyperphosphorylation, amyloid plaques formation and aggregation in the brain [38,46]. Inhibition of sodium glucose cotransporter 2 (SGLT2), facilitated by a constant glucose loss, is thought to restore the mTOR cycle via nutrient-driven, nocturnal periods of transient mTOR inhibition (catabolism) interferes by transient mTOR activation (anabolism) during daily accompanying nutrition. Thus, a flexible dynamic of mTOR is reinstated, preventing or arresting AD progression. The current paper aims to discuss the possible implications of SGLT2 inhibition on chronic activation of mTOR as a common pathogenic mechanism between AD and diabetes, according to the recent research findings.

## 2. Pharmacological Approaches Able of Impacting Alzheimer's Disease and Its Progression

Given the poor epidemiological forecast and the increasing number of experimental and clinical evidence that send the manifestations of AD beyond the brain, there is a major research interest in expanding testing of new hypotheses to attack the disease from different angles to provide insights into novel therapeutic strategies. Three such hypotheses are diabetes type 3, the mitochondrial cascade hypothesis and the endo-lysosomal dysfunction hypothesis. They provide a basis for therapeutic approaches to restore AD-related metabolic, mitochondrial and endo-lysosomal dysfunctions; changes that occur early in the progression of the disease in relation to tau and Aβ deposition, which means that they are viable factors of AD development [34,35].

In AD patients, factors related to mitochondrial functions have been severely compromised. Such factors include mitochondrial morphology, oxidative phosphorylation, $Ca^{2+}$ buffering, mitochondrial biogenesis and transport along the neuronal axon. These processes could lead to negative consequences for neurons as well as for the whole structure of the brain. Mitochondria are organelles that are defined as the powerhouse of the cell due to the fact that cells in the human body rely on them to provide energy for vital functions. Neurons depend on the presence of mitochondria especially at the synapses where these organelles produce adenosine triphosphate (ATP) while also buffering calcium ($Ca^{2+}$) ion concentration. Thus, the high number of mitochondria located in the synaptic area is justified, compared to other parts of neurons [27,47]. The activity of enzymes involved in mitochondrial energy production is decreased in AD brains, thus contributing to the compromise of the mitochondrial ATP production. In line with this observation is the fact that mild cognitive impairment which is one of the early stages in AD chronology is associated with an increased level of oxidative stress markers and a decreased level of antioxidants in the brain and peripheral compartments [27,48]. This suggests there is a strong connection between oxidative stress and mitochondrial dysfunction. The oxidation of ATP synthase, a mitochondrial enzyme involved in oxidative phosphorylation has been found in isolated lymphocytes from AD peripheral blood as well as in AD brains, thus explaining the compromised activity of the ATP synthase and the reduction of ATP levels in AD. Another mitochondrial factor that is modified in AD is related to the dynamics of the mitochondria and processes such as fusion and fission. The unbalance of these processes led to compromised morphology and distribution of the mitochondria in neurons, fragmented mitochondria being observed in fibroblasts and brains from AD patients [27]. Due to their involvement in production of reactive oxygen species (ROS), mitochondria developed a system that can cope with damage done by ROS to its contents. The degradation at the organelle level is realized through a process called mitophagy. Studies have shown that inadequate mitophagy activity in eliminating increased number of damaged mitochondria led to disturbance in mitochondrial homeostasis, thus showing the involvement of the mitophagy process in AD [26].

The endo-lysosomal dysfunction hypothesis refers to the endo-lysosomal and autophagy system which is involved in maintaining protein homeostasis in cells. This system consists of endosomes, retromers, autophagosomes and lysosomes, each with its specific set of functions. One of AD's vulnerable brain regions is the hippocampus. It is here that different factors related to the endo-lysosomal and autophagy system have been reported: increased number of endosomal compartments, abnormal accumulation of autophagic vacuoles and altered expression levels of protein degradation key regulators [49]. Abnormal functions of the endo-lysosomal and autophagic networks are common in AD due to their implication in the homeostasis of Aβ and tau [50]. Lysosomes are involved in degrading and recycling macromolecules, thus leading to generation of nutrients. They are the last step to degrading organelles, macromolecules or protein aggregates by the endocytic and autophagic pathway [51,52]. Being one of the main mechanisms of cellular waste removal, it is expected that genes that facilitate lysosomal degradation are linked to a broad number of diseases and factors such as enzymatic dysfunction and positioning regarding lysosomes are involved in neurodegenerative disorders. A common histopathological feature of AD is swollen, dystrophic neurites, with lysosomes accumulated within the axonal swellings, these swellings being located in regions proximal to Aβ plaques in patient brains [51,53,54]. Studies suggest that amyloid accumulation can be actively determined by abnormal lysosome axonal transport. Impaired lysosomal positioning may be a contributing factor in AD, this being confirmed by evidence of accumulation of axonal lysosomes, increased amyloid plaque burden and lysosome dysfunction [51]. Disruption of the endo-lysosomal system is one of the earliest detectable histopathological features of AD, abnormal transport and positioning of lysosomes being contributors to the pathogenesis of the disease [55].

The third hypothesis refers to AD as "diabetes type 3" due to the implications of insulin resistance within the brain and its impact on neuro-cognition, thus contributing to neurodegenerative diseases [56,57]. It seems that the metabolic dysfunction that characterizes obesity, type 2 diabetes mellitus and metabolic syndrome determines susceptibility for individuals to develop AD [58,59]. To understand the relationship between diabetes and neurodegenerative diseases it is important to know the role of energy homeostasis in diabetes. Differentiated neurons do not have the ability to regenerate. Lack of ATP moieties, energy crisis or oxidative stress will lead to their death or degeneration, causing neurodegenerative diseases [60]. Another important aspect is that more than 40% of ATP is used to maintain neurons viable or alive. Impaired glucose uptake is a result of compromised glucose metabolism in the brain, this eventually leading to glucose homeostasis alteration, which is an important factor in the pathogenesis of AD. Reduced levels of insulin in the central nervous system can determine overproduction and impaired clearance of Aβ and reduced levels of anti-amylogenic proteins [56]. Brain insulin resistance is the failure of brain cells to respond to insulin, this leading to insulin deficiency and impaired glucose transport inside the neurons. Insulin resistance in the central nervous system correlates with peripheral insulin resistance. Therefore, without the protective effect of insulin, neurons could be more susceptible to neurotoxic insults [61,62]. Insulin resistance in AD and diabetes can lead to hyperinsulinemia. Therefore, the insulin-degrading enzymes (IDE) can be saturated which can lead to defects in regulating levels of insulin, Aβ protein and amyloid precursor protein (APP), IDE being involved in the regulation of Aβ protein and APP levels [56,63]. In addition to its peripheral actions, insulin is involved in other processes such as inducing dendritic sprouting, cell growth and repair, neuronal stem cell activation. It appears that the neuroprotective effects of insulin are due to the regulation of phosphorylated tau levels. An increased level of insulin resistance is also associated with high levels of proinflammatory cytokines which are linked to Aβ depositions in the brains [64]. In diabetes, insulin resistance causes mitochondrial dysfunction, triggering inflammatory response with increased levels of cytokines such as interleukin (Il)-1β, Il-6, Il-8, tumor necrosis factor-alpha (TNF-α), alpha-1-antichymotrypsin (ACT) and C-reactive protein (CRP), the same mechanism being triggered in AD [65]. The common situation for both type 1 and 2 diabetes is chronic hyperglycemia, considered a risk factor for AD. Regarding AD, type 1 diabetes insulin deficiency seems to be the main factor for increased tau phosphorylation, while hyperglycemia-induced tau cleavage with insulin disturbances could be the factor that leads to tau pathology in type 2 diabetes [66]. The underlying mechanism that links these three hypotheses may be chronically-activated mTOR signaling, which influences mitochondrial dynamics, biogenesis and processes such as autophagy, mitophagy and proteostasis [47]. This activation is associated with physical inactivity and over-nutrition, which leads to chronic anabolic signaling driven by increased levels of glucose, amino acids and growth signaling factors prevalent in patients with metabolic conditions. By caloric restriction, increased activity, intermittent fasting or pharmacological agents capable of mimicking the interventions above-mentioned, the beneficial influence it would have on mTOR could lead to a positive impact on the progression of AD [58,67].

## 3. Implications of Restoring Metabolic Health in the Therapy of Alzheimer's Disease

Energy production in the brain depends largely on glucose metabolism, as the disruption of its homeostasis would endanger neuronal cells. Both hyperglycemia and hypoglycemia affect the integrity of the brain, especially the cognitive functions. Cerebral glucose metabolism consists of glucose transport and intracellular oxidative catabolism, as the damage of this metabolism favors the appearance of metabolic abnormalities highlighted in the brain of patients suffering from AD. In this regard, it appears that glucose transport abnormalities may be related to insulin resistance [68], the defects in glucose transporters and glycogenolysis [43].

Metabolic dysfunction is a well-recognized risk factor for dementia, and particularly patients with diabetes seem to have an increased risk of AD [69]. This risk may be due to a shared pathogenic mechanism between AD and diabetes involving hyperinsulinemia and hyperglycemia, which raises the question of whether the use of antidiabetic compounds could impact the risk of dementia, and whether these agents may be used to prevent or treat AD [70]. Acetylcholinesterase (AChE) inhibitors, as primary targets for Alzheimer's therapy, still offer symptomatic relief only, with no slowing of AD progression [71]. Thus, some recent studies explored the extent to which antidiabetic treatments could influence brain pathology, mainly AD characteristics (Table 1), with a majority of them targeting possible benefits on neuroinflammation, amyloid pathology, tau pathology, cognitive function, neurogenesis, oxidative stress or synapses [72–75]. A current nested case control research evaluating the implications of a range of antidiabetic drugs in dementia has shown that sulphonylureas/glinides, insulin, and thiazolidinediones (TZDs) had no positive impact on development of dementia. In contrast, dipeptidyl peptidase-4 (DPP-4) inhibitors, metformin, SGLT2 inhibitors and glucagon-like peptide-1 (GLP1) agonists showed benefit, with metformin barely reaching significance, whereas both SGLT2 inhibitors and GLP1 agonists use displayed a 42% decrease in dementia risk [76]. Metformin, a widely used biguanide, crosses the BBB and can improve various cognitive functions. An in vivo study of a diabetic mouse model treated with metformin found that it reduces hippocampal apoptosis, increases the expression of p- adenosine 5'mmonophosphate-activated protein kinase (AMPK), a protein involved in regulating energy metabolism, reduces vascular permeability, and stimulates endothelial nitric oxide synthesis [77]. Another study relates the neuromodulatory action of metformin, by activating various molecular signaling pathways with improved cognitive function such as memory in a streptozocin-induced diabetic rat model. After 8 weeks of treatment, the cognitive decline of diabetic rats was ameliorated and some of the therapeutic success would be due to the hypoglycemic effect of metformin [78].

**Table 1.** Classes of antidiabetic compounds as potential therapies for Alzheimer's disease.

| Antidiabetic Drugs | Experimental Model | Findings | References |
|---|---|---|---|
| Insulin | rat model of intracerebroventricular streptozotocin (STZ) injection-induced cognitive dysfunction, intraventricular delivery of 0.5 units = 12 nmol of detemir | rescued STZ-induced cognitive decline | [79] |
| | patients with early AD or moderate cognitive impairment; intranasal delivery of 20 or 40 IU insulin | improved attention, verbal memory and functional status; modulation of Aβ peptide | [80–83] |
| | healthy volunteers, intranasal administration of 4 × 40 IU of insulin | improvement in memory and mood, increase regional cerebral blood flow in the putamen and the insular cortex | [84–86] |
| Metformin | neuronal cell lines under prolonged hyperinsulinemic conditions, various concentrations of metformin (0.4–3.2 mM) | insulin signaling resensitization, prevention of the molecular and pathological changes observed in AD neurons | [87] |
| | murine primary neurons (from tau transgenic mice and wild type), different concentration of metformin (2.5 mM or 10 nM) | reduction of tau phosphorylation | [88] |
| | transgenic mouse model of AD intraperitoneal delivery of 200 mg/kg metformin; or 350 mg/kg/day metformin delivered in drinking water for several months | amelioration of cognitive deficits, reduce Aβ plaque deposition attenuation of memory impairment | [73] [89] |
| | in older adults with an incident diagnosis of AD; 1–9, 10–29, 30–59, or ≥60 metformin prescriptions | more than 60 prescriptions were correlated with a slightly increased risk of developing AD | [72] |
| Thiazolidinediones | transgenic AD mouse model 0.03 mg/kg/day of leptin intranasal delivery + intraperitoneal administration of 10 mg/kg/day pioglitazone for 2 weeks | reduce brain Aβ levels and spatial memory impairments | [71] |
| | 7 days gavage therapy with 40 mg/kg/day of pioglitazone | decrease glial inflammation and soluble Aβ1–42 peptide levels by 27% | [90] |
| | control trial in patients with AD and diabetes, doses of 15–30 mg pioglitazone for 6 months | cognitive deficits amelioration and stabilization of the disease in diabetics with AD | [91] |
| | pilot trial with AD patients without diabetes; daily 45 mg of pioglitazone | no important efficacy data were detected | [92] |
| | clinical trials; 2 to 8 mg of rosiglitazone, as adjunct therapy in AD patients | pro-cognitive effects | [93] |
| Glucagon-like peptide-1 receptor agonists | transgenic mouse model of AD intraperitoneal injection with 1 or 10 nmol/kg of lixisenatide for 10 weeks | prevented memory impairment, neuronal loss, and deterioration of synaptic plasticity reduction of amyloid plaques and neurofibrillary tangles | [94] [95] |
| | 10 nmol/kg lixisenatide for 60 days intraperitoneal injection with 2.5 or 25 nmol/kg of liraglutide for 10 weeks | reduce Aβ deposition by 40–50%, and decrease inflammatory response | [96] |
| | a pilot clinical trial in AD patients; daily subcutaneously injections of 0.6 mg liraglutide in the first week; hereafter 1.2 mg daily for another week before finally increasing to 1.8 mg daily (week 26) | brain glucose metabolism decline prevention; no important cognitive changes compared with placebo group | [97] |

Table 1. *Cont.*

| Antidiabetic Drugs | Experimental Model | Findings | References |
|---|---|---|---|
| Dipeptidyl Peptidase-4 Inhibitors | transgenic mouse models of AD 20 mg/kg/day of sitagliptin for an 8-weeks period | pro-cognitive effects, reduction of Aβ deposits | [98] |
| | daily gavage of 5, 10 and 20 mg/kg sitagliptin for 12 weeks | diminution of nitrosative stress and inflammation markers, reduction of Aβ deposition | [99] |
| | daily oral administration of 5, 10, and 20 mg/kg linagliptin for 8 weeks | amelioration of cognitive deficits, diminution of Aβ42 levels, reduction of tau phosphorylation and neuroinflammation | [100] |
| | STZ-induced rat model of AD; 0.25, 0.5 and 1 mg/kg of saxagliptin in gavage delivery for 60 days | reduction of Aβ formation, a marked decrease of Aβ42 level and tau phosphorylation | [101] |
| | STZ-induced rat model of AD; daily orally doses of 2.5, 5 and 10 mg/kg vildagliptin for 30 days | attenuation of tau phosphorylation, Aβ and inflammatory markers | [102] |
| Sodium-glucose cotransporter 2 inhibitors | scopolamine-induced rat model of memory impairment; daily oral gavage of 10 mg/kg canagliflozin for 14 days | improvement of memory dysfunction | [103] |

STZ, intracerebroventricular streptozotocin; AD, Alzheimer's disease; Aβ, amyloid β.

Insulin resistance has also been associated with elevated levels of proinflammatory cytokines (Il-1, Il-6, TNF-α). Insulin signaling involves the brain to take up glucose and synthesize the insulin-degrading enzyme and is also involved in the degradation of β amyloid. In diabetes, due to the change in insulin signaling, a low synthesis of the enzyme involved in its degradation takes place, thus reducing the process of degradation of β-amyloid with abnormal accumulation in the brain [46,64,104,105]. Insulin and insulin-like growth factor (IGF) are hormones that regulate cell metabolism. These hormones in the brain are needed for the synaptic activity, neurogenesis, neuronal survival and memory. Synthesized in the pancreas, they cross the BBB and reach the brain, bind to insulin receptors and its growth factor followed by autophosphorylation under the action of kinases, affecting a number of cellular signaling pathways including PI3K/AKT, MAPK/ERK. S6, a downstream target of mTOR acts as negative feedback, phosphorylates and deactivates insulin growth factor substrates [46]. Recent studies have focused on the effects of insulin and its growth factor on β-amyloid accumulation. Some studies show that reduced signaling of insulin growth factor has a protective effect against the accumulation of beta amyloid while other studies have shown that in the brains of patients with postmortem AD, insulin resistance and reduced insulin signaling have been correlated with increased risk of dementia and AD [106,107]. Although the physiological role of insulin in the brain is incompletely understood, the intranasal insulin-based therapy began to attract attention in AD research, when small human studies described improved knowledge without a change in blood glucose or insulin levels in healthy volunteers [85,108]. Therapeutically, antidiabetic agents such as rosiglitazone and pioglitazone have been recommended, peroxisome proliferator-activated receptors (PPARγ) agonists used to treat diabetes in order to improve the pathogenesis of insulin resistance and hyperglycemia [109]. PPARγ is a nuclear receptor with an essential role as a transcription factor in the control of inflammatory genes; PPARg agonists can inhibit these proinflammatory genes, as demonstrated in animal models of AD transgenic mice. These agonists reduced microglial inflammation and favored Aβ phagocytosis followed by improved cognitive function. The effectiveness of pioglitazone was demonstrated in a diabetic mouse model when the inflammatory responses present in AD were reduced. However, Phase III clinical trials for rosiglitazone and pioglitazone approved for the treatment of type 2 diabetes have failed due to lack of efficacy in AD, both of which have no impact on the disease [46,110]. Currently, type 2 diabetes therapy aims to reduce plasma glucose levels during the day by constantly discharging glucose into the urine and modifying sodium in the kidneys, SGLT2 inhibitors demonstrate a positive impact on anabolic/catabolic cycle restoration, a new way to treat AD [106]. SGLT2 inhibitors target the sodium-glucose cotransporter 2, the major glucose transporter in the kidney, responsible for the reabsorption of 90% of glucose from primary urine. Inhibition of SGLT2 decreases glucose reabsorption and thus increases urinary glucose excretion, leading to a reduction in both fasting and postprandial hyperglycemia; preventing glucotoxicity and hyperglycemia-induced damage [43]. The first clinical trial exploring the SGLT2 inhibition effects on AD patients is ongoing and focuses on brain energy metabolism impact following therapy with the SGLT2 inhibitor dapagliflozin [111]. Canagliflozin (known as Invokana) is SGLT2 targeting drug. A recent research discussed the canagliflozin effects on cerebral AChE activity in obese diabetic rats [103], while an enzoinformatics study was suggested as AChE inhibitor [112]. Recently, a new SGLT2i mechanistic theory was approached, which claims that the loss of glucose through urine directed by SGLT2 inhibitors restores the diurnal switching between anabolic and catabolic states caused by mTOR signaling [67].

mTOR is a serine/threonine (289 kDa) protein kinase with large dimensions present in all cell types, a protein named after rapamycin, a compound isolated in 1972 from *Streptomyces hygroscopicus* structurally related to lipid kinases such as phosphatidylinositol-3-OH kinase (PI3K), with a key role in multiple cellular processes such as glucose metabolism, apoptosis, proliferation, transcription and cell migration [113–115]. mTOR kinases function as a hub for switching between anabolic and catabolic processes, consisting of 2 complexes called mTORC1 and mTORC2, with different cellular functions and essential for life. mTOR binds to specific proteins in each complex (Raptor and Rictor), mTOR complex (mTORC)1 being activated by the availability of nutrients, especially amino acids and coordinates protein synthesis and degradation and mTORC2 being receptive especially to insulin, promoting stress responses, mediates conversation between pathways insulin signaling and mTOR signaling [116,117]. The target of mTOR is a protein kinase with an essential role in controlling protein synthesis, cellular functions and autophagic regulation, as the disorder of this major regulator is associated with the pathogenesis of various human diseases such as AD by Aβ deposition, deterioration of the metabolic state of the cell with the onset of diabetes and obesity, the inactivation of mTOR signaling being initiated in the early stages of AD [107].

Diabetes and AD are both linked to a condition of chronically activated mTOR, resulting in chronic inhibition of autophagic and lysosomal processes that affect the long-term functioning of the brain, pancreas, heart, kidney, and other organs [118–120]. Identifying which compound, if any, is ideal for the treatment of AD and whether these drugs would be optimal in association use, remains to be tested.

## 4. Impact of SGLT2 Inhibition on Chronic mTOR Activation: Is the Brain a Target?

mTOR activity is indispensable in terms of the normal cognitive process, while mTOR hyperactivity can be damaging to brain function [121–123]. The interrelation between neuropathological hallmarks of AD and mTOR has been studied extensively, highlighting a preclinical picture that often revealed contradictory-appearing data [124,125]. Figure 2 shows schematically the implications of mTOR hyperactivity in the normal cognitive process and AD.

Analyzing the changes of mTOR signaling in AD transgenic mouse models, Lafay-Chebassier et al. [126] reported lower mTOR signaling and an important alteration of mTOR phosphorylation in the cerebellum of 12-month-old APP/PS1 mice than controls, contradicting a previous study that revealed hyperactive mTOR signaling in 9-month-old APP/PS1 mice. The hyperactivity of mTOR has been described when the mice have extensive Aβ plaque deposits [127]. In a study that explored the correlation between the mTOR pathway and Aβ-induced synaptic dysfunction, which is considered to be critical in the AD pathogenesis; mTOR signaling was downregulated in young pre-pathological Tg2576 mice. In contrast, in elderly Tg2575 mice with established Aβ pathology, mTOR activity was comparable to that of wild-type mice of the same age [128]. Using 3xTg-AD mice, other studies have shown an age- and cerebral region-dependent increase in mTOR activity. The results showed that the formation of Aβ plaques preceded mTOR hyperactivity and was most likely due to high levels of soluble Aβ. Genetic or immunological prevention of Aβ formation and deposition was sufficient to decrease mTOR signaling to wild-type levels [129–131]. The findings were in agreement with reports exhibiting an upregulation in mTOR signaling in postmortem human brains affected by AD [132–136]. Chronic inhibition of mTOR by rapamycin therapy when it began in the early stage of Aβ deposition and in the absence of microtubule-associated protein tau (MAPT) pathology improved learning and memory function in transgenic mice modeling the disease [114,137].

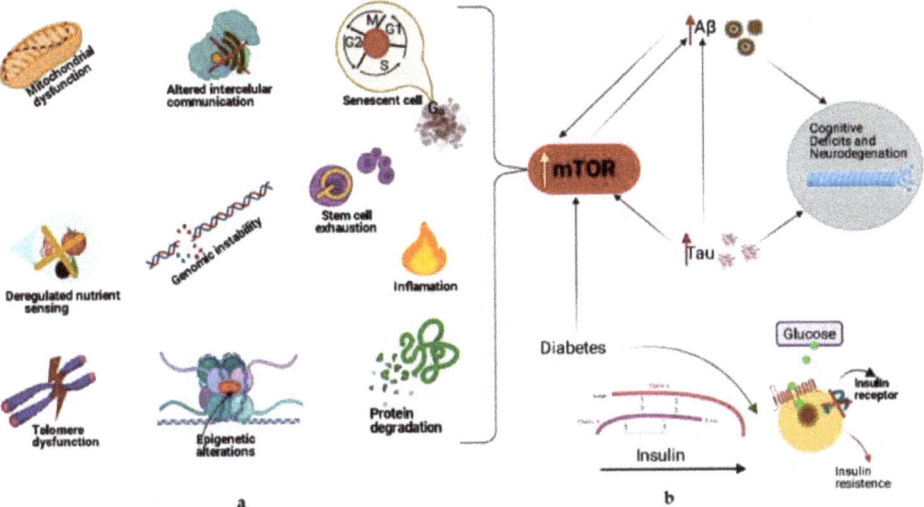

**Figure 2.** Schematic representation of mTOR hyperactivity in cognitive aging and AD. (**a**) Left—The implications of mTOR in main processes of aging. These features of aging, to different degrees, lead to an increased risk for AD, as well as cognitive decline during normal aging. Rapamycin and other pharmacological approaches that decrease mTOR activity may be valuable for delaying AD progression. (**b**) Right—The interrelation between neuropathological hallmarks of AD and mTOR. Hyperactive mTOR increases the production of Aβ and tau; and many factors including diabetes may influence the crosstalk of these proteins, and the aberrant cycle it creates contributes to the pathogenesis of AD.

Rapamycin administration both early and late in AD pathogenesis has been shown to delay, but not reverse accumulation of Aβ and MAPT tangles, as well as cognitive deficits in transgenic mouse models [122]. Although the data indicate that rapamycin treatment has unwanted side effects in the elderly population, therapies in which the compound is utilized in on-off programs may be designed for early or moderate AD stages. Additionally, research using agents other than rapamycin that inhibit the mTOR pathway and lack its side effects may be justified. While it is difficult to dissect the underlying causes of these divergent findings, the strain and age of animals, as well as variable Aβ levels may have differential effects on mTOR. Recent data suggests that, just as Aβ affects mTOR, mTOR similarly affects Aβ. This indicates that these proteins are closely correlated with each other and clarification of the mechanism of this relationship may reveal previously unknown features of AD pathogenesis [45].

Protein synthesis and their degradation controlled by the autophagy process, the mechanistic target of mTOR, is a main switch that integrates growth factors and the state of cellular nutrients that influence metabolism, modulate aging [133,138]. Reduced mTOR signaling may be a mechanism by which dietary restriction leads to increased longevity, compensating for reduced aging time [116,117,139]. Autophagy is a lysosome-dependent homeostatic process by which toxic compounds, damaged organelles and mitochondria, misfolded proteins are sequestered in autophagosomes, with vital roles in various physiological and pathological processes such as cell death and the elimination of pathogenic microorganisms or protein accumulation in cells followed by neurodegeneration [140–142]. The mTOR signaling pathway seems to be involved in both type 1 and type 2 diabetes, insulin production being reduced in type 1 diabetes due to the destruction of pancreatic β cells while insulin resistance occurs in type 2. The survival of β cells depends on the regulation of the insulin receptor substrate -2 (IRS), the chronic exposure of these cells to glucose and an increased phosphorylation of Ser/Thr being correlated with the decrease in the level of the IRS-2. Insulin-induced protein proliferation and glucose- and amino acid-induced growth are dependent on mTOR signaling in pancreatic cells, as chronic mTOR activation results in insulin resistance characterized by hyperglycemia, and the onset of type 2 diabetes [143] (Figure 3).

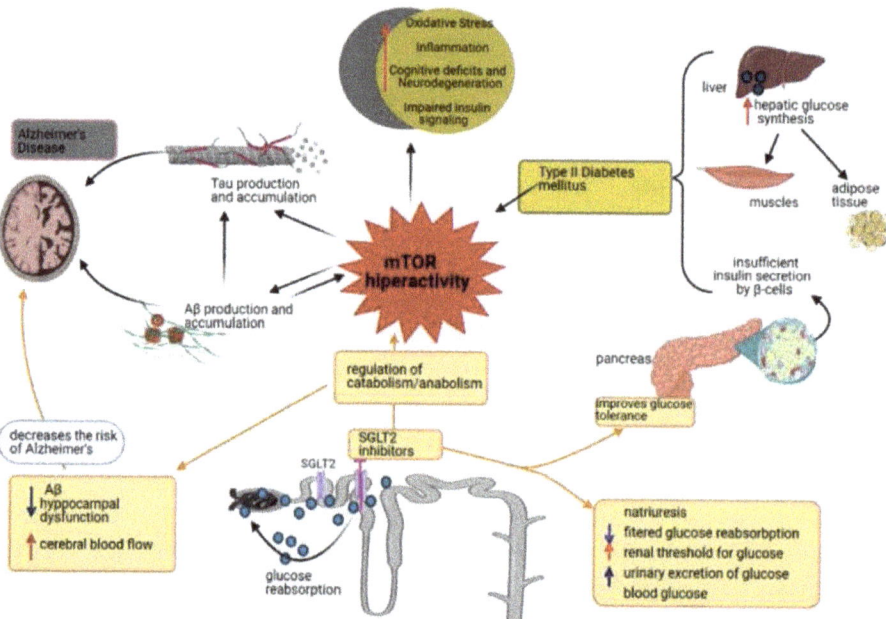

**Figure 3.** Type 2 diabetes is characterized by insulin resistance caused by uncontrolled hepatic glucose synthesis and by reduced uptake of glucose by muscle and adipose tissue. The pancreas contains functional β cells, but the variable secretion of insulin affects the maintenance of glucose homeostasis because β cells are gradually reduced. AD is characterized by increased synthesis and accumulation of tau and β-amyloid proteins. Aβ plaques may induce insulin resistance. Cerebral glucose metabolism consists of glucose transport and intracellular oxidative catabolism, affecting this metabolism favoring the appearance of metabolic abnormalities highlighted in the brains of patients with AD. Chronic activation of mTOR may be responsible for as endo-lysosomal, mitochondrial and metabolic dysfunctions in AD. High glucose intake causes hyperactivation of mTOR with abnormal insulin signaling accompanied by accelerated progression and symptoms similar to AD and with hyperglycemia and the appearance of type 2 diabetes. In patients with type 2 diabetes and AD it occurs: increased oxidative stress, inflammation, cognitive deficit and insulin resistance. Type 2 diabetes therapies based on type 2 co-transport inhibitors for sodium and glucose promotes: natriuresis, reduced filtered glucose reabsorption, decreased renal threshold for glucose, increased urinary glucose excretion followed by reduced plasma glucose levels. These compounds have a positive impact on the restoration of the anabolic/catabolic cycle and represent a new way to treat AD. AD, Alzheimer's disease; Aβ, amyloid β; SGLT2, sodium glucose cotransporter 2; mTOR, mechanistic target of rapamycin.

In therapy with SGLT2 inhibitors, the uric acid levels decrease early in conjunction with other inflammatory markers, such as high-sensitive CRP, suggesting an early influence on oxidative stress/inflammation-associated processes. Uric acid is recognized as a mediator of endothelial dysfunction and inflammation through its activation of the nod-like receptor pyrin domain containing 3 (NLRP3) inflammasome [144–146]. Activation of NLRP3 in the microglia is a key stress-induced innate immune mechanism that leads to AD pathology [147,148]. The detailed mechanism by which SGLT2 inhibitors decrease uric acid is currently unknown, but it is interesting that its elevated levels have been shown to indirectly activate mTOR [149]. Its rapid and persistent decrease caused by SGLT2 inhibitors, in patients with elevated uric acid levels, offers another possible mechanism to reduce chronically activated mTOR signaling. Even so, the role of uric acid in the development of neurodegenerative diseases is not clearly defined. Higher uric acid levels can positively influence cognitive function and reduce the risk of AD onset and progression [150,151].

A growing body of evidence suggests that reduced nitric oxide (NO) signaling is involved in AD-related pathological processes [152,153]. The NO production is diminished via endothelial (e) nitric oxide synthase (NOS) phosphorylation, resulting in uncoupling of NO production [154]. It has been shown that mTOR hyperactivity uncouples NO production through eNOS phosphorylation, thus increasing superoxide generation. With a key role in maintaining endothelial function, chronic disruption of NO production can lead to inflammation, oxidative stress and endothelial dysfunction [154,155]. Dietary rapamycin supplementation has been shown to reverse age-related vascular endothelial dysfunction and oxidative stress accompanied by a decrease in superoxide production similar to levels in younger animals [156]. These results suggest the potential for SGLT2-driven mTOR inhibition in endothelial cells at the BBB level to modulate the dysfunction and oxidative stress linked with chronic mTOR activation and to reinstate properly endothelial function and NO production.

The most essential amino acids that activate mTOR in order to prevent the formation of autophagosomes are leucine, glutamine and arginine. A decrease in the level of these amino acids also seems to drive the lysosomal acidification process critical for protein degradation independent of autophagy activation [157]. Remarkably, amino acid starvation appears to be a faster and stronger activator of lysosomal/autophagy degradation than rapamycin, a direct pharmacological inhibitor of mTOR, making SGLT2 inhibitors potentially superior options to rapamycin in treating disorders characterized by chronic mTOR activation [158]. Clinical data showing an increase in amino acid catabolism during use of SGLT2 inhibitors is suggested by the increased oxidation of proteins, which is evident following 3 months of dapagliflozin therapy [159]. The increase in urea and urea cycle metabolites evident in a study in diabetic patients treated for 30 days with empagliflozin also suggests that there is a growth in protein catabolism [160].

Moreover, recent data evaluating the post-mortem status of mTOR in the brain of the patient with AD revealed concurrent phosphorylation/activation of both AMPK and mTOR which were co-localized with hyperphosphorylated tau. The results of this study suggest that the concurrent dysregulated AMPK activity that causes chronic mTOR activation is critical for genesis and progression of AD, and fundamentally driven by a lack of constant periods of fasting amino acids flux to the liver to support gluconeogenesis [161]. The striking parallelism of these molecular, cellular, and clinical profiles occurring along the path towards AD could be beneficially impacted by restoration of circadian SGLT2 inhibition mTOR modulation.

## 5. Concluding Remarks

Precision therapies for AD, in which genetic, environmental, neuroendocrine, biochemical and immune data are included to design specific prevention and treatment strategies, lagged behind other areas such as neoplastic diseases. This gap is partly due to the fact that there is no strong consensus on which therapeutic approaches might be effective. With the emergence of new pharmaceutical options and the increasing availability of large sets of metabolic data, the targeted approaches are expected to become more feasible.

Activation/inhibition of mTOR activity may be a shared pathogenic link between all metabolic and mitochondrial dysfunctions in AD, influencing metabolic dynamics, mitochondrial activity and biogenesis (fusion/fission), and essential housekeeping processes (proteostatis, mitophagy and autophagy) facilitated via circadian nutrient flux.

These circadian anabolic and catabolic fluxes, specific to healthy people, are disturbed by aging, physical inactivity, over-nutrition and metabolic diseases leading to the idea that improvements in metabolic flow through either intermittent fasting, increased activity, caloric restriction or pharmacological compounds able of mimicking the physiology of intermittent fasting/exercise/caloric restriction on mTOR may play a critical role in AD progression.

The multifarious nature of metabolic/remodeling role in AD and related disorders will require further research. It is likely that various aspects of the restoration of circadian SGLT2-mTOR modulation, such as its effects on anabolic (cell growth, protein synthesis,) and catabolic (lysosomal function, autophagy) processes are responsible for sustaining metabolic dysfunction in AD. Restoring metabolic health is an attractive avenue to facilitate future therapies for the prevention and treatment of AD, as well as to promote the preservation of healthy brain and body aging throughout life.

**Author Contributions:** Conceptualization, G.D.S.; writing-original draft preparation, G.D.S., D.C.A., V.B., R.N.R., L.E.F.; writing-review and editing, G.D.S., B.-I.T.; supervision, B.-I.T., project administration, G.D.S.; funding acquisition, G.D.S. All authors have read and agreed to the published version of the manuscript.

**Funding:** This research was funded by "Grigore T. Popa" University of Medicine and Pharmacy, grant number 4715/25.02.2021.

**Institutional Review Board Statement:** Not applicable.

**Informed Consent Statement:** Not applicable.

**Data Availability Statement:** No new data were created or analyzed in this study. Data sharing is not applicable to this article.

**Conflicts of Interest:** The authors declare no conflict of interest. The funders had no role in the design of the study; in the collection, analyses, or interpretation of data; in the writing of the manuscript, or in the decision to publish the results.

## Abbreviations

| | |
|---|---|
| AD | Alzheimer's disease |
| Aβ | amyloid β |
| mTOR | mechanistic target of rapamycin kinase |
| SGLT2 | sodium glucose cotransporter 2 |
| APP/PS1 mice | double transgenic mouse model of Alzheimer's disease over expressing amyloid precursor protein, encoding the Swedish mutations at amino acids 595/596 and an exon-9-deleted human PS1 |
| Tg2576 mice | transgenic mouse model, which express a 695-aa residue splice form of human amyloid precursor protein modified by the Swedish Familial AD double mutation K670N-M671L |
| 3xTg-AD mice | triple-transgenic mouse model harboring PS1M146V, APPSwe, and tauP301L transgenes |
| ATP | adenosine triphosphate |
| MAPT | microtubule associated protein tau |
| ROS | reactive oxygen species |
| IDE | insulin-degrading enzymes |
| APP | amyloid precursor protein |
| TZDs | thiazolidinediones |
| GLP1 | glucagon-like peptide-1 |
| DPP-4 | dipeptidyl peptidase-4 |
| IGF-1 | insulin-like growth factor-1 |
| PS1 | presenilin 1 |

| | |
|---|---|
| PS 2 | presenilin 2 |
| APOE | Apolipoprotein E |
| PPARs | peroxisome proliferator-activated receptors |
| AChE | acetylcholinesterase |
| AMPK | adenosine 5'mmonophosphate-activated protein kinase |
| PPARs | peroxisome proliferator-activated receptors |
| PI3K | phosphatidylinositol-3-OH kinase |
| IRS-2 | insulin receptor-2 |
| NLRP3 | nod-like receptor pyrin domain containing 3 |

## References

1. Deture, M.A.; Dickson, D.W. The neuropathological diagnosis of Alzheimer's disease. *Mol. Neurodegener.* **2019**, *5*, 1–18. [CrossRef] [PubMed]
2. Stanciu, G.D.; Bild, V.; Ababei, D.C.; Rusu, R.N.; Cobzaru, A.; Paduraru, L.; Bulea, D. Link between diabetes and Alzheimer's disease due to the shared amyloid aggregation and deposition involving both neurodegenerative changes and neurovascular damages. *J. Clin. Med.* **2020**, *9*, 1713. [CrossRef]
3. Alzheimer's Association. 2019 Alzheimer's disease facts and figures. *Alzheimer's Dement.* **2019**, *15*, 321–387. [CrossRef]
4. Müller, U.C.; Deller, T.; Korte, M. Not just amyloid: Physiological functions of the amyloid precursor protein family. *Nat. Rev. Neurosci.* **2017**, *18*, 281–298. [CrossRef] [PubMed]
5. Mattson, M.P. Pathways towards and away from Alzheimer's disease. *Nature* **2004**, *430*, 631–639. [CrossRef]
6. Ferreira-Vieira, T.; Guimaraes, I.; Silva, F.; Ribeiro, F. Alzheimer's disease: Targeting the cholinergic system. *Curr. Neuropharmacol.* **2016**, *14*, 101–115. [CrossRef] [PubMed]
7. Tolar, M.; Abushakra, S.; Sabbagh, M. The path forward in Alzheimer's disease therapeutics: Reevaluating the amyloid cascade hypothesis. *Alzheimer's Dement.* **2020**. [CrossRef]
8. Wallin, K.; Boström, G.; Kivipelto, M.; Gustafson, Y. Risk factors for incident dementia in the very old. *Int. Psychogeriatr.* **2013**, *25*, 1135–1143. [CrossRef]
9. Stanciu, G.D.; Luca, A.; Rusu, R.N.; Bild, V.; Chiriac, S.I.B.; Solcan, C.; Bild, W.; Ababei, D.C. Alzheimer's disease pharmacotherapy in relation to cholinergic system involvement. *Biomolecules* **2020**, *10*, 40. [CrossRef]
10. Selkoe, D.J.; Hardy, J. The amyloid hypothesis of Alzheimer's disease at 25 years. *EMBO Mol. Med.* **2016**, *8*, 595–608. [CrossRef]
11. Zhang, X.; Fu, Z.; Meng, L.; He, M.; Zhang, Z. The early events that initiate β-amyloid aggregation in Alzheimer's disease. *Front. Aging Neurosci.* **2018**, *10*, 1–13. [CrossRef]
12. Chen, G.F.; Xu, T.H.; Yan, Y.; Zhou, Y.R.; Jiang, Y.; Melcher, K.; Xu, H.E. Amyloid beta: Structure, biology and structure-based therapeutic development. *Acta Pharmacol. Sin.* **2017**, *38*, 1205–1235. [CrossRef] [PubMed]
13. Hampel, H.; Mesulam, M.M.; Cuello, A.C.; Farlow, M.R.; Giacobini, E.; Grossberg, G.T.; Khachaturian, A.S.; Vergallo, A.; Cavedo, E.; Snyder, P.J.; et al. The cholinergic system in the pathophysiology and treatment of Alzheimer's disease. *Brain* **2018**, *141*, 1917–1933. [CrossRef]
14. Chen, X.Q.; Mobley, W.C. Exploring the pathogenesis of Alzheimer disease in basal forebrain cholinergic neurons:Converging insights from alternative hypotheses. *Front. Neurosci.* **2019**, *13*, 446. [CrossRef] [PubMed]
15. Lippens, G.; Sillen, A.; Landrieu, I.; Amniai, L.; Sibille, N.; Barbier, P.; Leroy, A.; Hanoulle, X.; Wieruszeski, J.M. Tau aggregation in Alzheimer's disease: What role for phosphorylation? *Prion* **2007**, *1*, 21–25. [CrossRef] [PubMed]
16. Liu, M.; Dexheimer, T.; Sui, D.; Hovde, S.; Deng, X.; Kwok, R.; Bochar, D.A.; Kuo, M.H. Hyperphosphorylated tau aggregation and cytotoxicity modulators screen identified prescription drugs linked to Alzheimer's disease and cognitive functions. *Sci. Rep.* **2020**, *10*, 1–14. [CrossRef] [PubMed]
17. Huang, W.J.; Zhang, X.; Chen, W.W. Role of oxidative stress in Alzheimer's disease. *Biomed. Rep.* **2016**, *4*, 519–522. [CrossRef]
18. Teixeira, J.P.; Castro, A.A.D.; Soares, F.V.; Cunha, E.F.F.D.; Ramalho, T.C. Future therapeutic perspectives into the Alzheimer's disease targeting the oxidative stress hypothesis. *Molecules* **2019**, *24*, 4410. [CrossRef]
19. Kinney, J.W.; Bemiller, S.M.; Murtishaw, A.S.; Leisgang, A.M.; Salazar, A.M.; Lamb, B.T. Inflammation as a central mechanism in Alzheimer's disease. *Alzheimer's Dement. Transl. Res. Clin. Interv.* **2018**, *4*, 575–590. [CrossRef]
20. Wyss-Coray, T.; Rogers, J. Inflammation in Alzheimer disease—A brief review of the basic science and clinical literature. *Cold Spring Harb. Perspect. Med.* **2012**, *2*, a006346. [CrossRef] [PubMed]
21. Bolós, M.; Perea, J.R.; Avila, J. Alzheimer's disease as an inflammatory disease. *Biomol. Concepts* **2017**, *8*, 37–43. [CrossRef]
22. Funk, K.E.; Kuret, J. Lysosomal fusion dysfunction as a unifying hypothesis for alzheimers disease pathology. *Int. J. Alzheimer's Dis.* **2012**, *2012*. [CrossRef]
23. Van Acker, Z.P.; Bretou, M.; Annaert, W. Endo-lysosomal dysregulations and late-onset Alzheimer's disease: Impact of genetic risk factors. *Mol. Neurodegener.* **2019**, *14*, 1–20. [CrossRef]
24. Cacace, R.; Sleegers, K.; Van Broeckhoven, C. Molecular genetics of early-onset Alzheimer's disease revisited. *Alzheimer's Dement.* **2016**, *12*, 733–748. [CrossRef]
25. Swerdlow, R.H.; Burns, J.M.; Khan, S.M. The Alzheimer's disease mitochondrial cascade hypothesis: Progress and perspectives. *Biochim. Biophys. Acta Mol. Basis Dis.* **2014**, *1842*, 1219–1231. [CrossRef] [PubMed]

26. Wang, W.; Zhao, F.; Ma, X.; Perry, G.; Zhu, X. Mitochondria dysfunction in the pathogenesis of Alzheimer's disease: Recent advances. *Mol. Neurodegener.* **2020**, *15*, 1–22. [CrossRef] [PubMed]
27. Cenini, G.; Voos, W. Mitochondria as potential targets in Alzheimer disease therapy: An update. *Front. Pharmacol.* **2019**, *10*, 902. [CrossRef]
28. Bell, S.M.; Barnes, K.; Marco, M.D.; Shaw, P.J.; Ferraiuolo, L.; Blackburn, D.J.; Venneri, A.; Mortiboys, H. Mitochondrial dysfunction in Alzheimer's disease: A biomarker of the future? *Biomedicines* **2021**, *9*, 63. [CrossRef]
29. Morgen, K.; Frölich, L. The metabolism hypothesis of Alzheimer's disease: From the concept of central insulin resistance and associated consequences to insulin therapy. *J. Neural. Transm.* **2015**, *122*, 499–504. [CrossRef] [PubMed]
30. Argentati, C.; Tortorella, I.; Bazzucchi, M.; Emiliani, C.; Morena, F.; Martino, S. The other side of Alzheimer's disease: Influence of metabolic disorder features for novel diagnostic biomarkers. *J. Pers. Med.* **2020**, *10*, 115. [CrossRef]
31. Paroni, G.; Bisceglia, P.; Seripa, D. Understanding the amyloid hypothesis in Alzheimer's disease. *J. Alzheimer's Dis.* **2019**, *68*, 493–510. [CrossRef] [PubMed]
32. Hillen, H. The beta amyloid dysfunction (BAD) hypothesis for Alzheimer's disease. *Front. Neurosci.* **2019**, *13*, 1154. [CrossRef] [PubMed]
33. Stanciu, G.D.; Ababei, D.C.; Bild, V.; Bild, W.; Paduraru, L.; Gutu, M.M.; Tamba, B.-I. Renal contributions in the pathophysiology and neuropathological substrates shared by chronic kidney disease and Alzheimer's disease. *Brain Sci.* **2020**, *10*, 563. [CrossRef]
34. Swerdlow, R.H. Mitochondria and mitochondrial cascades in Alzheimer 's disease. *J. Alzheimer's Dis.* **2018**, *62*, 1403–1416. [CrossRef] [PubMed]
35. Nixon, R.A. Amyloid precursor protein & endosomal-lysosomal dysfunction in Alzheimer's disease: Inseparable partners in a multifactorial disease. *FASEB J.* **2017**, *31*, 2729–2743.
36. Lie, P.P.Y.; Nixon, R.A. Lysosome trafficking and signaling in health and neurodegenerative diseases. *Neurobiol. Dis.* **2019**, *122*, 94–105. [CrossRef]
37. Carosi, J.M.; Sargeant, T.J. Rapamycin and Alzheimer disease: A double-edged sword? *Autophagy* **2019**, *15*, 1460–1462. [CrossRef]
38. Talboom, J.S.; Velazquez, R.; Oddo, S. The mammalian target of rapamycin at the crossroad between cognitive aging and Alzheimer's disease. *NPJ Aging Mech. Dis.* **2015**, *1*, 1–7. [CrossRef]
39. Barbagallo, M. Type 2 diabetes mellitus and Alzheimer's disease. *World J. Diabetes* **2014**, *5*, 889. [CrossRef]
40. Janson, J.; Laedtke, T.; Parisi, J.E.; O'Brien, P.; Petersen, R.C.; Butler, P.C. Increased risk of type 2 diabetes in Alzheimer disease. *Diabetes* **2004**, *53*, 474–481. [CrossRef] [PubMed]
41. Mosconi, L. Glucose metabolism in normal aging and Alzheimer's disease: Methodological and physiological considerations for PET studies. *Clin. Transl. Imaging* **2013**, *1*, 217–233. [CrossRef] [PubMed]
42. Sivanesan, S.; Mundugaru, R.; Rajadas, J. Possible clues for brain energy translation via endolysosomal trafficking of APP-CTFs in Alzheimer's disease. *Oxid. Med. Cell. Longev.* **2018**, *2018*, 1–12. [CrossRef]
43. An, Y.; Varma, V.R.; Varma, S.; Casanova, R.; Dammer, E.; Pletnikova, O.; Chia, C.W.; Egan, J.M.; Ferrucci, L.; Troncoso, J.; et al. Evidence for brain glucose dysregulation in Alzheimer's disease. *Alzheimer's Dement.* **2018**, *14*, 318–329. [CrossRef] [PubMed]
44. Mueed, Z.; Tandon, P.; Maurya, S.K.; Deval, R.; Kamal, M.A.; Poddar, N.K. Tau and mTOR: The hotspots for multifarious diseases in Alzheimer's development. *Front. Neurosci.* **2019**, *13*, 1017. [CrossRef]
45. Oddo, S. The role of mTOR signaling in Alzheimer disease. *Front. Biosci.* **2012**, *4*, 941–952. [CrossRef] [PubMed]
46. Uddin, M.S.; Rahman, M.A.; Kabir, M.T.; Behl, T.; Mathew, B.; Perveen, A.; Barreto, G.E.; Bin-Jumah, M.N.; Abdel-Daim, M.M.; Ashraf, G.M. Multifarious roles of mTOR signaling in cognitive aging and cerebrovascular dysfunction of Alzheimer's disease. *IUBMB Life* **2020**, *72*, 1843–1855. [CrossRef]
47. Stanciu, G.D.; Solcan, G. Acute idiopathic polyradiculoneuritis concurrent with acquired myasthenia gravis in a West Highland white terrier dog. *BMC Vet. Res.* **2016**, *12*, 111. [CrossRef]
48. Praticò, D.; Clark, C.M.; Liun, F.; Lee, V.Y.M.; Trojanowski, J.Q. Increase of brain oxidative stress in mild cognitive impairment: A possible predictor for Alzheimer disease. *Arch. Neurol.* **2002**, *59*, 972–976. [CrossRef]
49. Cao, J.; Zhong, M.B.; Toro, C.A.; Zhang, L.; Cai, D. Endo-lysosomal pathway and ubiquitin-proteasome system dysfunction in Alzheimer's disease pathogenesis. *Neurosci. Lett.* **2019**, *703*, 68–78. [CrossRef] [PubMed]
50. Wang, C.; Telpoukhovskaia, M.A.; Bahr, B.A.; Chen, X.; Gan, L. Endo-lysosomal dysfunction: A converging mechanism in neurodegenerative diseases. *Curr. Opin. Neurobiol.* **2018**, *48*, 52–58. [CrossRef]
51. Malik, B.R.; Maddison, D.C.; Smith, G.A.; Peters, O.M. Autophagic and endo-lysosomal dysfunction in neurodegenerative disease. *Mol. Brain* **2019**, *12*, 1–21. [CrossRef]
52. Huotari, J.; Helenius, A. Endosome maturation. *EMBO J.* **2011**, *30*, 3481–3500. [CrossRef]
53. Cataldo, A.M.; Hamilton, D.J.; Nixon, R.A. Lysosomal abnormalities in degenerating neurons link neuronal compromise to senile plaque development in Alzheimer disease. *Brain Res.* **1994**, *640*, 68–80. [CrossRef]
54. Nixon, R.A.; Wegiel, J.; Kumar, A.; Yu, W.H.; Peterhoff, C.; Cataldo, A.; Cuervo, A.M. Extensive involvement of autophagy in Alzheimer disease: An immuno-electron microscopy study. *J. Neuropathol. Exp. Neurol.* **2005**, *64*, 113–122. [CrossRef] [PubMed]
55. Cataldo, A.M.; Peterhoff, C.M.; Troncoso, J.C.; Gomez-Isla, T.; Hyman, B.T.; Nixon, R.A. Endocytic pathway abnormalities precede amyloid β deposition in sporadic Alzheimer's disease and down syndrome: Differential effects of APOE genotype and presenilin mutations. *Am. J. Pathol.* **2000**, *157*, 277–286. [CrossRef]

56. Nguyen, T.T.; Ta, Q.T.H.; Nguyen, T.K.O.; Nguyen, T.T.D.; Giau, V.V. Type 3 diabetes and its role implications in Alzheimer's disease. *Int. J. Mol. Sci.* **2020**, *21*, 3165. [CrossRef] [PubMed]
57. Pardeshi, R.; Bolshette, N.; Gadhave, K.; Ahire, A.; Ahmed, S.; Cassano, T.; Gupta, V.B.; Lahkar, M. Insulin signaling: An opportunistic target to minify risk of Alzheimer's disease. *Psychoneuroendocrinology* **2017**, *83*, 159–171. [CrossRef] [PubMed]
58. Esterline, R.; Oscarsson, J.; Burns, J. A Role for Sodium Glucose Cotransporter 2 Inhibitors (SGLT2is) in the Treatment of Alzheimer's Disease? In *International Review of Neurobiology*; Academic Press Inc.: Cambridge, MA, USA, 2020; Volume 155, pp. 113–140. ISBN 9780128231210.
59. Mao, Z.; Zhang, W. Role of mTOR in glucose and lipid metabolism. *Int. J. Mol. Sci.* **2018**, *19*, 2043. [CrossRef]
60. Herrup, K.; Yang, Y. Cell cycle regulation in the postmitotic neuron: Oxymoron or new biology? *Nat. Rev. Neurosci.* **2007**, *8*, 368–378. [CrossRef]
61. Mielke, J.G.; Taghibiglou, C.; Liu, L.; Zhang, Y.; Jia, Z.; Adeli, K.; Wang, Y.T. A biochemical and functional characterization of diet-induced brain insulin resistance. *J. Neurochem.* **2005**, *93*, 1568–1578. [CrossRef]
62. Hardigan, T.; Ward, R.; Ergul, A. Cerebrovascular complications of diabetes: Focus on cognitive dysfunction. *Clin. Sci.* **2016**, *130*, 1807–1822. [CrossRef]
63. Calabrò, M.; Rinaldi, C.; Santoro, G.; Crisafulli, C. The biological pathways of Alzheimer disease: A review. *AIMS Neurosci.* **2021**, *8*, 86–132. [CrossRef] [PubMed]
64. Femminella, G.D.; Livingston, N.R.; Raza, S.; Van der Doef, T.; Frangou, E.; Love, S.; Busza, G.; Calsolaro, V.; Carver, S.; Holmes, C.; et al. Does insulin resistance influence neurodegeneration in non-diabetic Alzheimer's subjects? *Alzheimer's Res. Ther.* **2021**, *13*, 47. [CrossRef]
65. Kandimalla, R.; Thirumala, V.; Reddy, P.H. Is Alzheimer's disease a Type 3 Diabetes? A critical appraisal. *Biochim. Biophys. Acta Mol. Basis Dis.* **2017**, *1863*, 1078–1089. [CrossRef]
66. Rorbach-Dolata, A.; Piwowar, A. Neurometabolic evidence supporting the hypothesis of increased incidence of type 3 diabetes mellitus in the 21st century. *Biomed. Res. Int.* **2019**, *2019*. [CrossRef]
67. Esterline, R.L.; Vaag, A.; Oscarsson, J.; Vora, J. SGLT2 inhibitors: Clinical benefits by restoration of normal diurnal metabolism? *Eur. J. Endocrinol.* **2018**, *178*, R113–R125. [CrossRef] [PubMed]
68. Perluigi, M.; Domenico, F.D.; Butterfield, D.A. mTOR signaling in aging and neurodegeneration: At the crossroad between metabolism dysfunction and impairment of autophagy. *Neurobiol. Dis.* **2015**, *84*, 39–49. [CrossRef] [PubMed]
69. Zhang, J.; Chen, C.; Hua, S.; Liao, H.; Wang, M.; Xiong, Y.; Cao, F. An updated meta-analysis of cohort studies: Diabetes and risk of Alzheimer's disease. *Diabetes Res. Clin. Pract.* **2017**, *124*, 41–47. [CrossRef]
70. Ninomiya, T. Diabetes mellitus and dementia. *Curr. Diab. Rep.* **2014**, *14*, 1–9. [CrossRef] [PubMed]
71. Fernandez-Martos, C.M.; Atkinson, R.A.K.; Chuah, M.I.; King, A.E.; Vickers, J.C. Combination treatment with leptin and pioglitazone in a mouse model of Alzheimer's disease. *Alzheimer's Dement. Transl. Res. Clin. Interv.* **2017**, *3*, 92–106. [CrossRef] [PubMed]
72. Imfeld, P.; Bodmer, M.; Jick, S.S.; Meier, C.R. Metformin, other antidiabetic drugs, and risk of Alzheimer's disease: A population-based case-control study. *J. Am. Geriatr. Soc.* **2012**, *60*, 916–921. [CrossRef]
73. Ou, Z.; Kong, X.; Sun, X.; He, X.; Zhang, L.; Gong, Z.; Huang, J.; Xu, B.; Long, D.; Li, J.; et al. Metformin treatment prevents amyloid plaque deposition and memory impairment in APP/PS1 mice. *Brain. Behav. Immun.* **2018**, *69*, 351–363. [CrossRef] [PubMed]
74. Stanciu, G.D.; Bild, V.; Ababei, D.C.; Rusu, R.N.; Beschea Chiriac, S.I.; Resus, E.; Luca, A. Relevance of surface neuronal protein autoantibodies as biomarkers in seizures-associated disorders 2019, 20, 4529. *Int. J. Mol. Sci.* **2019**, *20*, 4529. [CrossRef] [PubMed]
75. Yaribeygi, H.; Ashrafizadeh, M.; Henney, N.C.; Sathyapalan, T.; Jamialahmadi, T.; Sahebkar, A. Neuromodulatory effects of anti-diabetes medications: A mechanistic review. *Pharmacol. Res.* **2020**, *152*, 104611. [CrossRef] [PubMed]
76. Wium-Andersen, I.K.; Osler, M.; Jørgensen, M.B.; Rungby, J.; Wium-Andersen, M.K. Antidiabetic medication and risk of dementia in patients with type 2 diabetes: A nested case-control study. *Eur. J. Endocrinol.* **2019**, *181*, 499–507. [CrossRef]
77. Oliveira, W.H.D.; Nunes, A.K.D.S.; França, M.E.R.D.; Santos, L.A.D.; Lós, D.B.; Rocha, S.W.S.; Barbosa, K.P.D.S.; Rodrigues, G.B.; Peixoto, C.A. Effects of metformin on inflammation and short-term memory in streptozotocin-induced diabetic mice. *Brain Res.* **2016**, *1644*, 149–160. [CrossRef]
78. Mousavi, F.; Eidi, A.; Khalili, M.; Roghani, M. Metformin ameliorates learning and memory deficits in streptozotocin-induced diabetic rats. *J. Basic Clin. Pathophysiol.* **2018**, *6*, 17–22.
79. Shingo, A.S.; Kanabayashi, T.; Kito, S.; Murase, T. Intracerebroventricular administration of an insulin analogue recovers STZ-induced cognitive decline in rats. *Behav. Brain Res.* **2013**, *241*, 105–111. [CrossRef]
80. Reger, M.A.; Watson, G.S.; Frey, W.H.; Baker, L.D.; Cholerton, B.; Keeling, M.L.; Belongia, D.A.; Fishel, M.A.; Plymate, S.R.; Schellenberg, G.D.; et al. Effects of intranasal insulin on cognition in memory-impaired older adults: Modulation by APOE genotype. *Neurobiol. Aging* **2006**, *27*, 451–458. [CrossRef]
81. Reger, M.A.; Watson, G.S.; Green, P.S.; Wilkinson, C.W.; Baker, L.D.; Cholerton, B.; Fishel, M.A.; Plymate, S.R.; Breitner, J.C.S.; DeGroodt, W.; et al. Intranasal insulin improves cognition and modulates β-amyloid in early AD. *Neurology* **2008**, *70*, 440–448. [CrossRef]

82. Craft, S.; Baker, L.D.; Montine, T.J.; Minoshima, S.; Watson, G.S.; Claxton, A.; Arbuckle, M.; Callaghan, M.; Tsai, E.; Plymate, S.R.; et al. Intranasal insulin therapy for Alzheimer disease and amnestic mild cognitive impairment: A pilot clinical trial. *Arch. Neurol.* **2012**, *69*, 29–38. [CrossRef] [PubMed]
83. Claxton, A.; Baker, L.D.; Hanson, A.; Trittschuh, E.H.; Cholerton, B.; Morgan, A.; Callaghan, M.; Arbuckle, M.; Behl, C.; Craft, S. Long-acting intranasal insulin detemir improves cognition for adults with mild cognitive impairment or early-stage Alzheimer's Disease dementia. *J. Alzheimer's Dis.* **2015**, *44*, 897–906. [CrossRef] [PubMed]
84. Schilling, T.M.; Ferreira de Sá, D.S.; Westerhausen, R.; Strelzyk, F.; Larra, M.F.; Hallschmid, M.; Savaskan, E.; Oitzl, M.S.; Busch, H.P.; Naumann, E.; et al. Intranasal insulin increases regional cerebral blood flow in the insular cortex in men independently of cortisol manipulation. *Hum. Brain Mapp.* **2014**, *35*, 1944–1956. [CrossRef]
85. Benedict, C.; Hallschmid, M.; Hatke, A.; Schultes, B.; Fehm, H.L.; Born, J.; Kern, W. Intranasal insulin improves memory in humans. *Psychoneuroendocrinology* **2004**, *29*, 1326–1334. [CrossRef] [PubMed]
86. Benedict, C.; Hallschmid, M.; Schmitz, K.; Schultes, B.; Ratter, F.; Fehm, H.L.; Born, J.; Kern, W. Intranasal insulin improves memory in humans: Superiority of insulin aspart. *Neuropsychopharmacology* **2007**, *32*, 239–243. [CrossRef]
87. Gupta, A.; Bisht, B.; Dey, C.S. Peripheral insulin-sensitizer drug metformin ameliorates neuronal insulin resistance and Alzheimer's-like changes. *Neuropharmacology* **2011**, *60*, 910–920. [CrossRef]
88. Kickstein, E.; Krauss, S.; Thornhill, P.; Rutschow, D.; Zeller, R.; Sharkey, J.; Williamson, R.; Fuchs, M.; Köhler, A.; Glossmann, H.; et al. Biguanide metformin acts on tau phosphorylation via mTOR/protein phosphatase 2A (PP2A) signaling. *Proc. Natl. Acad. Sci. USA* **2010**, *107*, 21830–21835. [CrossRef] [PubMed]
89. DiTacchio, K.A.; Heinemann, S.F.; Dziewczapolski, G. Metformin treatment alters memory function in a mouse model of Alzheimer's disease. *J. Alzheimer's Dis.* **2015**, *44*, 43–48. [CrossRef] [PubMed]
90. Heneka, M.T.; Sastre, M.; Dumitrescu-Ozimek, L.; Hanke, A.; Dewachter, I.; Kuiperi, C.; O'Banion, K.; Klockgether, T.; Van Leuven, F.; Landreth, G.E. Acute treatment with the PPARgamma agonist pioglitazone and ibuprofen reduces glial inflammation and Abeta1–42 levels in APPV717I transgenic mice. *Brain* **2005**, *128*, 1442–1453. [CrossRef] [PubMed]
91. Sato, T.; Hanyu, H.; Hirao, K.; Kanetaka, H.; Sakurai, H.; Iwamoto, T. Efficacy of PPAR-γ agonist pioglitazone in mild Alzheimer disease. *Neurobiol. Aging* **2011**, *32*, 1626–1633. [CrossRef]
92. Geldmacher, D.S.; Fritsch, T.; McClendon, M.J.; Landreth, G. A randomized pilot clinical trial of the safety of pioglitazone in treatment of patients with alzheimer disease. *Arch. Neurol.* **2011**, *68*, 45–50. [CrossRef] [PubMed]
93. Cao, B.; Rosenblat, J.D.; Brietzke, E.; Park, C.; Lee, Y.; Musial, N.; Pan, Z.; Mansur, R.B.; McIntyre, R.S. Comparative efficacy and acceptability of antidiabetic agents for Alzheimer's disease and mild cognitive impairment: A systematic review and network meta-analysis. *Diabetes Obes. Metab.* **2018**, *20*, 2467–2471. [CrossRef] [PubMed]
94. Cai, H.Y.; Yang, J.T.; Wang, Z.J.; Zhang, J.; Yang, W.; Wu, M.N.; Qi, J.S. Lixisenatide reduces amyloid plaques, neurofibrillary tangles and neuroinflammation in an APP/PS1/tau mouse model of Alzheimer's disease. *Biochem. Biophys. Res. Commun.* **2018**, *495*, 1034–1040. [CrossRef]
95. McClean, P.L.; Hölscher, C. Lixisenatide, a drug developed to treat type 2 diabetes, shows neuroprotective effects in a mouse model of Alzheimer's disease. *Neuropharmacology* **2014**, *86*, 241–258. [CrossRef] [PubMed]
96. Duarte, A.I.; Candeias, E.; Alves, I.N.; Mena, D.; Silva, D.F.; Machado, N.J.; Campos, E.J.; Santos, M.S.; Oliveira, C.R.; Moreira, P.I. Liraglutide protects against brain amyloid-$\beta_{1-42}$ accumulation in female mice with early Alzheimer's disease-like pathology by partially rescuing oxidative/nitrosative stress and inflammation. *Int. J. Mol. Sci.* **2020**, *21*, 1746. [CrossRef]
97. Gejl, M.; Gjedde, A.; Egefjord, L.; Møller, A.; Hansen, S.B.; Vang, K.; Rodell, A.; Brændgaard, H.; Gottrup, H.; Schacht, A.; et al. In Alzheimer's disease, 6-month treatment with GLP-1 analog prevents decline of brain glucose metabolism: Randomized, placebo-controlled, double-blind clinical trial. *Front. Aging Neurosci.* **2016**, *8*, 108. [CrossRef]
98. Dong, Q.; Teng, S.W.; Wang, Y.; Qin, F.; Li, Y.; Ai, L.L.; Yu, H. Sitagliptin protects the cognition function of the Alzheimer's disease mice through activating glucagon-like peptide-1 and BDNF-TrkB signalings. *Neurosci. Lett.* **2019**, *696*, 184–190. [CrossRef] [PubMed]
99. D'Amico, M.; Filippo, C.D.; Marfella, R.; Abbatecola, A.M.; Ferraraccio, F.; Rossi, F.; Paolisso, G. Long-term inhibition of dipeptidyl peptidase-4 in Alzheimer's prone mice. *Exp. Gerontol.* **2010**, *45*, 202–207. [CrossRef]
100. Kosaraju, J.; Holsinger, R.M.D.; Guo, L.; Tam, K.Y. Linagliptin, a dipeptidyl peptidase-4 inhibitor, mitigates cognitive deficits and pathology in the 3×Tg-AD mouse model of Alzheimer's disease. *Mol. Neurobiol.* **2017**, *54*, 6074–6084. [CrossRef]
101. Kosaraju, J.; Gali, C.C.; Khatwal, R.B.; Dubala, A.; Chinni, S.; Holsinger, R.M.D.; Madhunapantula, V.S.R.; Nataraj, S.K.M.; Basavan, D. Saxagliptin: A dipeptidyl peptidase-4 inhibitor ameliorates streptozotocin induced Alzheimer's disease. *Neuropharmacology* **2013**, *72*, 291–300. [CrossRef]
102. Kosaraju, J.; Murthy, V.; Khatwal, R.B.; Dubala, A.; Chinni, S.; Nataraj, S.K.M.; Basavan, D. Vildagliptin: An anti-diabetes agent ameliorates cognitive deficits and pathology observed in streptozotocin-induced Alzheimer's disease. *J. Pharm. Pharmacol.* **2013**, *65*, 1773–1784. [CrossRef] [PubMed]
103. Arafa, N.M.S.; Ali, E.H.A.; Hassan, M.K. Canagliflozin prevents scopolamine-induced memory impairment in rats: Comparison with galantamine hydrobromide action. *Chem. Biol. Interact.* **2017**, *277*, 195–203. [CrossRef]
104. Felice, F.G.D.; Vieira, M.N.N.; Bomfim, T.R.; Decker, H.; Velasco, P.T.; Lambert, M.P.; Viola, K.L.; Zhao, W.Q.; Ferreira, S.T.; Klein, W.L. Protection of synapses against Alzheimer's-linked toxins: Insulin signaling prevents the pathogenic binding of Aβ oligomers. *Proc. Natl. Acad. Sci. USA* **2009**, *106*, 1971–1976. [CrossRef] [PubMed]

105. Khoury, N.B.E.; Gratuze, M.; Papon, M.A.; Bretteville, A.; Planel, E. Insulin dysfunction and Tau pathology. *Front. Cell. Neurosci.* **2014**, *8*, 22. [CrossRef]
106. Bryan, M.R.; Bowman, A.B. Manganese and the Insulin-IGF Signaling Network in Huntington's Disease and Other Neurodegenerative Disorders. In *Advances in Neurobiology*; Springer: New York, NY, USA, 2017; Volume 18, pp. 113–142.
107. Hossain, M.F.; Wang, N.; Chen, R.; Li, S.; Roy, J.; Uddin, M.G.; Li, Z.; Lim, L.W.; Song, Y.Q. Exploring the multifunctional role of melatonin in regulating autophagy and sleep to mitigate Alzheimer's disease neuropathology. *Ageing Res. Rev.* **2021**, *67*, 101304. [CrossRef]
108. Born, J.; Lange, T.; Kern, W.; McGregor, G.P.; Bickel, U.; Fehm, H.L. Sniffing neuropeptides: A transnasal approach to the human brain. *Nat. Neurosci.* **2002**, *5*, 514–516. [CrossRef]
109. Femminella, G.D.; Bencivenga, L.; Petraglia, L.; Visaggi, L.; Gioia, L.; Grieco, F.V.; Lucia, C.D.; Komici, K.; Corbi, G.; Edison, P.; et al. Antidiabetic drugs in Alzheimer's disease: Mechanisms of action and future perspectives. *J. Diabetes Res.* **2017**, *2017*. [CrossRef]
110. Sarkar, S. Regulation of autophagy by mTOR-dependent and mTOR-independent pathways: Autophagy dysfunction in neurodegenerative diseases and therapeutic application of autophagy enhancers. *Biochem. Soc. Trans.* **2013**, *41*, 1103–1130. [CrossRef]
111. Burns, J. Dapagliflozin In Alzheimer's Disease—Full Text View—ClinicalTrials. Available online: https://clinicaltrials.gov/ct2/show/NCT03801642 (accessed on 19 April 2021).
112. Rizvi, S.; Shakil, S.; Biswas, D.; Shakil, S.; Shaikh, S.; Bagga, P.; Kamal, M. Invokana (canagliflozin) as a dual inhibitor of acetylcholinesterase and sodium glucose co-transporter 2: Advancement in Alzheimer's disease—Diabetes type 2 linkage via an enzoinformatics study. *CNS Neurol. Disord. Drug Targets* **2014**, *13*, 447–451. [CrossRef]
113. O'Neill, C. PI3-kinase/Akt/mTOR signaling: Impaired on/off switches in aging, cognitive decline and Alzheimer's disease. *Exp. Gerontol.* **2013**, *48*, 647–653. [CrossRef] [PubMed]
114. Lin, A.L.; Zheng, W.; Halloran, J.J.; Burbank, R.R.; Hussong, S.A.; Hart, M.J.; Javors, M.; Shih, Y.Y.I.; Muir, E.; Solano Fonseca, R.; et al. Chronic rapamycin restores brain vascular integrity and function through NO synthase activation and improves memory in symptomatic mice modeling Alzheimer's disease. *J. Cereb. Blood Flow Metab.* **2013**, *33*, 1412–1421. [CrossRef]
115. Gureev, A.P.; Popov, V.N.; Starkov, A.A. Crosstalk between the mTOR and Nrf2/ARE signaling pathways as a target in the improvement of long-term potentiation. *Exp. Neurol.* **2020**, *328*, 113285. [CrossRef]
116. Laplante, M.; Sabatini, D.M. mTOR signaling at a glance. *J. Cell Sci.* **2009**, *122*, 3589–3594. [CrossRef]
117. Stanfel, M.N.; Shamieh, L.S.; Kaeberlein, M.; Kennedy, B.K. The TOR pathway comes of age. *Biochim. Biophys. Acta Gen. Subj.* **2009**, *1790*, 1067–1074. [CrossRef]
118. Garza-Lombó, C.; Schroder, A.; Reyes-Reyes, E.M.; Franco, R. mTOR/AMPK signaling in the brain: Cell metabolism, proteostasis and survival. *Curr. Opin. Toxicol.* **2018**, *8*, 102–110. [CrossRef]
119. Guillén, C.; Benito, M. MTORC1 overactivation as a key aging factor in the progression to type 2 diabetes mellitus. *Front. Endocrinol.* **2018**, *9*, 621. [CrossRef]
120. Sciarretta, S.; Forte, M.; Frati, G.; Sadoshima, J. New insights into the role of mtor signaling in the cardiovascular system. *Circ. Res.* **2018**, *122*, 489–505. [CrossRef] [PubMed]
121. Johnson, S.C.; Rabinovitch, P.S.; Kaeberlein, M. MTOR is a key modulator of ageing and age-related disease. *Nature* **2013**, *493*, 338–345. [CrossRef] [PubMed]
122. Majumder, S.; Richardson, A.; Strong, R.; Oddo, S. Inducing autophagy by rapamycin before, but not after, the formation of plaques and tangles ameliorates cognitive deficits. *PLoS ONE* **2011**, *6*, e25416. [CrossRef] [PubMed]
123. Cai, Z.; Zhao, B.; Li, K.; Zhang, L.; Li, C.; Quazi, S.H.; Tan, Y. Mammalian target of rapamycin: A valid therapeutic target through the autophagy pathway for alzheimer's disease? *J. Neurosci. Res.* **2012**, *90*, 1105–1118. [CrossRef]
124. Liu, G.Y.; Sabatini, D.M. mTOR at the nexus of nutrition, growth, ageing and disease. *Nat. Rev. Mol. Cell Biol.* **2020**, *21*, 183–203. [CrossRef] [PubMed]
125. Kaeberlein, M.; Galvan, V. Rapamycin and Alzheimer's disease: Time for a clinical trial? *Sci. Transl. Med.* **2019**, *11*, eaar4289. [CrossRef] [PubMed]
126. Lafay-Chebassier, C.; Paccalin, M.; Page, G.; Barc-Pain, S.; Perault-Pochat, M.C.; Gil, R.; Pradier, L.; Hugon, J. mTOR/p70S6k signalling alteration by Aβ exposure as well as in APP-PS1 transgenic models and in patients with Alzheimer's disease. *J. Neurochem.* **2005**, *94*, 215–225. [CrossRef]
127. Zhou, X.W.; Tanila, H.; Pei, J.J. Parallel increase in p70 kinase activation and tau phosphorylation (S262) with Aβ overproduction. *FEBS Lett.* **2008**, *582*, 159–164. [CrossRef]
128. Ma, T.; Hoeffer, C.A.; Capetillo-Zarate, E.; Yu, F.; Wong, H.; Lin, M.T.; Tampellini, D.; Klann, E.; Blitzer, R.D.; Gouras, G.K. Dysregulation of the mTOR pathway mediates impairment of synaptic plasticity in a mouse model of Alzheimer's disease. *PLoS ONE* **2010**, *5*, e12845. [CrossRef]
129. Caccamo, A.; Maldonado, M.A.; Majumder, S.; Medina, D.X.; Holbein, W.; Magrí, A.; Oddo, S. Naturally secreted amyloid-β increases mammalian target of rapamycin (mTOR) activity via a PRAS40-mediated mechanism. *J. Biol. Chem.* **2011**, *286*, 8924–8932. [CrossRef] [PubMed]
130. Caccamo, A.; Majumder, S.; Richardson, A.; Strong, R.; Oddo, S. Molecular interplay between mammalian target of rapamycin (mTOR), amyloid-β, and Tau: Effects on cognitive impairments. *J. Biol. Chem.* **2010**, *285*, 13107–13120. [CrossRef] [PubMed]

131. Caccamo, A.; Magrì, A.; Medina, D.X.; Wisely, E.V.; López-Aranda, M.F.; Silva, A.J.; Oddo, S. mTOR regulates tau phosphorylation and degradation: Implications for Alzheimer's disease and other tauopathies. *Aging Cell* **2013**, *12*, 370–380. [CrossRef]
132. Onuki, R.; Bando, Y.; Suyama, E.; Katayama, T.; Kawasaki, H.; Baba, T.; Tohyama, M.; Taira, K. An RNA-dependent protein kinase is involved in tunicamycin-induced apoptosis and Alzheimer's disease. *EMBO J.* **2004**, *23*, 959–968. [CrossRef]
133. Tramutola, A.; Triplett, J.C.; Domenico, F.D.; Niedowicz, D.M.; Murphy, M.P.; Coccia, R.; Perluigi, M.; Butterfield, D.A. Alteration of mTOR signaling occurs early in the progression of Alzheimer disease (AD): Analysis of brain from subjects with pre-clinical AD, amnestic mild cognitive impairment and late-stage AD. *J. Neurochem.* **2015**, *133*, 739–749. [CrossRef]
134. Griffin, R.J.; Moloney, A.; Kelliher, M.; Johnston, J.A.; Ravid, R.; Dockery, P.; O'Connor, R.; O'Neill, C. Activation of Akt/PKB, increased phosphorylation of Akt substrates and loss and altered distribution of Akt and PTEN are features of Alzheimer's disease pathology. *J. Neurochem.* **2005**, *93*, 105–117. [CrossRef] [PubMed]
135. Pei, J.J.; Björkdahl, C.; Zhang, H.; Zhou, X.; Winblad, B. p70 S6 kinase and tau in Alzheimer's disease. *J. Alzheimer's Dis.* **2008**, *14*, 385–392. [CrossRef]
136. An, W.L.; Cowburn, R.F.; Li, L.; Braak, H.; Alafuzoff, I.; Iqbal, K.; Iqbal, I.G.; Winblad, B.; Pei, J.J. Up-regulation of phosphorylated/activated p70 S6 kinase and its relationship to neurofibrillary pathology in Alzheimer's disease. *Am. J. Pathol.* **2003**, *163*, 591–607. [CrossRef]
137. Jiang, T.; Yu, J.T.; Zhu, X.C.; Tan, M.S.; Wang, H.F.; Cao, L.; Zhang, Q.Q.; Shi, J.Q.; Gao, L.; Qin, H.; et al. Temsirolimus promotes autophagic clearance of amyloid-β and provides protective effects in cellular and animal models of Alzheimer's disease. *Pharmacol. Res.* **2014**, *81*, 54–63. [CrossRef]
138. Domenico, F.D.; Tramutola, A.; Foppoli, C.; Head, E.; Perluigi, M.; Butterfield, D.A. mTOR in Down syndrome: Role in Aβ and tau neuropathology and transition to Alzheimer disease-like dementia. *Free Radic. Biol. Med.* **2018**, *114*, 94–101. [CrossRef] [PubMed]
139. Sabatini, D.M. Twenty-five years of mTOR: Uncovering the link from nutrients to growth. *Proc. Natl. Acad. Sci. USA* **2017**, *114*, 11818–11825. [CrossRef] [PubMed]
140. Wolfe, D.M.; Lee, J.H.; Kumar, A.; Lee, S.; Orenstein, S.J.; Nixon, R.A. Autophagy failure in Alzheimer's disease and the role of defective lysosomal acidification. *Eur. J. Neurosci.* **2013**, *37*, 1949–1961. [CrossRef] [PubMed]
141. Glick, D.; Barth, S.; Macleod, K.F. Autophagy: Cellular and molecular mechanisms. *J. Pathol.* **2010**, *221*, 3–12. [CrossRef]
142. Rubinsztein, D.C.; Mariño, G.; Kroemer, G. Autophagy and aging. *Cell* **2011**, *146*, 682–695. [CrossRef]
143. Briaud, I.; Dickson, L.M.; Lingohr, M.K.; McCuaig, J.F.; Lawrence, J.C.; Rhodes, C.J. Insulin receptor substrate-2 proteasomal degradation mediated by a mammalian target of rapamycin (mTOR)-induced negative feedback down-regulates protein kinase B-mediated signaling pathway in β-cells. *J. Biol. Chem.* **2005**, *280*, 2282–2293. [CrossRef] [PubMed]
144. Bailey, C.J. Uric acid and the cardio-renal effects of SGLT2 inhibitors. *Diabetes Obes. Metab.* **2019**, *21*, 1291–1298. [CrossRef] [PubMed]
145. Bonnet, F.; Scheen, A.J. Effects of SGLT2 inhibitors on systemic and tissue low-grade inflammation: The potential contribution to diabetes complications and cardiovascular disease. *Diabetes Metab.* **2018**, *44*, 457–464. [CrossRef]
146. Ferrannini, E.; Baldi, S.; Frascerra, S.; Astiarraga, B.; Heise, T.; Bizzotto, R.; Mari, A.; Pieber, T.R.; Muscelli, E. Shift to fatty substrate utilization in response to sodium-glucose cotransporter 2 inhibition in subjects without diabetes and patients with type 2 diabetes. *Diabetes* **2016**, *65*, 1190–1196. [CrossRef] [PubMed]
147. Heneka, M.T. Inflammasome activation and innate immunity in Alzheimer's disease. *Brain Pathol.* **2017**, *27*, 220–222. [CrossRef]
148. White, C.S.; Lawrence, C.B.; Brough, D.; Rivers-Auty, J. Inflammasomes as therapeutic targets for Alzheimer's disease. *Brain Pathol.* **2017**, *27*, 223–234. [CrossRef]
149. Joosten, L.A.B.; Crişan, T.O.; Bjornstad, P.; Johnson, R.J. Asymptomatic hyperuricaemia: A silent activator of the innate immune system. *Nat. Rev. Rheumatol.* **2020**, *16*, 75–86. [CrossRef]
150. Tana, C.; Ticinesi, A.; Prati, B.; Nouvenne, A.; Meschi, T. Uric acid and cognitive function in older individuals. *Nutrients* **2018**, *10*, 975. [CrossRef] [PubMed]
151. Verhaaren, B.F.J.; Vernooij, M.W.; Dehghan, A.; Vrooman, H.A.; Boer, R.D.; Hofman, A.; Witteman, J.C.M.; Niessen, W.J.; Breteler, M.M.B.; Van Der Lugt, A.; et al. The relation of uric acid to brain atrophy and cognition: The rotterdam scan study. *Neuroepidemiology* **2013**, *41*, 29–34. [CrossRef] [PubMed]
152. Giannitsi, S.; Maria, B.; Bechlioulis, A.; Naka, K. Endothelial dysfunction and heart failure: A review of the existing bibliography with emphasis on flow mediated dilation. *JRSM Cardiovasc. Dis.* **2019**, *8*, 204800401984304. [CrossRef] [PubMed]
153. Venturelli, M.; Pedrinolla, A.; Galazzo, I.B.; Fonte, C.; Smania, N.; Tamburin, S.; Muti, E.; Crispoltoni, L.; Stabile, A.; Pistilli, A.; et al. Impact of nitric oxide bioavailability on the progressive cerebral and peripheral circulatory impairments during aging and Alzheimer's disease. *Front. Physiol.* **2018**, *9*, 169. [CrossRef] [PubMed]
154. Decker, B.; Pumiglia, K. mTORc1 activity is necessary and sufficient for phosphorylation of eNOSS1177. *Physiol. Rep.* **2018**, *6*, 13733. [CrossRef]
155. Van Skike, C.E.; Jahrling, J.B.; Olson, A.B.; Sayre, N.L.; Hussong, S.A.; Ungvari, Z.; Lechleiter, J.D.; Galvan, V. Inhibition of mTOR protects the blood-brain barrier in models of Alzheimer's disease and vascular cognitive impairment. *Am. J. Physiol. Heart Circ. Physiol.* **2018**, *314*, H693–H703. [CrossRef] [PubMed]

156. Lesniewski, L.A.; Seals, D.R.; Walker, A.E.; Henson, G.D.; Blimline, M.W.; Trott, D.W.; Bosshardt, G.C.; LaRocca, T.J.; Lawson, B.R.; Zigler, M.C.; et al. Dietary rapamycin supplementation reverses age-related vascular dysfunction and oxidative stress, while modulating nutrient-sensing, cell cycle, and senescence pathways. *Aging Cell* **2017**, *16*, 17–26. [CrossRef] [PubMed]
157. Nwadike, C.; Williamson, L.E.; Gallagher, L.E.; Guan, J.-L.; Chan, E.Y.W. AMPK inhibits ULK1-dependent autophagosome formation and lysosomal acidification via distinct mechanisms. *Mol. Cell. Biol.* **2018**, *38*. [CrossRef]
158. Wong, P.M.; Feng, Y.; Wang, J.; Shi, R.; Jiang, X. Regulation of autophagy by coordinated action of mTORC1 and protein phosphatase 2A. *Nat. Commun.* **2015**, *6*, 1–11. [CrossRef] [PubMed]
159. Mudaliar, S.; Henry, R.R.; Boden, G.; Smith, S.; Chalamandaris, A.G.; Duchesne, D.; Iqbal, N.; List, J. Changes in insulin sensitivity and insulin secretion with the sodium glucose cotransporter 2 inhibitor dapagliflozin. *Diabetes Technol. Ther.* **2014**, *16*, 137–144. [CrossRef]
160. Kappel, B.A.; Lehrke, M.; Schütt, K.; Artati, A.; Adamski, J.; Lebherz, C.; Marx, N. Effect of empagliflozin on the metabolic signature of patients with type 2 diabetes mellitus and cardiovascular disease. *Circulation* **2017**, *136*, 969–972. [CrossRef]
161. Majd, S.; Power, J.H.T. Oxidative stress and decreased mitochondrial superoxide dismutase 2 and peroxiredoxins 1 and 4 based mechanism of concurrent activation of AMPK and mTOR in Alzheimer's disease. *Curr. Alzheimer Res.* **2018**, *15*, 764–776. [CrossRef]

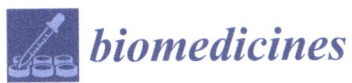 

Article

# The Insulin Receptor: A Potential Target of Amarogentin Isolated from *Gentiana rigescens* Franch That Induces Neurogenesis in PC12 Cells

Lihong Cheng [1], Hiroyuki Osada [2], Tianyan Xing [3], Minoru Yoshida [4,5], Lan Xiang [1,*] and Jianhua Qi [1,*]

1. College of Pharmaceutical Sciences, Zhejiang University, Hangzhou 310058, China; clh83787711@zju.edu.cn
2. Chemical Biology Research Group, RIKEN Center for Sustainable Resource Science, Wako-shi, Saitama 351-0198, Japan; hisyo@riken.jp
3. School of Pharmacy, Hubei University of Chinese Medicine, Wuhan 430065, China; tongsherry@sina.cn
4. Chemical Genomics Research Group, RIKEN Center for Sustainable Resource Science, Wako-shi, Saitama 351-0198, Japan; yoshidam@riken.jp
5. Department of Biotechnology and Collaborative Research Institute for Innovative Microbiology, The University of Tokyo, Bunkyo-ku, Tokyo 113-0033, Japan
* Correspondence: lxiang@zju.edu.cn (L.X.); qijianhua@zju.edu.cn (J.Q.); Tel.: +86-571-88-208-627 (J.Q.)

**Citation:** Cheng, L.; Osada, H.; Xing, T.; Yoshida, M.; Xiang, L.; Qi, J. The Insulin Receptor: A Potential Target of Amarogentin Isolated from *Gentiana rigescens* Franch That Induces Neurogenesis in PC12 Cells. *Biomedicines* **2021**, *9*, 581. https://doi.org/10.3390/biomedicines9050581

Academic Editor: Lorenzo Falsetti

Received: 7 April 2021
Accepted: 11 May 2021
Published: 20 May 2021

**Publisher's Note:** MDPI stays neutral with regard to jurisdictional claims in published maps and institutional affiliations.

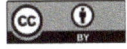

**Copyright:** © 2021 by the authors. Licensee MDPI, Basel, Switzerland. This article is an open access article distributed under the terms and conditions of the Creative Commons Attribution (CC BY) license (https:// creativecommons.org/licenses/by/ 4.0/).

**Abstract:** Amarogentin (AMA) is a secoiridoid glycoside isolated from the traditional Chinese medicine, *Gentiana rigescens* Franch. AMA exhibits nerve growth factor (NGF)-mimicking and NGF-enhancing activities in PC12 cells and in primary cortical neuron cells. In this study, a possible mechanism was found showing the remarkable induction of phosphorylation of the insulin receptor (INSR) and protein kinase B (AKT). The potential target of AMA was predicted by using a small-interfering RNA (siRNA) and the cellular thermal shift assay (CETSA). The AMA-induced neurite outgrowth was reduced by the siRNA against the INSR and the results of the CETSA suggested that the INSR showed a significant thermal stability-shifted effect upon AMA treatment. Other neurotrophic signaling pathways in PC12 cells were investigated using specific inhibitors, Western blotting and PC12(rasN17) and PC12(mtGAP) mutants. The inhibitors of the glucocorticoid receptor (GR), phospholipase C (PLC) and protein kinase C (PKC), Ras, Raf and mitogen-activated protein kinase (MEK) significantly reduced the neurite outgrowth induced by AMA in PC12 cells. Furthermore, the phosphorylation reactions of GR, PLC, PKC and an extracellular signal-regulated kinase (ERK) were significantly increased after inducing AMA and markedly decreased after treatment with the corresponding inhibitors. Collectively, these results suggested that AMA-induced neuritogenic activity in PC12 cells potentially depended on targeting the INSR and activating the downstream Ras/Raf/ERK and PI3K/AKT signaling pathways. In addition, the GR/PLC/PKC signaling pathway was found to be involved in the neurogenesis effect of AMA.

**Keywords:** neurodegenerative disease; aging; Alzheimer's disease; insulin receptor; target identification

## 1. Introduction

Alzheimer's disease (AD) is a type of progressive neurodegenerative disease that accounts for 60–70% of dementia cases and its symptoms include an initial memory loss, later visual, language and cognitive disorders and a decline in the executive capacity in daily life [1]. The World Alzheimer Report 2019 states that over 50 million people are estimated to live with dementia worldwide and the number of patients will increase to 152 million by 2050. Additionally, the current yearly expenditure of dementia is estimated to reach USD 1 trillion, which will double by 2030 [2]. Currently, several drugs on the market such as tacrine, rivastigmine, huperzine A, donepezil, galantamine and memantine are used to treat AD. However, only the symptoms are mitigated and the efficacy of the drugs is not ideal, implying that a new strategy is needed for an effective AD treatment [3].

The nerve growth factor (NGF), the first recognized neurotrophic factor that plays a very important role in the survival, growth and maintenance of neuron cells, has become a drug candidate [4]. Nevertheless, with its high polarity and large molecule weight, the NGF cannot pass through the blood-brain barrier (BBB) and is difficult to apply as a drug [5]. This finding indicates that discovering a small molecule with an NGF-mimicking activity may be a potential alternative for AD treatment.

Given the characteristic of exhibiting sympathetic neuron-like phenotypes under the stimulation of the NGF, the PC12 cell line, which is derived from rat pheochromocytoma cells, is widely used as a model to screen small molecules with NGF-mimicking activities [6]. In previous studies, under the guidance of a PC12 cell bioassay system, several small molecules with NGF-mimicking activities were isolated from traditional Chinese medicines (TCMs) such as *Gentiana rigescens* Franch, *Lindernia crustacean* and *Desmodium sambuense* and the mechanism of the action studies was also identified [7–12].

The genus *Gentiana* is a major group in the Gentianaceae family and its major constituents include iridoids and secoiridoids, which are responsible for various biological activities, and other important molecules such as essential oils, xanthones and terpenoids [13]. *G. rigescens* Franch (Jian Long Dan in Chinese), a well-known TCM that is widely distributed in the Yunnan Province, southwest China, is generally utilized for hepatitis, rheumatism, cholecystitis and inflammation treatment [14]. This TCM is praised with its anti-aging activity and cognition-improving effect in 'Sheng Nong's Herbal Classic', a classic book on TCM material medica. In previous studies, gentisides A–K, which are 11 novel neuritogenic benzoate-type molecules, were isolated from *G. rigescens* and their mixture was confirmed to alleviate the impaired memory of an AD model [7,8,15].

In the present study, a secoiridoid-type compound was isolated from *G. rigescens* Franch. The chemical structure was determined as amarogentin (AMA) (Figure 1a). AMA was previously reported by our group to be a molecule with anti-aging and neuroprotection effects by an anti-oxidative stress activity [16]. Herein, the NGF-mimicking and NGF-enhancing activities of AMA were revealed and the mechanism of the action of the neurite outgrowth induced by AMA was investigated by using specific inhibitors in combination with Western blotting assays. Furthermore, the potential target was predicted using the cellular thermal shift assay (CETSA) and a small-interfering RNA (siRNA) analysis. The results indicated that AMA potentially targeted the insulin receptor and activated the PI3K/AKT and Ras/Raf/MEK/ERK signaling pathways. In addition, the GR/PLC/PKC was also involved in the neuritogenic activity of AMA in PC12 cells.

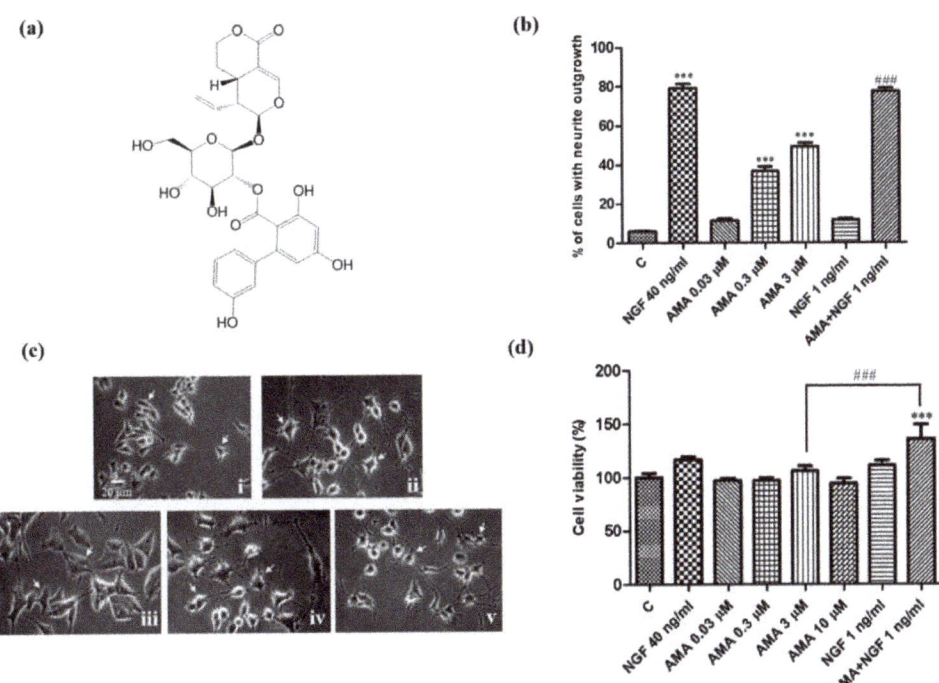

**Figure 1.** Neurogenesis effect of AMA in PC12 cells. (**a**) Chemical structure of AMA. (**b**) Percentage of PC12 cells with neurite outgrowth after treatment with AMA at different doses or AMA combined with a low dose of the NGF. (**c**) Morphological changes in PC12 cells under an inverted optical microscope at 48 h after treatment with (**i**) control (0.5% DMSO); (**ii**) NGF (40 ng/mL); (**iii**) NGF (1 ng/mL); (**iv**) AMA (3 µM); (**v**) AMA (3 µM) + NGF (1 ng/mL). (**d**) Cell viability analysis results of PC12 cells after treatment with various doses of AMA or AMA combined with the NGF. Each experiment was repeated three times. The data were expressed as a mean ± SEM. *** indicates significant differences at $p < 0.001$ compared with the negative control and ### indicates a significant difference at $p < 0.001$ compared with the 3 µM AMA group.

## 2. Experimental Section

### 2.1. Chemicals and Reagents

TrkA (k252a), GR (RU486), PI3K (LY294002), MEK/ERK (U0126) and PKC (Go6983) inhibitors, DMSO and NGF were purchased from Sigma—Aldrich Co. (St. Louis, MO, USA). The Ras inhibitor (farnesylthiosalicylic acid) was purchased from Cayman Chemical (Ann Arbor, MI, USA). The INSR (HNMPA-[AM]$_3$), PLC (U73343) and Raf (AZ628) inhibitors were purchased from Santa Cruz Biotechnology (Dallas, TX, USA). The TrkB inhibitor (ANA-12) was purchased from Selleck (Shanghai, China) (see the details in Supplementary Table S1). Insulin and demethylasterriquinone B1 were purchased from YEASEN Biotech Co. Ltd. (Shanghai, China) and GlpBio Technology (Shanghai, China), respectively.

### 2.2. Preparation of the AMA

AMA was isolated from the roots of *G. rigescens* and the chemical structure was determined by comparing the $^1$H NMR and $^{13}$C NMR spectra with the reported literature (Figure 1a). The detailed separation and structure elucidation steps were reported in a previous study [16].

### 2.3. Evaluation of the Neuritogenic Activity

The neuritogenic activity was evaluated as described in our previous paper [12]. Briefly, in each well of a 24-well microplate, around 50,000 PC12 cells were seeded and cultured under humidified conditions with 5% $CO_2$ at 37 °C for 24 h. After 24 h, 1 mL of serum-free Dulbecco's modified eagle medium (DMEM) containing a test sample or DMSO (0.5%) was used to replace the previous medium in each well. An NGF (40 ng/mL) was used as the positive control. Approximately 100 cells were counted thrice from a randomly selected area. Cells with a neurite outgrowth longer than the diameter of its body were counted as positive cells. The percentage of the positive cells in the selected area was regarded as the activities and the results were expressed as a mean ± SEM.

In the inhibitor test, the cells in each well of a 24-well microplate were first pretreated with 500 μL of the culture medium containing the specific inhibitor for 30 min. After this, 500 μL of the culture medium containing the sample or DMSO (0.5%) was added. The morphological changes in the cells were observed after 48 h.

In addition, the wide-type of the PC12 cell lines and corresponding mutants (PC12(ras-N17), PC12(mtGAP)) were provided by Prof. Hiroyuki Osada (RIKEN Center for Sustainable Resource Science, Japan).

*2.4. Analysis of the Cell Viability by Using the MTT Assay*

The cell viability was determined in accordance with the mitochondria-dependent reduction of MTT to purple formazan. Briefly, cells with AMA at concentrations of 0, 0.03, 0.3, 3 and 10 μM or AMA (3 μM) combined with a low dose of NGF were incubated for 48 h. The medium was removed carefully by aspiration. Afterward, 0.5 mL of fresh medium containing MTT (200 μg/mL) was added to each well and plates were incubated at 37 °C for 2 h. The medium in each well was then completely replaced with 0.2 mL DMSO to solubilize the formazan crystals. The resultant formazan was detected using a plate reader at 570 nm. All experiments were repeated at least three times.

*2.5. Primary Culture of Mouse Cortical Neuron Cells*

According to a previous study, primary cortical neuron cultures were prepared from the brains of C57BL/6J mice at embryonic day 17 [12]. Briefly, the cortex was digested in 0.5% trypsin in a 5% $CO_2$ incubator at 37 °C for 20 min. Around $6 \times 10^4$ neurons were seeded into the poly-L-lysine-coated 24-well plates in a serum-free neurobasal medium (Gibco, Grand Island, NY, USA). Samples with different concentrations (AMA at 0.1, 0.3, 1 and 3 μM; 0.1 μM AMA together with 1 ng/mL NGF) were added to each well and incubated for 24 h and 0.5% DMSO and NGF were used as negative and positive control samples, respectively. After 72 h of treatment with samples, 500 nM of NeuO were added to the cultures for 1 h. Fluorescence microscopy at an excitation/emission wavelength of 430/560 nm was then used to image the neurons. Image J software (National Institutes of Health, Bethesda, MD, USA) was used to measure the relative length of the neurite outgrowth of the neurons. The results were expressed as a mean ± SEM.

*2.6. Western Blot Analysis*

A Western blot analysis was performed in accordance with previous studies [12]. Briefly, in each 60 mm culture dish containing 5 mL DMEM, approximately $2 \times 10^6$ PC12 cells were seeded and incubated for 24 h. For the time-dependent study of AMA, AMA (3 μM) was supplemented to the dishes, which were incubated for specific time periods. For the study of the inhibitors, AMA (3 μM) or AMA (3 μM) with a low dose of the NGF (1 ng/mL) were added to the dishes, which were then incubated for a certain period (2 h for GR, p-GR, PLC and p-PLC; 8 h for the INSR and p-INSR; 24 h for AKT and p-AKT; 48 h for ERK1/2, p-ERK1/2, PKC and p-PKC). Sodium dodecyl sulphate polyacrylamide gel electrophoresis was used to separate the proteins (15 μg) and transfer them onto a PVDF membrane. The membranes were incubated with primary antibodies and secondary antibodies (see the details in Supplementary Table S2). The antigens were visualized using a high sensitivity chemiluminescence detection kit (Beijing Cowin Biotech Company, Beijing, China). The primary antibodies used for immunoblotting were as follows: anti-insulin receptor antibody, anti-phospho-insulin receptor (Tyr1150/1151) antibody, anti-phospho-

AKT (Ser473), anti-AKT antibody, anti-phospho-p44/42 MAPK (ERK1/2) (Thr202/Tyr204) antibody, anti-44/42 MAPK (ERK1/2) antibody, anti-phospho-PLC γ antibody, anti-PLC antibody, anti-phospho-PKC antibody, anti-PKC antibody (Cell Signaling Technology, Boston, MA, USA), anti-phospho-GR antibody (Affinity BioReagents, OH, USA) and anti-GR antibody (Santa Cruz, CA, USA) and GAPDH antibody (Beijing Cowin Biotech Company, Beijing, China). The secondary antibodies used in this study were as follows: horseradish peroxidase-linked anti-rabbit and anti-mouse IgGs (Beijing Cowin Biotech Company, Beijing, China). The bands were quantitatively measured using ImageJ software (National Institutes of Health, Bethesda, MD, USA).

*2.7. Cellular Thermal Shift Assay*

A CETSA was performed as described in other reports [17]. First, in 60 mm dishes containing 5 mL DMEM, $2 \times 10^6$ cells were separately added and incubated for 24 h. In each plate, AMA was added at a final concentration of 3 µM. After a continuous incubation for 8 h, cells were collected and heated at temperatures ranging from 46 °C to 66 °C. Finally, a Western blot analysis was used to detect the changes in the INSR protein and GR protein.

*2.8. RNA Interference*

PC12 cells were transfected with different concentrations of FAM-labelled siRNA to evaluate the transfection efficiency. Finally, 150 nM was decided as the final concentration to perform the experiment at which 90% of the transfection efficiency was obtained. The following primer sequences were used to generate siRNAs that knocked down the INSR and the negative control (Sangon Biotech Co. Ltd., Shanghai, China): for INSR-4295, sense: 5′-GUG AAG AGC UGG AGA UGG ATT-3′, anti-sense: 5′-UCC AUC UCC AGC UCU UCA CTT-3′; for the negative control, sense: 5′-UUC UCC GAA CGU GUC ACG UTT-3′, anti-sense: 5′-ACG UGA CAC GUU CGG AGA ATT-3′.

The transfection of PC12 cells with an siRNA was performed on the basis of the manufacturer's instructions. Briefly, in each well of 24-well plates, $5 \times 10^4$ cells were seeded and allowed to reach 70–90% confluence in a growth medium without antibiotics one day before the transfection. SiRNA against the INSR or the negative control siRNA were then used at a concentration of 150 nM with Lipofectamine 2000 (Invitrogen) as the transfection agent. After 6 h of transfection, the fresh medium containing 3 µM AMA or AMA combined with a low dose of the NGF was used to replace the previous medium in the plates and the plate was then incubated for another 24 h. The cell morphological features were observed and recorded using an inverted microscope fitted with a camera. The percentage of the cells with a neurite outgrowth was expressed as the mean ± SEM. Finally, a Western blot analysis was used to detect the changes in the INSR protein.

*2.9. Statistical Analysis*

Data were presented as a mean ± SEM of three independent experiments in triplicate. Data were subjected to a one-way ANOVA and a Tukey's post hoc analysis by using the GraphPad Prism software. $p < 0.05$ was considered statistically significant.

## 3. Results

*3.1. AMA-Induced Neuritogenic Effect in PC12 Cells and in Primary Cortical Neuron Cells*

The neuritogenic activity of AMA was first detected in PC12 cells. PC12 cells were treated with different concentrations of AMA (0.03, 0.3 and 3 µM) for 48 h. The results showed that AMA induced neurite outgrowth in PC12 cells in a dose-dependent manner. The percentages of the cells with a neurite outgrowth after treatment with 0, 0.03, 0.3 and 3 µM of AMA were 6.0% ± 0.6%, 11.3% ± 1.2%, 36.7% ± 2.3% ($p < 0.001$) and 53.0% ± 2.1% ($p < 0.001$), respectively (Figure 1b). Interestingly, AMA with a low dose of the NGF (1 ng/mL) significantly increased the percentage of PC12 cells with neurite outgrowth from 53.0% ± 2.1% to 77.3% ± 1.3% ($p < 0.001$, Figure 1b). The morphological changes in PC12 cells after treatment with 3 µM of AMA and AMA combined with 1 ng/mL of NGF are displayed in Figure 1c. These results indicated that AMA exhibited NGF-mimicking and NGF-enhancing activities in PC12 cells. The effect of AMA in PC12 cell viability was then determined using the 3-(4,5-dimethylthiazol-2-yl)-2,5-diphenyl tetrazolium bromide (MTT) analysis. The viabilities of PC12 cells were 96.9% ± 2.3%, 97.3% ± 2.4%, 106.1% ± 4.4% and 94.0% ± 4.9% after treatment with AMA at doses of 0.03, 0.3, 3 and 10 µM, respectively (Figure 1d). None of these concentrations produced considerable cytotoxicity as detected by the MTT assay. Furthermore, the viability of PC12 cells in the 3 µM AMA-treated group was significantly increased to 135.7% ± 13.4% after adding a low dose of the NGF (1 ng/mL, $p < 0.001$, Figure 1d). These results suggested that AMA showed no cytotoxicity at a dose of 10 µM and that the low-dose NGF could increase the cell viability of AMA in PC12 cells.

In addition, the neuritogenic effect of AMA was further estimated in the primary cortical neuron cells. As shown in Figure 2, the neurite outgrowth was increased significantly after treatment with different concentrations of AMA and AMA with the NGF. The morphological changes in the primary cortical neurons are shown in Figure 2a. The average of the neurite length and primary dendrite number are displayed in Figure 2b,c, respectively. Treatment with AMA at 0.1, 0.3 and 1 µM significantly increased the neurite length from 41.7 ± 1.2 µm to 61.7 ± 3.2 µm ($p < 0.05$), 69.3 ± 2.2 µm ($p < 0.01$) and 80.9 ± 5.7 µm ($p < 0.001$), respectively. Moreover, 0.1 µM AMA combined with 1 ng/mL of NGF increased the neurite length to a level that was comparable with the effect of the NGF at 10 ng/mL ($p < 0.01$). Collectively, these results demonstrated that AMA exhibited significant neuritogenic activity in PC12 cells and in primary cortical neuron cells.

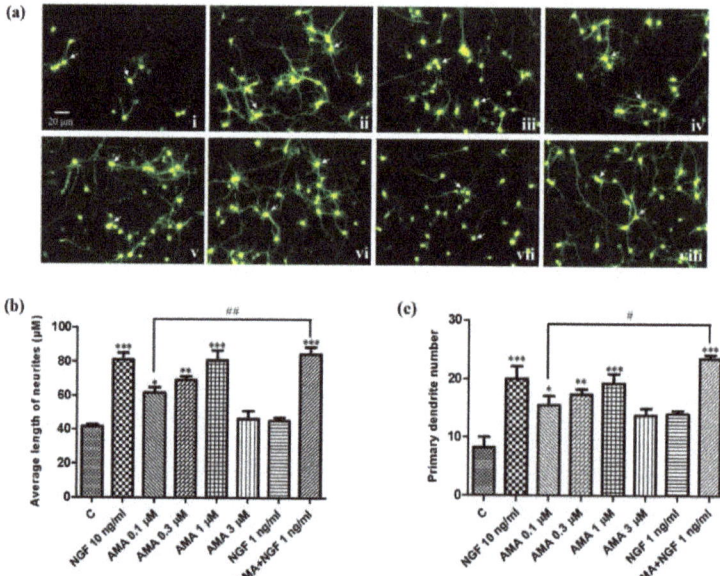

**Figure 2.** Neurogenesis effect of AMA in primary cortical neuron cells. (**a**) Micrographs of primary cortical neuron cells at 48 h after treatment with (**i**) control (0.5% DMSO); (**ii**) NGF (10 ng/mL); (**iii**) NGF (1 ng/mL); (**iv**) AMA (0.1 µM); (**v**) AMA (0.3 µM); (**vi**) AMA (1 µM); (**vii**) AMA (3 µM); (**viii**) AMA (0.1 µM) + NGF (1 ng/mL). (**b**) Average length of neurite outgrowth of the indicated groups in the primary cortical neuron cells. (**c**) Average primary dendrite number in each group. Each experiment was repeated three times. The data were expressed as a mean ± SEM. *, ** and *** indicate significant differences at $p < 0.05$, $p < 0.01$ and $p < 0.001$ compared with the negative control; #, ## indicate a significant difference at $p < 0.05$ and $p < 0.01$ compared with the 0.1 µM AMA group.

## 3.2. Effect of AMA on the Ras/Raf/MEK/ERK Signaling Pathway

Different neurotrophic factors such as NGF and BDNF specifically bind to the transmembrane receptors TrkA and TrkB and activate several kinases to stimulate the function of differentiation and survival in neuron cells [18,19]. Therefore, the mechanism of the action of AMA was first investigated using the inhibitors of TrkA and TrkB. However, the neurite outgrowth induced by AMA or AMA combined with the NGF did not change after the treatment with the inhibitor of TrkA, K252a (Figure 3a). Similarly, the inhibitor of TrkB, ANA-12, did not affect the NGF-mimicking or NGF-enhancing effect of AMA in PC12 cells (Figure 3b).

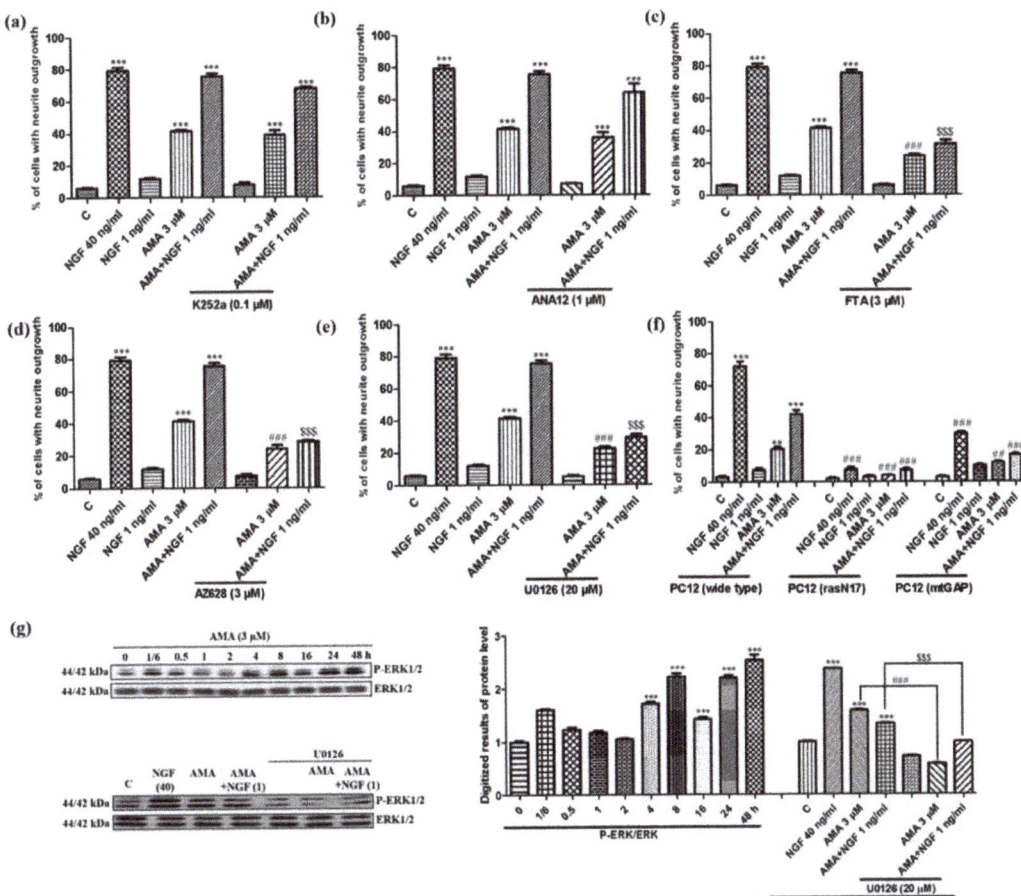

**Figure 3.** Effect of AMA on the Ras/Raf/MEK/ERK signaling pathway in PC12 cells. (**a**,**b**) Effect of TrkA inhibitor K252a and TrkB inhibitor ANA-12 on the neurite outgrowth induced by AMA and AMA combined with the NGF. (**c**–**e**) Effects of Ras, Raf and MEK inhibitors on the neurogenesis activity of AMA and AMA combined with the NGF. (**f**) Percentage of the neurite outgrowth induced by AMA and AMA combined with the NGF for 48 h in wide-type or Ras mutant PC12 cells. (**g**) Phosphorylation of ERK at different time points induced by AMA. The ERK phosphorylation was reduced by the inhibitor of MEK and quantified using Western blots through ImageJ software. Each experiment was repeated three times. ** and *** indicate significant differences at $p < 0.01$ and $p < 0.001$ compared with the negative control; ##, ### indicate a significant difference at $p < 0.01$ and $p < 0.001$ compared with the 3 μM AMA group; $$$ indicates a significant difference at $p < 0.001$ compared with the AMA-combined NGF group.

Ras/Raf//MEK/ERK was believed to be the major cascade for the NGF-stimulated differentiation in PC12 cells [20]. Therefore, the effect of these signaling pathways was investigated using specific inhibitors, mutants and a Western blot analysis. As displayed in Figure 3c–e, after adding the inhibitors of Ras (farnesylthiosalicylic acid, FTA), Raf (AZ628) and MEK (U0126), the neurite outgrowth induced by AMA was significantly reduced from $53.0\% \pm 2.1\%$ to $24.0\% \pm 1.2\%$ ($p < 0.001$), $22.3\% \pm 1.2\%$ ($p < 0.001$) and $21.0\% \pm 1.0\%$ ($p < 0.001$), respectively. Similarly, the neuritogenic activity of AMA combined with the NGF was decreased by these above mentioned inhibitors from $75.3\% \pm 1.9\%$ to $31.3\% \pm 2.4\%$ ($p < 0.001$), $28.3\% \pm 0.9\%$ ($p < 0.001$) and $29.3\% \pm 1.7\%$ ($p < 0.001$), respectively (Figure 3c–e).

Furthermore, the Ras mutant types of PC12 cells including the membrane-targeted PC12(mtGAP) or the dominant inhibitory mutant PC12(rasN17) were used to detect the effect of AMA on the Ras protein. AMA or AMA combined with the NGF failed to induce the neurite outgrowth on the Ras mutant cell lines due to the inhibition of the Ras function. This finding suggested that the Ras signaling was involved in the effect of AMA (Figure 3f, Supplementary Figure S1).

The effect of AMA on ERK phosphorylation at the protein level was studied. The phosphorylation of ERK was increased from 4 h and peaked at 48 h (Figure 3g, Supplementary Figure S2). Meanwhile, the ERK phosphorylation in the AMA-treated group or the AMA with a low dose of NGF-treated group was diminished by the inhibitor of MEK, U0126 (Figure 3g). These results indicated that TrkA and TrkB were not involved in the neurogenesis effect of AMA. However, the Ras/Raf/MEK/ERK signaling pathway took an important role in the neurogenesis effect of AMA.

### 3.3. Effect of AMA on the INSR/PI3K/AKT Signaling Pathway

Growing evidence shows that insulin plays an important role in brain functions such as cognitive and memory improvement. Insulin binds to the INSR and activates the PI3K/AKT pathway, thereby enhancing the cell growth and survival [21]. Therefore, the inhibitor of the INSR, HNMPA-(AM)$_3$, was used to study the mechanism of the action of AMA. After treatment with HNMPA-(AM)$_3$, the AMA-induced neurite outgrowth was significantly decreased from $53.0\% \pm 2.1\%$ to $11.7\% \pm 0.9\%$ ($p < 0.001$) (Figure 4a). Moreover, the neurite outgrowth induced by AMA was reduced after treatment with the inhibitor of PI3K, LY294002, from $53.0\% \pm 2.1\%$ to $22.3\% \pm 1.2\%$ ($p < 0.001$) (Figure 4b). The neurite outgrowth of PC12 cells induced by AMA combined with the NGF was also decreased by HNMPA-(AM)$_3$ and LY294002 (Figure 4a,b).

Subsequently, the phosphorylation of the INSR and AKT induced by AMA were investigated in a time-dependent manner. The INSR phosphorylation increased at 1 h and peaked at 8 h after treatment with AMA (Figure 4c, Supplementary Figure S3). Furthermore, the phosphorylation of AKT after the treatment with AMA was increased at 2 h and peaked at 24 h (Figure 4c). The increase in the phosphorylation of the INSR and downstream protein AKT and ERK in the AMA with or without 1 ng/mL of NGF were significantly decreased by HNMPA-(AM)$_3$ (Figure 4d, Supplementary Figure S3). In addition, the phosphorylation of AKT induced by AMA and AMA combined with the NGF were also reduced by the inhibitor of PI3K, LY294002 (Figure 4e, Supplementary Figure S3). These results suggested that the INSR/PI3K/AKT signaling pathway exerted an important effect on the AMA-induced neurite outgrowth in PC12 cells.

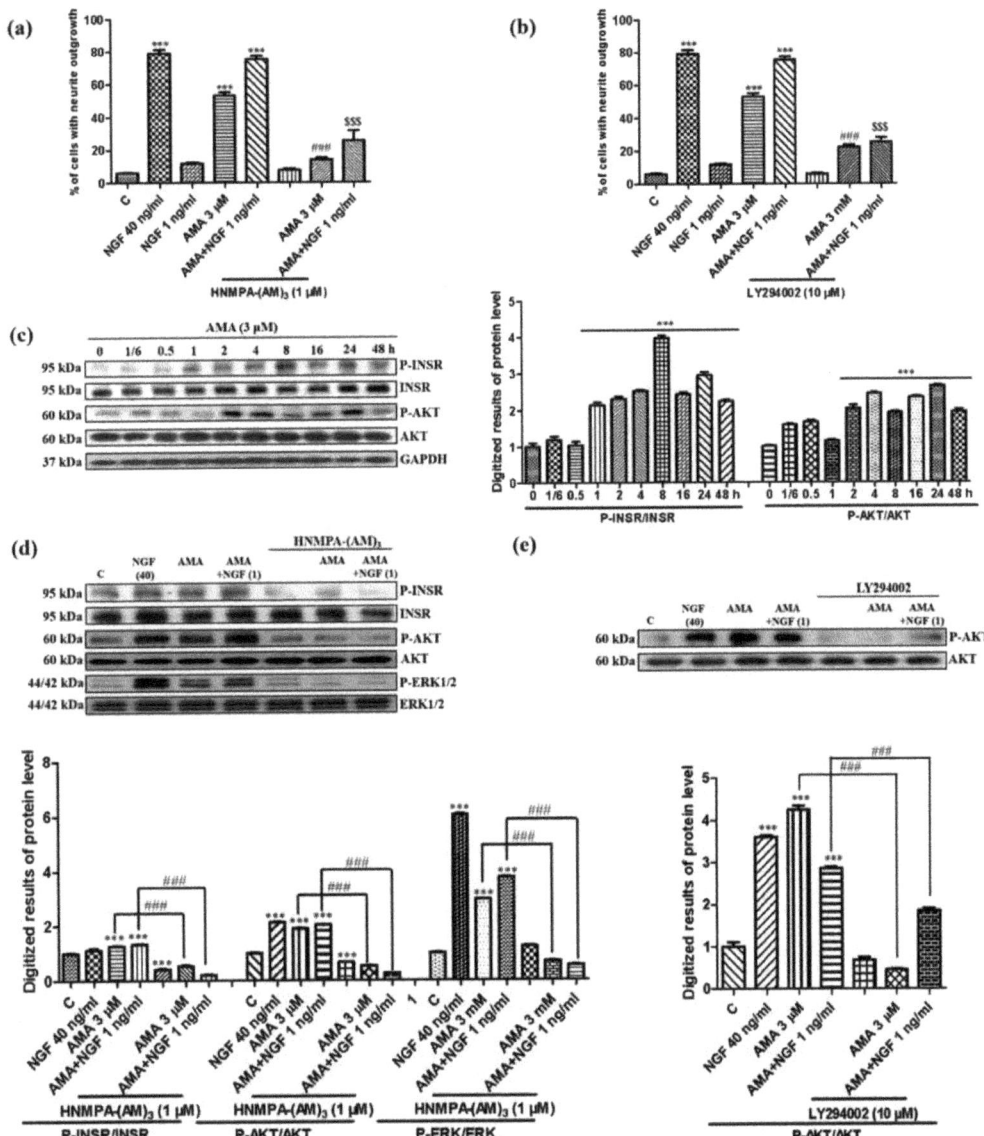

**Figure 4.** Effect of amarogentin on the insulin receptor/PI3K/AKT signaling pathway in PC12 cells. (**a**,**b**) Effect of the insulin receptor inhibitor HNMPA-(AM)3 and PI3K inhibitor LY294002 on the neurite outgrowth induced by AMA and AMA combined with the NGF. (**c**) AMA-induced phosphorylation of the insulin receptor and AKT in a time-dependent manner and quantification of the Western blots by using ImageJ software. (**d**) Phosphorylation of the insulin receptor, AKT and ERK induced by AMA or AMA combined with the NGF was decreased by the inhibitor HNMPA-(AM)3. (**e**) Phosphorylation of AKT induced by AMA or AMA combined with the NGF was decreased by the inhibitor LY294002. Each experiment was repeated three times. *** indicates significant differences at $p < 0.001$ compared with the negative control; ### indicates a significant difference at $p < 0.001$ compared with the 3 µM AMA group and $^{\$\$\$}$ indicates a significant difference at $p < 0.001$ compared with the AMA-combined NGF group.

## 3.4. Effect of AMA on the GR/PLC/PKC Signaling Pathway

GR has been reported to regulate a series of genes important for neuronal structure and plasticity and is involved in the neuritogenic activity in PC12 cells [22,23]. Therefore, the inhibitor of GR, RU486, was used to elucidate the mechanism of the action of AMA. The percentage of cells with a neurite outgrowth was significantly decreased from 53.0% ± 2.1% to 28.3% ± 1.2% ($p < 0.001$) after treatment with RU486 (Figure 5a). Given that the PLC/PKC signaling pathway is located at the downstream of GR and plays an important role in cell survival and differentiation [24], the inhibitors of PLC (U73343) and PKC (Go6983) were used to examine the effect of AMA. The neurite outgrowth of AMA was diminished from 53.0% ± 2.1% to 16.3% ± 2.0% and 17.7% ± 1.6% ($p < 0.001$) after the addition of U73343 and Go6983, respectively (Figure 5b,c). Similarly, the effect of AMA combined with a low dose of the NGF was also inhibited by RU486, U73343 and Go6983 (Figure 5a–c).

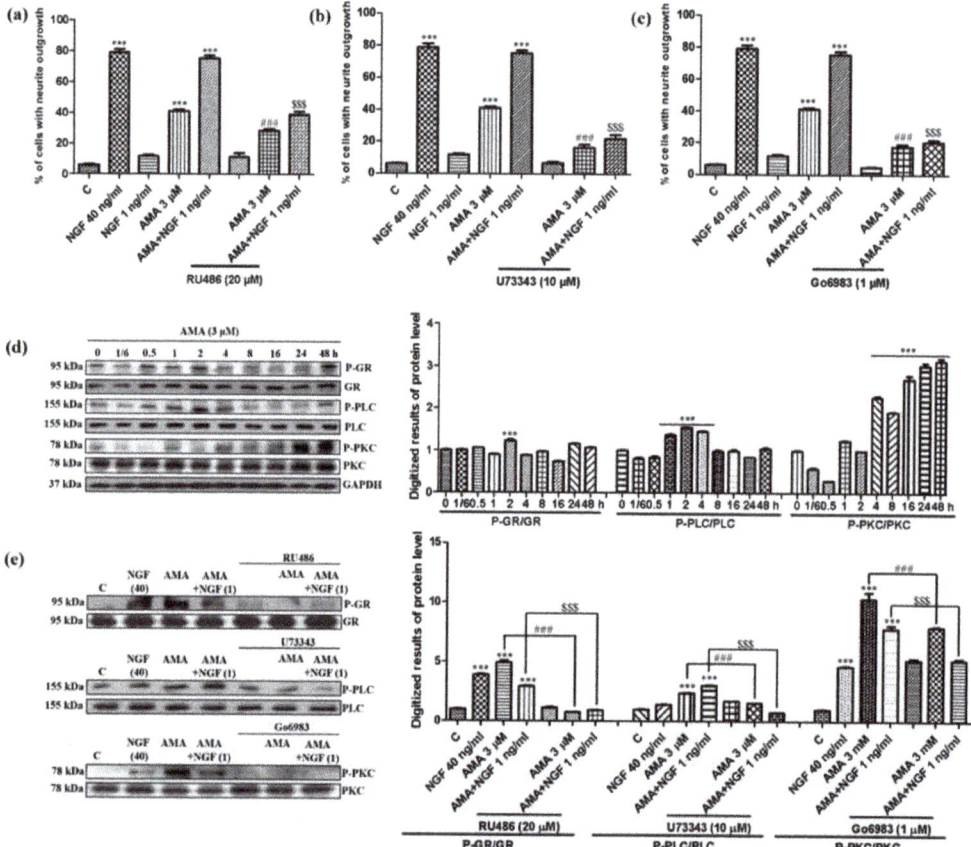

**Figure 5.** Effect of AMA on the GR/PLC/PKC signaling pathway in PC12 cells. (**a–c**) Effect of GR (RU486), PLC (U73343) and PKC (Go6983) inhibitors on the neurite outgrowth induced by AMA and AMA combined with the NGF. (**d**) AMA-stimulated phosphorylation of GR, PLC and PKC proteins in a time-dependent manner and the quantification of Western blots by using ImageJ software. (**e**) Phosphorylation of GR, PLC and PKC induced by AMA or AMA combined with the NGF reduced by the corresponding inhibitors and quantified using Western blots through ImageJ software. Each experiment was repeated three times. *** indicates significant differences at $p < 0.001$ compared with the negative control; ### indicates a significant difference at $p < 0.001$ compared with the 3 μM AMA group and $^{\$\$\$}$ indicates a significant difference at $p < 0.001$ compared with the AMA-combined NGF group.

The phosphorylation of GR/PLC/PKC was then determined at the protein level by using a Western blot analysis. The GR phosphorylation peaked at 2 h and was reduced by RU486 (Figure 5d,e, Supplementary Figure S4). The PLC phosphorylation was increased from 1 h, peaked at 2 h and decreased by the inhibitor of PLC, U73343 (Figure 5d,e). Furthermore, the phosphorylation of PKC peaked at 48 h and was reduced by Go6983, the inhibitor of PKC (Figure 5d,e). The AMA combined with the NGF group changed in a similar way (Figure 5d,e). These results demonstrated that the AMA-induced neuritogenic activity in PC12 cells was related to the GR/PLC/PKC signaling pathway.

*3.5. Identification of the Target Protein for AMA by Using siRNA Analysis and CETSA*

Considering that TrkA and TrkB are not involved in the neurogenesis effect of AMA, we predicted that the INSR or GR protein might be the potential target of AMA. Given that the inhibition effect of the INSR for AMA was stronger than that of GR, the INSR was first considered as the potential target of AMA. The 5-carboxyfluorescein (FAM)-labelled siRNA was initially used to confirm the optimal transfection concentration of siRNA and whether AMA targeted the INSR. Approximately 90% of the PC12 cells produced fluorescence after treatment with 150 nM of the FAM-labelled siRNA and 150 nM of the INSR siRNA was used to perform the transfection (Supplementary Figure S5). The INSR siRNA was transfected into PC12 cells for 6 h and treated with 3 μM AMA or AMA combined with the NGF. After the treatment of the PC12 cells with the INSR siRNA, the percentage of cells with a neurite outgrowth induced by AMA with or without a low dose of the NGF for 48 h was significantly decreased (Figure 6a,b). In addition, the total and the phosphorylation protein levels of the INSR were significantly decreased by the treatment with the INSR siRNA regardless of the AMA treatment ($p < 0.001$, Figure 6c, Supplementary Figure S6). Hence, these results indicated that the INSR might be the target protein of AMA.

A CETSA was used to discover the target protein of molecules on the basis of the thermal stabilization of proteins upon ligand binding [17]. Therefore, a CETSA was used to detect the binding correlations between the INSR and AMA to further confirm the potential target of AMA. After treating the PC12 cells with dimethyl sulfoxide (DMSO) or AMA and heating at temperature ranging from 46 °C to 66 °C, the immunoblotting analysis was conducted using a specific antibody for the INSR. The results suggested a significant thermal stabilization of the INSR protein upon AMA treatment (Figure 6d, Supplementary Figure S6). At the same time, the change of GR at the protein level was detected using the same method. As expected, the GR protein did not show the thermal stability-shifted effect after the AMA treatment (Figure 6e, Supplementary Figure S6). Furthermore, other known insulin agonists such as insulin and demethylasterriquinone B1 (DB1) were selected to detect whether they exhibited a similar neurogenesis as AMA in PC12 cells [25]. The results indicated that both showed a significant NGF-mimicking and NGF-enhancing activity in the PC12 cells (Figure 6f, Supplementary Figure S7). These results indicated that AMA might target the INSR to produce the NGF-mimicking activity.

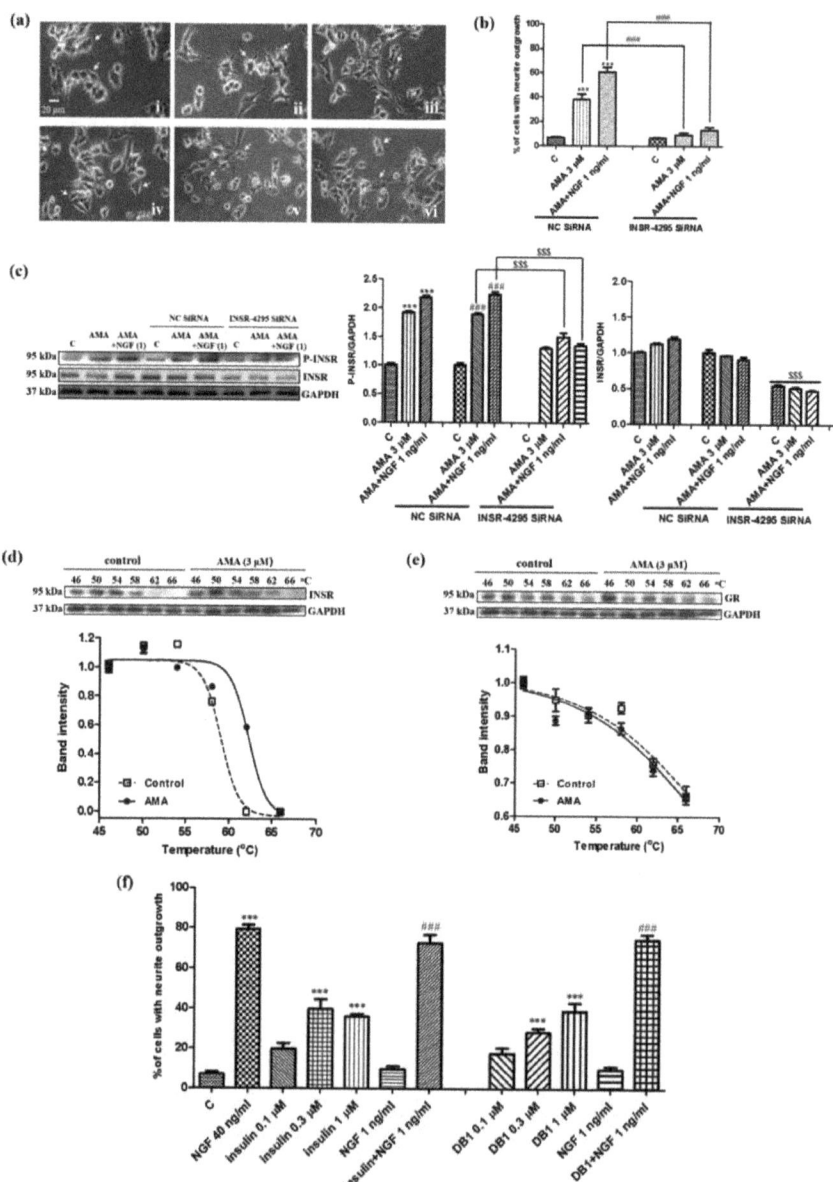

**Figure 6.** Target prediction of AMA in PC12 cells by using siRNA and a CETSA assay. (**a**) Microphotographs of PC12 cells after treatment with siRNA and AMA or AMA combined with the NGF: (**i**) negative control siRNA, control (0.5% DMSO); (**ii**) negative control siRNA, AMA (3 μM); (**iii**) negative control siRNA, AMA (3 μM) + NGF (1 ng/mL); (**iv**) insulin receptor siRNA, control (0.5% DMSO); (**v**) insulin receptor siRNA, AMA (3 μM); (**vi**) insulin receptor siRNA, AMA (3 μM) + NGF (1 ng/mL). (**b**) Percentage of cells with a neurite outgrowth after treatment with siRNA and AMA or AMA combined with the NGF. (**c**) Western blot analysis for the insulin receptor after transfection with negative siRNA or insulin receptor siRNA and treatment with AMA or AMA combined with the NGF. Cells were transfected with Lipofectamine 2000 and 150 nM siRNA for 6 h and treated with AMA or AMA combined with the NGF. (**d**,**e**) CETSA of PC12 cells on the insulin receptor or GR protein and corresponding fitting curves. (**f**) Neuritogenic activity of insulin and demethylasterriquinone B1 in PC12 cells. ***, ### and $$$ indicate significant differences at $p < 0.001$ compared with the corresponding groups.

## 4. Discussion

Aging is a major risk factor for age-related diseases such as Parkinson's disease and AD [26]. We speculated that if we prevent or delay aging, we can prevent the occurrence of AD or cure AD. Our laboratory began to screen small anti-aging molecules from food and TCMs ten years ago to verify this hypothesis. To date, we have found more than 30 anti-aging compounds with different types of chemical structures such as sterols, benzoquinones, phenols and terpenes [27–30]. Furthermore, we have indicated that cucurbitacin B with an anti-aging effect can improve the memory of APP/PS1 mice via the target cofilin and the regulation of GR signaling pathways [23,31]. These results indicate that anti-aging substances may prevent and treat AD.

*G. rigescens* Franch is a TCM used to treat hepatitis, rheumatism, cholecystitis and inflammation in China [14]. In our previous study, we discovered gentisides A–K with a novel NGF-mimicking effect from the nonpolar extract of this plant and indicated that a mixture of benzoates could alleviate the impaired memory of AD model mice induced by scopolamine [15]. We have also focused on the water layer of *G. rigescens* Franch to isolate active molecules under the guidance of PC12 cells and a yeast replicative lifespan assay to understand whether the small molecules of the polar part have the same function. We have found that AMA produces anti-aging effects on yeasts and neuron protection in PC12 cells via anti-oxidative stress [16]. In the present study, we used PC12 cells and primary cortical neuron cells to investigate the neurogenesis effect of AMA. The morphological changes of PC12 cells and primary cortical neuron cells after AMA treatment suggested that AMA had a neurogenesis effect on PC12 cells and primary cortical neuron cells (Figures 1 and 2). These results were consistent with those of our previous reports [12,23].

The target protein identification has an important role in drug development and can provide strong evidence for the elucidation of the mechanism of the action, safety evaluation and targeted treatment of a disease [32]. Therefore, we first focused on the target protein discovery of AMA to perform deep research with specific inhibitors, siRNA, a CETSA and a Western blot analysis. The results of the specific inhibitors for TrkA, TrkB, INSR, GR, PI3K, PLC, PKC and MEK and the Western blot analysis in Figures 3–6 indicated that AMA induced neuritogenic activity in PC12 cells by activating the INSR and regulating the PI3K/AKT/Ras/Raf/ERK and GR/PLC/PKC signaling pathways. Interestingly, the mechanism of the action of AMA for its NGF-mimicking effect was different from that of previously reported compounds (such as ABG-001, lindersin B, 3beta,23,28-trihydroxy-12-oleanene 3beta-caffeate and CuB). Tetradecyl 2,3-dihydroxybenzoate (ABG-001) was designed and synthesized as a lead compound in accordance with the gentiside series to induce neurogenesis in PC12 cells by the IGF-1R/PI3K/MAPK signaling pathway [9,10]. Lindersin B from *L. crustacea* induced neuritogenic activity through the activation of the TrkA/PI3K/ERK signaling pathway [11]. 3beta,23,28-trihydroxy-12-oleanene 3beta-caffeate from *D. sambuense* induced neurogenesis in PC12 cells mediated by the ER stress and BDNF-TrkB signaling pathways [12] and CuB induced neuritogenic activity by targeting cofilin and regulating the GR TrkA signaling pathways [23]. These molecules possess different structures but exhibit neurogenesis effects by activating various related signaling pathways. AMA was the first compound we discovered to target the INSR for the NGF-mimicking activity in PC12 cells. These results provided insights into the combination that the use of these molecules may have in increasing the therapy effect for AD.

TrkA and TrkB are specific transmembrane receptors that bind to neurotrophic factors such as NGF and BDNF [18,19]. Therefore, the effects of these two proteins were investigated. We found that TrkA and TrkB were not involved in the neurogenesis effect of AMA (Figure 3b). We focused on the INSR and GR to determine the target protein. The results of the INSR knockdown experiment, a CETSA and a Western blot analysis for the INSR and GR in Figure 6 revealed that the INSR was the potential target protein of AMA. Furthermore, known insulin agonists including insulin and DB1 showed similar neurogenesis effects as AMA in PC12 cells, which confirmed the INSR as the potential target of AMA (Figure 6). It was different from the target proteins of CuB, cofilin and

3beta,23,28-trihydroxy-12-oleanene 3beta-caffeate and ER stress [11,23]. AMA may have effects for diabetes and inflammation because of the involvement of insulin and GR signaling pathways [33,34].

In conclusion, AMA from *Gentiana rigescens* Franch showed significant neuritogenic activity in PC12 cells and in primary cortical neuron cells. The neuritogenic activity induced by AMA in PC12 cells was through the targeting of the INSR and the regulation of the PI3K/AKT/Ras/Raf/ERK and GR/PLC/PKC signaling pathways (Figure 7). This study indicated the potential applications of AMA for its neurogenesis effect and provided evidence for the treatment of neurodegenerative diseases and anti-aging. Furthermore, the structure-activity relationship of AMA should be studied to discover the novel leading compounds and elucidate the underlying mechanism in animal levels and also applied to clinical trials.

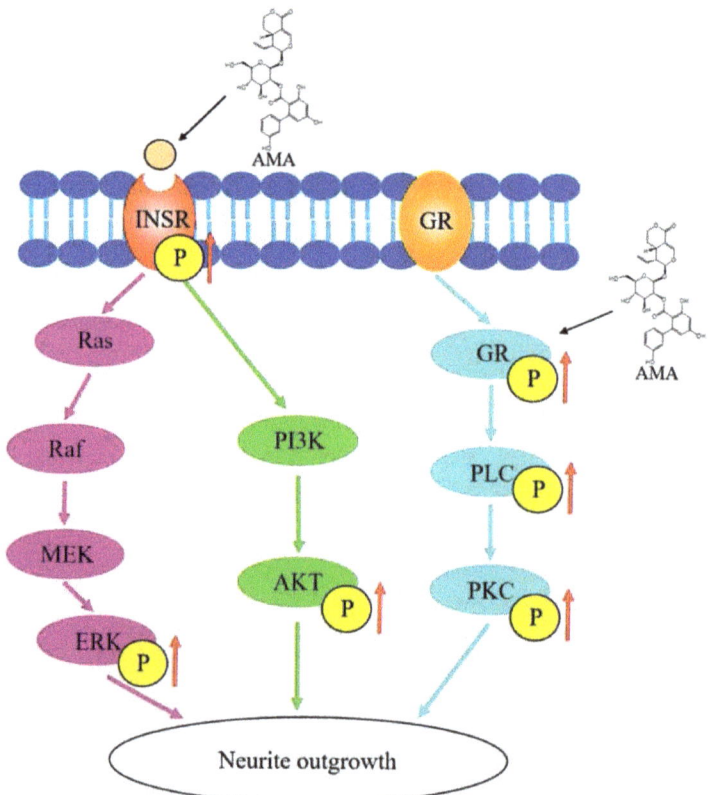

**Figure 7.** Proposed mechanism of the action of AMA in the neuritogenic activity in PC12 cells.

**Supplementary Materials:** The following are available online at https://www.mdpi.com/article/10.3390/biomedicines9050581/s1, Figure S1: Differentiation of PC12 cells expressing dominant negative Ras (PC12(rasN17)) or membrane-targeted GAP (PC12(mtGAP)) induced by AMA or AMA combined with NGF, Figure S2: Origin data of Western blot analysis in Figure 3g, Figure S3: Origin data of Western blot analysis in Figure 4c–e, Figure S4: Origin data of Western blot analysis in Figure 5d,e, Figure S5: Microphotograph of PC12 cells after transfection with different concentrations of FAM-siRNA (50 nM, 100 nM and 150 nM), Figure S6: Origin data of Western blot analysis in Figure 6c–e, Figure S7: Microphotograph of PC12 cells after treatment with insulin and Demethylasterriquinone B1, Table S1: List of inhibitors used in this study, Table S2: List of antibodies used in this study.

**Author Contributions:** L.C. performed the bioassay, mechanism study and data analysis as well as writing the original draft; T.X. provided assistance with editing; H.O., M.Y., L.X. and J.Q. contributed to designing the overall research strategy, supervision and revision of the manuscript. All authors have read and agreed to the published version of the manuscript.

**Funding:** Publication of this paper. This research was funded by the National Key R&D Program of China (Grant No. 2017YFE0117200, Grant No. 2019YFE0100700) and the National Natural Science Foundation of China (Grant No. 21877098, 21661140001).

**Institutional Review Board Statement:** This study did not involve humans or animals experiments.

**Informed Consent Statement:** Not applicable.

**Data Availability Statement:** All figures and data used to support this study are included within this article.

**Acknowledgments:** This work was financially supported by the National Key R&D Program of China (Grant No. 2017YFE0117200, Grant No. 2019YFE0100700) and the National Natural Science Foundation of China (Grant No. 21877098, 21661140001). This work was inspired by the JSPS Asian Chemical Biology Initiative. The authors thank Young-Tae Chang (Pohang University of Science and Technology) for providing the NeuO reagent. We thank Julius Adam V. Lopez and Makoto Muroi for valuable comments on the manuscript.

**Conflicts of Interest:** The authors declare that there is no conflict of interest regarding publication of this paper.

## Abbreviations

Alzheimer's disease (AD); amarogentin (AMA); blood-brain barrier (BBB); cellular thermal shift assay (CETSA); demethylasterriquinone B1 (DB1); dimethyl sulfoxide (DMSO); extracellular signal-regulated kinase (ERK); glucocorticoid receptor (GR); insulin receptor (INSR); mitogen-activated protein kinase (MEK); nerve growth factor (NGF); phospholipase C (PLC); protein kinase B (AKT); protein kinase C (PKC); small-interfering RNA (siRNA); traditional Chinese medicines (TCMs).

## References

1. Huang, L.-K.; Chao, S.-P.; Hu, C.-J. Clinical trials of new drugs for Alzheimer disease. *J. Biomed. Sci.* **2020**, *27*, 1–13. [CrossRef] [PubMed]
2. Alzheimer's Disease International. *World Alzheimer Report 2019: Attitudes to Dementia*; Alzheimer's Disease International: London, UK, 2019.
3. Ng, Y.P.; Or, T.C.T.; Ip, N.Y. Plant alkaloids as drug leads for Alzheimer's disease. *Neurochem. Int.* **2015**, *89*, 260–270. [CrossRef] [PubMed]
4. Xu, C.-J.; Wang, J.-L.; Jin, W.-L. The Emerging Therapeutic Role of NGF in Alzheimer's Disease. *Neurochem. Res.* **2016**, *41*, 1211–1218. [CrossRef] [PubMed]
5. Aloe, L.; Rocco, M.L.; Balzamino, B.O.; Micera, A. Nerve Growth Factor: A Focus on Neuroscience and Therapy. *Curr. Neuropharmacol.* **2015**, *13*, 294–303. [CrossRef]
6. Greene, L.A.; Tischler, A.S. Establishment of a noradrenergic clonal line of rat adrenal pheochromocytoma cells which respond to nerve growth factor. *Proc. Natl. Acad. Sci. USA* **1976**, *73*, 2424–2428. [CrossRef]
7. Gao, L.; Li, J.; Qi, J. Gentisides A and B, two new neuritogenic compounds from the traditional Chinese medicine *Gentiana rigescens* Franch. *Bioorg. Med. Chem.* **2010**, *18*, 2131–2134. [CrossRef]
8. Gao, L.; Xiang, L.; Luo, Y.; Wang, G.; Li, J.; Qi, J. Gentisides C–K: Nine new neuritogenic compounds from the traditional Chinese medicine *Gentiana rigescens* Franch. *Bioorg. Med. Chem.* **2010**, *18*, 6995–7000. [CrossRef]
9. Wang, G.; Bian, L.; Zhang, H.; Wang, Y.; Gao, L.; Sun, K.; Xiang, L.; Qi, J. Synthesis and SAR Studies of Neuritogenic Gentiside Derivatives. *Chem. Pharm. Bull.* **2016**, *64*, 161–170. [CrossRef]
10. Tang, R.; Gao, L.; Kawatani, M.; Chen, J.; Cao, X.; Osada, H.; Xiang, L.; Qi, J. Neuritogenic Activity of Tetradecyl 2,3-Dihydroxybenzoate Is Mediated through the Insulin-Like Growth Factor 1 Receptor/Phosphatidylinositol 3 Kinase/Mitogen-Activated Protein Kinase Signaling Pathway. *Mol. Pharmacol.* **2015**, *88*, 326–334. [CrossRef]
11. Cheng, L.; Ye, Y.; Xiang, L.; Osada, H.; Qi, J. Lindersin B from *Lindernia crustacea* induces neuritogenesis by activation of tyrosine kinase A/phosphatidylinositol 3 kinase/extracellular signal-regulated kinase signaling pathway. *Phytomedicine* **2017**, *24*, 31–38. [CrossRef]
12. Cheng, L.; Muroi, M.; Cao, S.; Bian, L.; Osada, H.; Xiang, L.; Qi, J. 3β,23,28-Trihydroxy-12-oleanene 3β-Caffeate from *Desmodium sambuense*-Induced Neurogenesis in PC12 Cells Mediated by ER Stress and BDNF–TrkB Signaling Pathways. *Mol. Pharm.* **2019**, *16*, 1423–1432. [CrossRef] [PubMed]

13. Xu, Y.; Li, Y.; Maffucci, K.G.; Huang, L.; Zeng, R. Analytical Methods of Phytochemicals from the Genus Gentiana. *Molecules* **2017**, *22*, 2080. [CrossRef]
14. Xu, M.; Wang, D.; Zhang, Y.-J.; Yang, C.-R. Dammarane Triterpenoids from the Roots of *Gentiana rigescens*. *J. Nat. Prod.* **2007**, *70*, 880–883. [CrossRef] [PubMed]
15. Li, J.; Gao, L.; Sun, K.; Xiao, D.; Li, W.; Xiang, L.; Qi, J. Benzoate fraction from *Gentiana rigescens* Franch alleviates scopolamine-induced impaired memory in mice model in vivo. *J. Ethnopharmacol.* **2016**, *193*, 107–116. [CrossRef]
16. Disasa, D.; Cheng, L.; Manzoor, M.; Liu, Q.; Wang, Y.; Xiang, L.; Qi, J. Amarogentin from *Gentiana rigescens* Franch Exhibits Antiaging and Neuroprotective Effects through Antioxidative Stress. *Oxidative Med. Cell. Longev.* **2020**, *2020*, 1–15. [CrossRef] [PubMed]
17. Jafari, R.; Almqvist, H.; Axelsson, H.; Ignatushchenko, M.; Lundbäck, T.; Nordlund, P.; Molina, D.M. The cellular thermal shift assay for evaluating drug target interactions in cells. *Nat. Protoc.* **2014**, *9*, 2100–2122. [CrossRef] [PubMed]
18. Bothwell, M. NGF, BDNF, NT3, and NT4. *Organotypic Models Drug Dev.* **2014**, *220*, 3–15. [CrossRef]
19. Huang, E.J.; Reichardt, L.F. Neurotrophins: Roles in Neuronal Development and Function. *Annu. Rev. Neurosci.* **2001**, *24*, 677–736. [CrossRef]
20. Vaudry, D.; Stork, P.J.S.; Lazarovici, P.; Eiden, L.E. Signaling Pathways for PC12 Cell Differentiation: Making the Right Connections. *Science* **2002**, *296*, 1648–1649. [CrossRef]
21. De Sousa, R.A.L.; Harmer, A.R.; Freitas, D.A.; Mendonça, V.A.; Lacerda, A.C.R.; Leite, H.R. An update on potential links between type 2 diabetes mellitus and Alzheimer's disease. *Mol. Biol. Rep.* **2020**, *47*, 6347–6356. [CrossRef]
22. Polman, J.A.E.; Welten, J.E.; Bosch, D.S.; De Jonge, R.T.; Balog, J.; Van Der Maarel, S.M.; De Kloet, E.R.; Datson, N.A. A genome-wide signature of glucocorticoid receptor binding in neuronal PC12 cells. *BMC Neurosci.* **2012**, *13*, 118. [CrossRef] [PubMed]
23. Li, J.; Sun, K.; Muroi, M.; Gao, L.; Chang, Y.; Osada, H.; Xiang, L.; Qi, J. Cucurbitacin B induces neurogenesis in PC12 cells and protects memory in APP/PS1 mice. *J. Cell. Mol. Med.* **2019**, *23*, 6283–6294. [CrossRef]
24. Jozic, I.; Vukelic, S.; Stojadinovic, O.; Liang, L.; Ramirez, H.A.; Pastar, I.; Canic, M.T. Stress Signals, Mediated by Membranous Glucocorticoid Receptor, Activate PLC/PKC/GSK-3β/β-catenin Pathway to Inhibit Wound Closure. *J. Investig. Dermatol.* **2017**, *137*, 1144–1154. [CrossRef] [PubMed]
25. Webster, N.J.G.; Park, K.; Pirrung, M.C. Signaling Effects of Demethylasterriquinone B1, a Selective Insulin Receptor Modulator. *ChemBioChem* **2003**, *4*, 379–385. [CrossRef]
26. Rottenberg, H.; Hoek, J.B. The Mitochondrial Permeability Transition: Nexus of Aging, Disease and Longevity. *Cells* **2021**, *10*, 79. [CrossRef]
27. Sun, Y.; Lin, Y.; Cao, X.; Xiang, L.; Qi, J. Sterols from Mytilidae Show Anti-Aging and Neuroprotective Effects via Anti-Oxidative Activity. *Int. J. Mol. Sci.* **2014**, *15*, 21660–21673. [CrossRef] [PubMed]
28. Farooq, U.; Pan, Y.; Disasa, D.; Qi, J. Novel Anti-Aging Benzoquinone Derivatives from *Onosma bracteatum* Wall. *Molecules* **2019**, *24*, 1428. [CrossRef]
29. Cao, X.; Sun, Y.; Lin, Y.; Pan, Y.; Farooq, U.; Xiang, L.; Qi, J. Antiaging of Cucurbitane Glycosides from Fruits of *Momordica charantia* L. *Oxidative Med. Cell. Longev.* **2018**, *2018*, 1–10. [CrossRef]
30. Xiang, L.; Sun, K.; Lu, J.; Weng, Y.; Taoka, A.; Sakagami, Y.; Qi, J. Anti-Aging Effects of Phloridzin, an Apple Polyphenol, on Yeast via the SOD and Sir2 Genes. *Biosci. Biotechnol. Biochem.* **2011**, *75*, 854–858. [CrossRef]
31. Lin, Y.; Kotakeyama, Y.; Li, J.; Pan, Y.; Matsuura, A.; Ohya, Y.; Yoshida, M.; Xiang, L.; Qi, J. Cucurbitacin B Exerts Antiaging Effects in Yeast by Regulating Autophagy and Oxidative Stress. *Oxidative Med. Cell. Longev.* **2019**, *2019*, 15. [CrossRef]
32. Danese, S.; Fiocchi, C.; Panés, J. Drug development in IBD: From novel target identification to early clinical trials. *Gut* **2016**, *65*, 1233–1239. [CrossRef] [PubMed]
33. Zhao, C.; Zhao, C.; Zhao, H. Defective insulin receptor signaling in patients with gestational diabetes is related to dysregulated miR-140 which can be improved by naringenin. *Int. J. Biochem. Cell Biol.* **2020**, *128*, 105824. [CrossRef] [PubMed]
34. Rhen, T.; Cidlowski, J.A. Antiinflammatory Action of Glucocorticoids—New Mechanisms for Old Drugs. *N. Engl. J. Med.* **2005**, *353*, 1711–1723. [CrossRef] [PubMed]

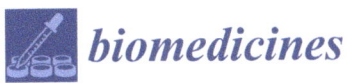 

Article

# Brain-Specific Gene Expression and Quantitative Traits Association Analysis for Mild Cognitive Impairment

Shao-Xun Yuan, Hai-Tao Li, Yu Gu and Xiao Sun *

State Key Laboratory of Bioelectronics, School of Biological Science and Medical Engineering, Southeast University, Nanjing 210096, China; 230159460@seu.edu.cn (S.-X.Y.); 230169443@seu.edu.cn (H.-T.L.); 230198583@seu.edu.cn (Y.G.)
* Correspondence: xsun@seu.edu.cn

**Abstract:** Transcriptome–wide association studies (TWAS) have identified several genes that are associated with qualitative traits. In this work, we performed TWAS using quantitative traits and predicted gene expressions in six brain subcortical structures in 286 mild cognitive impairment (MCI) samples from the Alzheimer's Disease Neuroimaging Initiative (ADNI) cohort. The six brain subcortical structures were in the limbic region, basal ganglia region, and cerebellum region. We identified 9, 15, and 6 genes that were stably correlated longitudinally with quantitative traits in these three regions, of which 3, 8, and 6 genes have not been reported in previous Alzheimer's disease (AD) or MCI studies. These genes are potential drug targets for the treatment of early–stage AD. Single–Nucleotide Polymorphism (SNP) analysis results indicated that cis–expression Quantitative Trait Loci (cis–eQTL) SNPs with gene expression predictive abilities may affect the expression of their corresponding genes by specific binding to transcription factors or by modulating promoter and enhancer activities. Further, baseline structure volumes and cis–eQTL SNPs from correlated genes in each region were used to predict the conversion risk of MCI patients. Our results showed that limbic volumes and cis–eQTL SNPs of correlated genes in the limbic region have effective predictive abilities.

**Keywords:** subcortical structure; quantitative trait; longitudinal stably correlated; mild cognitive impairment; conversion

Citation: Yuan, S.-X.; Li, H.-T.; Gu, Y.; Sun, X. Brain-Specific Gene Expression and Quantitative Traits Association Analysis for Mild Cognitive Impairment. *Biomedicines* **2021**, *9*, 658. https://doi.org/10.3390/biomedicines9060658

Academic Editor: Lorenzo Falsetti

Received: 24 May 2021
Accepted: 4 June 2021
Published: 8 June 2021

**Publisher's Note:** MDPI stays neutral with regard to jurisdictional claims in published maps and institutional affiliations.

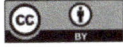

Copyright: © 2021 by the authors. Licensee MDPI, Basel, Switzerland. This article is an open access article distributed under the terms and conditions of the Creative Commons Attribution (CC BY) license (https://creativecommons.org/licenses/by/4.0/).

## 1. Introduction

Alzheimer's disease (AD) is a progressive and irreversible neurodegenerative disorder, accounting for more than 75% of all dementia events worldwide [1]. Approximately 35% of individuals over 80 years of age suffer from AD around the world [2]. Mild Cognitive Impairment (MCI) is the preclinical stage of AD and is clinically heterogeneous [3]. Genome–wide association studies (GWAS) have identified several susceptible single nucleotide polymorphisms (SNPs) for AD [4–7] and MCI [7]. However, GWAS can be used to understand which SNPs are associated with traits but cannot explain how the SNPs affect the traits. SNPs are likely to influence traits by regulating gene expression [8,9]. On the other hand, gene expression may be regulated by causal SNPs but not by the SNP with the lowest p-value within a linkage disequilibrium block.

Transcriptome sequencing can be used to study associations between whole transcription levels and traits in a specific tissue. Howevr, sampling for transcriptome sequencing is costly and difficult. Gusev et al. [10] proposed a new strategy, leveraging expression prediction to perform a transcriptome–wide association study (TWAS) to identify significant trait–expression associations. TWAS first fits tissue–specific models using reference data with both SNP genotype data and gene expression data available. Then, these models are used to predict gene expression in a new dataset with genotype data available. Finally, the predicted gene expression in each tissue is associated with corresponding traits. TWAS has been proved as an effective method to identify gene associations between gene expression and traits in specific tissues [11].

Several TWAS studies have identified multiple novel susceptibility genes for AD by combining Genotype–Tissue Expression Project (GTEx) gene expression models and genotype data of AD. Raj et al. [12] identified 21 genes with significant associations with AD in two cohorts, 8 of which were were novel. Hao et al. [13] combined TWAS and data from the International Genomics of Alzheimer's Project (IGAP) cohort and identified 29 potential disease–causing genes, 21 of which were new. Jung et al. [14] combined tissue specifically predicted gene expression levels and polygenic risk score from 207 AD cases and 239 cognitively normal controls and found that the inclusion of polygenic risk score and gene expression features provided better performance in AD classification. Gerring et al. [15] performed a multi–tissue TWAS of AD and observed associated genes in brain and skin tissue.

The aim of our study was to identify genes potentially related with specific brain structure quantitative traits in MCI samples, reveal possible relationships with biological mechanisms, and use them for conversion analyses. We performed TWAS between predicted gene expression and longitudinal quantitative traits in six brain subcortical structures to identify longitudinally stable correlated genes for MCI. First, gene expression prediction models provided by GTEx [16] were used to predict gene expression in amygdala, hippocampus, accumbens area, caudate, putamen, and cerebellum using 286 MCI samples from the Alzheimer's Disease Neuroimaging Initiative (ADNI) cohort. Second, the expression of genes in the above six structures was correlated with baseline and 12–month follow–up quantitative traits in the corresponding structures. Overlapping genes in baseline and 12–month follow–up were considered as longitudinally stable correlated genes in each structure. Third, fine–mapping analyses were performed on these longitudinally stable correlated genes and corresponding cis–eQTL SNPs to identify the potential regulation mechanisms. Finally, we further investigated the potentials of baseline quantitative traits and gene expression–determined cis–eQTL SNPs of longitudinally stable correlated genes for conversion analysis of MCI samples.

## 2. Materials and Methods

Data used in the preparation of this article were obtained from the ADNI database (adni.loni.usc.edu). ADNI was launched in 2003 as a public–private partnership, led by the Principal Investigator Michael W. Weiner, MD. The primary goal of ADNI is to test whether findings from serial magnetic resonance imaging (MRI), positron emission tomography (PET), other biological markers, and clinical and neuropsychological assessment can be combined to measure the progression of MCI and early AD.

### 2.1. Ethics Statement

We used the ADNI subject data collected from 50 clinic sites. The ADNI study was conducted according to Good Clinical Practice guidelines, US 21CFR Part 50—Protection of Human Subjects, and Part 56—Institutional Review Boards (IRBs)/Research Ethics Boards (REBs)—and pursuant to state and federal HIPAA regulations. Written informed consent was obtained from all participants after they had received a complete description before protocol–specific procedures were carried out based on the 1975 Declaration of Helsinki. IRBs were constituted according to applicable State and Federal requirements for each participating location. The protocols were submitted to appropriate Boards, and their written unconditional approval obtained and submitted to Regulatory Affairs at the Alzheimer's disease Neuroimaging Initiative Coordinating Center (ADNICC) prior to commencement of the study. We have obtained permission to use data from ADNI, and the approval date is 25 November 2019.

### 2.2. Samples

A total of 819 samples of European ancestry were recruited by the ADNI cohort, and 757 of them were run on the Human610–Quad BeadChip (Illumina Inc., San Diego, CA, USA) for genotyping. Among these 757 samples, 286 MCI samples were MPRAGE N3–Scaled sMRI data available at both baseline and 12–month follow-up. MRI images marked with "N3" and "scaled" in the file name were downloaded from the ADNI dataset; these files underwent B1 bias field correction and N3 intensity nonuniformity correction [17]. The following information was also collected from the the ADNI dataset for 286 selected samples: gender, age, education years, Clinical Dementia Rating Sum of Boxes (CDR-SB) score, Mini–Mental State Examination (MMSE) score, Functional Assessment Questionnaire (FAQ) and Alzheimer Disease Assessment Scale scores (ADAS, version 11, 13 and Q4).

*2.3. Genotype and Image Data Pre–Processing*

PLINK 1.9 software [18] (Boston, MA, USA) was used for quality control of genotype data for 286 MCI samples. SNPs with a call rate smaller than 90%, Minor Allele Frequency (MAF) smaller than 10%, or deviations from the Hardy–Weinberg Equilibrium ($5 \times 10^{-7}$) were removed from the original genotype data. After quality control, imputation was performed using impute2 software [19]. After quality control and imputation, 28,571,732 SNPs were retained from the 286 MCI samples.

Freesurfer 6.0 software (Boston, MA, USA) was applied for automated segmentation and volume measurement of subcortical structures and total intracranial volume (ICV) for all selected MCI samples from MRI image data at baseline and 12–month follow-up. Left and right volumes from the same structure were summed. Adjustments were performed for subcortical structure volumes using gender, age, and ICV, using the following formulas:

$$QT = a * AGE + b * GENDER + c * ICV + d \quad (1)$$

$$QT_{adj} = a * AGE_{mean} + b * GENDER_{mean} + c * ICV_{mean} + d + r \quad (2)$$

$QT$ and $QT_{adj}$ represent raw quantitative trait volumes extracted using Freesurfer and adjusted quantitative trait volumes of a subcortical structure across the 286 MCI samples. *AGE*, *GENDER*, and *ICV* represent age, gender, and ICV of all MCI samples, while $AGE_{mean}$, $GENDER_{mean}$, and $ICV_{mean}$ represent mean age, mean gender, and mean ICV across all MCI samples; *d* represents error, while *r* represents residual. We first calculated coefficients of age (*a*), gender (*b*), and ICV (*c*) from a mixed linear regression model (Equation (1)). Then, adjusted volumes were calculated using Equation (2). Adjusted volumes of each subcortical structure were used as quantitative traits.

*2.4. Correspondences among GTEx Models, Anatomical Regions, and Freesurfer–Defined Structures*

We defined correspondences the GTEx models, anatomical regions, and freesurfer-defined structures. The PredictDB Data Repository provides 49 gene–predicted models based on GTEx data (www.gtexportal.org, accessed on 5 September 2020), of which 13 are brain–related gene expression predictive models. Freesurfer software provides 35 brain subcortical structures according to the Desikan–Killiany (DK) atlas template. In our study, 6 one–to–one corresponding gene expression predictive model–subcortical structure pairs were selected and assigned to three regions (Table 1).

**Table 1.** Corresponence of GTEx models, anatomical regions, and subcortical structures.

| GTEx Model | Region | Subcortical Structures |
|---|---|---|
| Brain Amygdala | Limbic | Amygdala |
| Brain Hippocampus | | Hippocampus |
| Brain Caudate basal ganglia | Basal Ganglia | Caudate |
| Brain Putamen basal ganglia | | Putamen |
| Brain Nucleus accumbens basal ganglia | | Accumbens area |
| Brain Cerebellum | Cerebellum | Cerebellum cortex |

GTEx models were downloaded from http://predictdb.org/ (accessed on 5 September 2020); Subcortical structures were segmented by Freesurfer software according to the Desikan-Killiany (DK) atlas template.

## 2.5. Correlation between Predictive Gene Expression and Quantitative Traits

We utilized the PrediXcan software to predict gene expression based on the genotype data of all MCI samples. PrediXcan establishes a linear prediction model of gene expression in a dataset with both SNP genotype data and gene expression available (GTEx version 8) using a multivariate adaptive shrinkage regression (mashr) approach. Brain–specific gene expressions in 6 structures were predicted by combined prediction models and MCI genotype data. Brain–specific gene expression was determined by corresponding cis–eQTL SNPs from the LD reference files for the corresponding model in PredictDB Data Repository (http://predictdb.org/) (accessed on 5 September 2020).

We annotated the chromosomal locations of cis–eQTL SNPs in the corresponding genes using SNPnexus database [20] (accessed on 15 May 2021). Regulatory information for cis–eQTL SNPs were annotated using HaploReg database [21] (accessed on 15 May 2021) and RegulomeDB database [22] (accessed on 15 May 2021). HaploReg is a web–based tool for annotating SNPs, including chromosome number, protein binding, motif change. RegulomeDB can be used to predict whether an SNP affects transcription factor binding and gene expression. RegulomeDB provides a rank score of SNP, with a low score representing strong evidence of regulatory function. We used VARAdb database [23] to annotate the location of cis–eQTL SNPs in promoter or enhancer regions of corresponding genes (accessed on 15 May 2021). VARAdb determines promoters based on the basic gene annotation file release 33 from GENCODE (2 kb upstream of transcription start site) and determines super enhancers from 542 H3K27ac ChIP–seq samples from the human super–enhancer database [24].

Pearson correlation coefficients were used to calculate correlations between predicted gene expression and adjusted subcortical structure volumes in Table 1. The correlation matrix heatmaps were constructed using the *pheatmap* package (version 1.0.12) in R.

## 2.6. Conversion Analysis Based on Quantitative Traits and SNPs

The performances of quantitative traits and cis–eQTL SNPs were further evaluated in terms of their ability to determine the "time to progression" from MCI to AD via Kaplan–Meier analysis. For this evaluation of MCI samples in the ADNI dataset, the midpoint between the first follow–up with an AD diagnosis and the last follow–up without an AD diagnosis was considered as the conversion time point for MCI samples. The longest follow–up time was collected for samples who did not convert to AD, and these samples were regarded as non–conversion MCI samples [25]. First, quantitative trait volumes or genotypes of cis–eQTL SNPs were used as feature vectors to represent MCI samples and to calculate distances across all MCI samples through Euclidean distance. Hierarchical clustering was completed using stats package in R to cluster MCI samples into two subgroups. Then, we applied the "survfit" function in the *survival* package (version 3.2-7) in R and plotted Kaplan–Meier curves for the two subgroups. The median conversion time of MCI samples in the two subgroups was calculated; the group with a high medium time was regarded as a low–risk group, while the group with a low medium time was regarded as a high–risk group. A log rank test with a $p$-value less than 0.05 was considered statistically significant for median conversion time between risk groups [26].

## 3. Results

### 3.1. Sample Characteristics

The baseline characteristics of 286 MCI samples and their association with AD are shown in Table 2. The samples were obtained from patients with a mean (SD) age of 74.85 (6.97) years; 33.9% were female, 18.5% had less than 12 years of education. In accordance with their MCI diagnosis, the average scores of most neuropsychological tests were in the normal–to–low range. A total of 167 (58.4%) study participants converted to probable AD over a mean (SD) follow–up period of 25.05 (21.76) months. Of the 119 who did not convert, 45 had less than 36 months of follow–up data, whereas 71 were followed for more than 36 months. Three samples had only one follow–up visit.

Table 2. Baseline characteristics of 286 MCI samples.

| Characteristic | Number (%) or Mean ± SD |
|---|---|
| Demographic | |
| Age, years | 74.85 ± 6.97 |
| Gender, female | 97 (33.9) |
| Education, ≤12 years | 53 (18.5) |
| Neuropsychological measures | |
| CDRSB | 1.53 ± 0.85 |
| MMSE | 27.04 ± 1.78 |
| FAQ | 3.89 ± 4.49 |
| ADAS11 | 11.66 ± 4.40 |
| ASAS13 | 4.40 ± 6.38 |
| ADASQ4 | 18.91 ± 2.23 |
| Conversion MCI | 167 (58.4) |
| Conversion period | 25.05 ± 21.76 |
| Non–conversion MCI | 119 (41.6) |
| With <3 years of follow–up data | 45 (37.8) |
| With ≥3 years of follow–up data | 71 (59.7) |
| With only 1 follow–up visit | 3 (0.03) |

MCI, Mild Cognitive Impairment; CDRSB, Clinical Dementia Rating Sum of Boxes; MMSE, Mini–Mental State Examination; FAQ, Functional Assessment Questionnaire; ADAS, Alzheimer Disease Assessment Scale scores.

*3.2. Identification of Quantitative Traits–Related Genes*

PrediXcan software was applied to predict gene expression by integrating GTEx gene expression prediction models and ADNI genotype data. Correlations between quantitative traits and predicted gene expressions were computed by Pearson correlation across all selected samples at baseline and 12–month follow-up. The correlation heatmaps for all six structures at baseline and 12–month follow–up are shown in Figure 1. Gene–quantitative traits pairs with a correlation coefficient greater than 0.2 and lower than −0.2 are displayed in the heatmaps. Genes associated with quantitative traits were distinct across all structures at baseline (Figure 1A) and 12–month follow–up (Figure 1B).

We evaluated the overlapping correlated genes at baseline and 12–month follow–up. Table 3 shows overlapping genes associated with structure volumes at baseline and after 12 months across all MCI samples. In the limbic region, 10 and 8 amygdala–specific expressed genes were correlated with baseline and 12–month amygdala volume, while 9 and 10 hippocampal–specific expressed genes were correlated with baseline and 12–month hippocampal volume. Four amygdala–specific expressed genes were overlapping between baseline and 12–month follow–up, while five hippocampal–specific expressed genes were overlapping between baseline and 12–month follow–up. In addition, we identified 15 overlapping genes with basal ganglia structures, including accumbens area, caudate and putamen, and 9 overlapping genes with the cerebellum. We considered these overlapping genes as stably correlated longitudinally with the corresponding quantitative traits. We used GeneCards database to annotate these genes, to define whether they were related to AD or MCI. We found that six, seven, and three genes were related to AD or MCI, while three (*NOXRED1*, *MYL6B*, and *FAM162B*), eight (*RELCH*, *IRX3*, *RELL1*, *TMEM50A*, *SETD4*, *TMEM253*, *HPS3*, *SLC26A10*), and six (*SLC6A16*, *SLC10A5*, *ENSG00000272542*, *LINC00958*, *FCGRT*, *TRPM4*) genes were potentially correlated to AD or MCI in limbic region, basal ganglia region, and cerebellum region, respectively. We summarized the potential biologic mechanisms of all these longitudinally stable correlated genes (Table S1). Genes in the limbic region are involved in energy metabolism, regulation of cell growth, apoptosis, migration and invasion, and synaptic plasticity. Genes in the basal ganglia region are involved in the inflammatory response and signal transduction. Genes in the cerebellum region are involved in signal transduction, material transport, lipid metabolism, neuronal migration, and neuritic plaques.

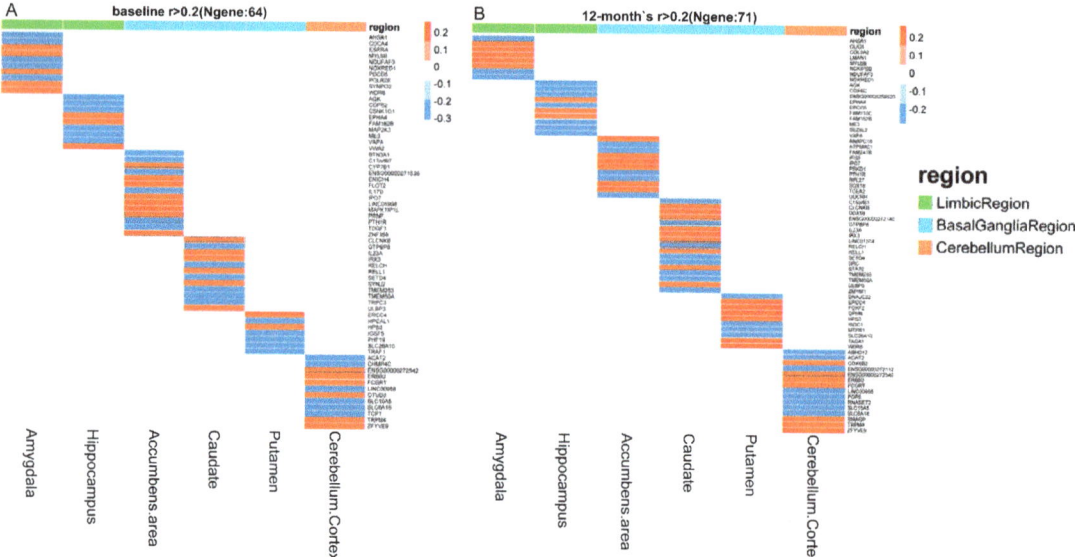

**Figure 1.** Heatmaps of correlations between predicted gene expressions and quantitative traits at baseline (**A**) and 12–month follow−up (**B**). Correlations with coefficient $r$ greater than 0.2 and less than −0.2 are displayed in the heatmaps. The red color represents positive correlations, while the blue color indicates negative correlations in heatmaps. Column annotations represent brain structures for correlation analyses. For annotations, limbic region, basal ganglia region, and cerebellum region are displayed in green, sky blue, and orange, respectively.

*3.3. Fine-Mapping Analyses of Gene Expression-Determined Cis-eQTL SNPs*

We annotated the 56 gene expression–determined cis–eQTL SNPs of all longitudinally stable correlated genes (Table 3) using SNPnexus, HaploReg, RegulomeDB, and VARAdb databases. In this study, 12, 26, and 18 SNPs were found in to 9, 15, and 9 longitudinally stable correlated genes in the limbic region, basal ganglia region, and cerebellum region, respectively. We annotated the locations of these SNPs in the corresponding genes using SNPnexus (Table S2). Among these 56 cis–eQTL SNPs, 54 SNPs (54/56, 96.4%) were in the intronic or untranslated regions of the various transcript isoforms of the genes. According to the annotation from the HaploReg database (Table S3), a total of 49 SNPs (49/56, 87.5%) can affect the corresponding genes through motifs changes, while 25 can affect the corresponding genes through proteins binding (25/56, 44.6%). According to the annotation from RegulomeDB (Table S3), 41 SNPs (41/56, 73.2%) had RegulomeDB rank scores smaller than 4, indicating transcription factor binding and location within a region of DNase hypersensitivity. We used the VARAdb database to annotate whether these cis–eQTL SNPs were located in promoters or enhancers of the corresponding genes. We found that 32 SNPs (32/56, 57.1%) were in the promoters of their corresponding genes (Table S4), while 22 SNPs were located in the forward strand, and 10 in the reverse strand. In addition, 25 SNPs (25/56, 44.6%) were enriched in super enhancers, with the corresponding genes being the closest genes (distance between the gene and the SNP was less than 1000 kb), while 13 SNPs (13/56, 23.2%) were enriched in super enhancers with the corresponding genes being the proximal genes (distance between the gene and the SNP was less than 50 kb) (Table S5). We inferred that cis–eQTL SNPs regulate the expression of the corresponding genes by affecting promoters or enhancers.

**Table 3.** Overlapping quantitative traits-correlated gene sets between baseline and 12-month follow-up in six subcortical structures.

| Structures | N | n | Overlap Genes | SNPs | Ranks | Annotations |
|---|---|---|---|---|---|---|
| **Limbic Region** | | | | | | |
| Amygdala | 10/8 | 4 | NDUFAF3 (−) | rs7100 | 1/1 | MCI |
| | | | NOXRED1 (−) | rs141260780 [a], rs11846861 [a] | 2/3 | - |
| | | | AHSA1 (−) | rs11845345 [a] | 5/4 | AD/MCI |
| | | | MYL6B (+) | rs3809134 [ab] | 9/2 | - |
| Hippocampus | 9/10 | 5 | VAPA (−) | rs4798889 [ab] | 1/5 | AD/MCI |
| | | | ME3 (−) | rs670736 [ab] | 2/1 | MCI |
| | | | AGK (−) | rs7790742 [a], rs7795885 [a] | 3/9 | AD/MCI |
| | | | FAM162B (+) | rs9387433, rs641338 [a] | 6/7 | - |
| | | | EPHA4 (+) | rs149636195 [ab] | 8/3 | AD/MCI |
| **Basal ganglia Region** | | | | | | |
| Accumbens Area | 14/11 | 2 | PTH1R (−) | rs2168442 [ab], rs144645644 [b] | 1/7 | AD/MCI |
| | | | IPO7 (+) | rs75955853 [ab], rs12363308 [b] | 3/1 | AD |
| Caudate | 12/17 | 10 | GTPBP8 (−) | rs114429530 [ab] | 1/1 | AD |
| | | | RELCH (−) | rs3752091 [a], rs9958695 | 2/8 | - |
| | | | IRX3 (+) | rs191251428 [ab] | 4/3 | - |
| | | | CLCNKB (+) | rs75909377 [ab] | 5/5 | MCI |
| | | | IL23A (+) | rs79824801 [ab] | 6/10 | AD/MCI |
| | | | RELL1 (+) | rs3832308, rs4832933 [ab] | 7/7 | - |
| | | | TMEM50A (−) | rs3093586 [b], rs3091243 [b], rs8876 [b] | 8/4 | - |
| | | | SETD4 (−) | rs2835263, rs142847892 [a] | 9/11 | - |
| | | | ULBP3 (+) | rs1537648 [a] | 10/16 | AD |
| | | | TMEM253 (−) | rs10872886 | 11/14 | - |
| Putamen | 7/10 | 3 | ERCC4 (+) | rs6498486 [a], rs3136042 [a], rs1799798 [a] | 1/1 | AD/MCI |
| | | | HPS3 (+) | rs13089410 [a], rs7643410 [a] | 3/4 | - |
| | | | SLC26A10 (−) | rs10747780, rs10437954 | 5/5 | - |
| **Cerebellum Region** | | | | | | |
| Cerebellum Cortex | 12/15 | 9 | SLC6A16 (−) | rs8102658 [a] | 1/1 | - |
| | | | SLC10A5 (−) | rs2955002, rs58379275, rs75348453 | 2/2 | - |
| | | | ACAT2 (−) | rs2025187 [ab] | 3/5 | AD/MCI |
| | | | ZFYVE9 (+) | rs627011 [ab] | 4/4 | MCI |
| | | | ENSG00000272542 (+) | rs1886087, rs9518861, rs9554903 | 5/3 | - |
| | | | ERBB2 (+) | rs2517955 [ab], rs75849983 [ab] | 7/6 | AD/MCI |
| | | | LINC00958 (−) | rs111880988, rs4756736 | 8/15 | - |
| | | | FCGRT (+) | rs2946865 [ab], rs1132990 [b] | 9/13 | - |
| | | | TRPM4 (+) | rs11882563 [ab], rs11083963 [b], rs73048855 | 12/9 | - |

N, number of correlated genes at baseline and 12-month follow-up; n, number of overlapping genes between baseline and 12-month follow-up (positive/negative correlation); Overlapping genes, overlapping genes between baseline and 12-month follow-up; SNPs, gene expression-determined cis-eQTL SNPs; Ranks, ranks of overlapping genes at baseline and 12-month follow-up; Annotations, annotations were performed using https://www.genecards.org/ (accessed on 20 March 2021). The lists of cis-eQTL SNPs of the corresponding genes were download from the LD reference file in PredictDB Data Repository (http://predictdb.org/) (accessed on 5 September 2020); SNPs with superscripts "a" and "b" indicate that these SNPs are in the promoters and enhancers of the corresponding genes, respectively.

To evaluate whether these 56 SNPs were associated with the volume of the corresponding subcortical structures, we performed quantitative traits–based GWAS analysis using SNPs directly, instead of using predicted gene expression (Figure 2). Among five cis–eQTL SNPs for longitudinally stable correlated genes in the amygdala, four SNPs (80.0%) were significantly associated only with amygdala volume at baseline and 12–month follow–up. Among seven cis–eQTL SNPs (71.4%) for longitudinally stable correlated genes in the hippocampus, five SNPs were significantly associated only with hippocampus volume at baseline and 12–month follow–up. In the basal ganglia region and cerebellum region, 58.3% and 71.4% of SNPs were significantly associated only with corresponding quantitative traits (Figures S1 and S2). The results indicated that the correlations between quantitative traits and predicted gene expression were reasonable. On the basis of our results, we speculated that these cis–eQTL SNPs can affect both promoters and enhancers, as well as the binding of transcription factors, which may alter the expression of their target genes.

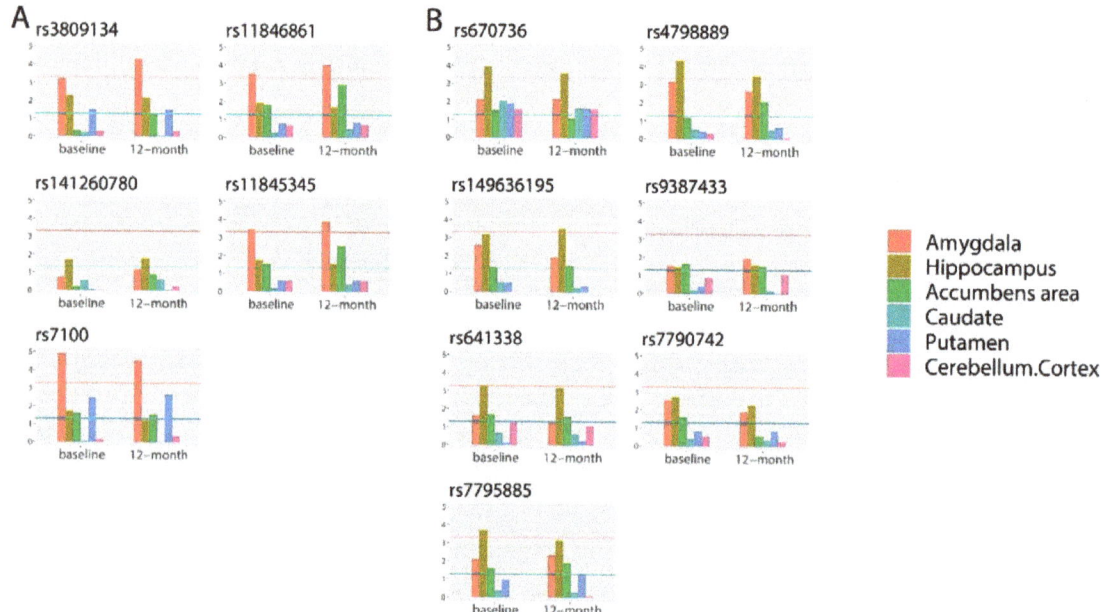

**Figure 2.** Bar plots of associations between 12 SNPs in the limbic region and 6 subcortical structures. (**A**) Five SNPs gene expression-determined SNPs in the amygdala. (**B**) Seven SNPs gene expression-determined SNPs in the hippocampus. The X-axis reports six subcortical structures (amygdala, hippocampus, accumbens area, caudate, putamen, and cerebellum cortex) at baseline and 12-month follow-up. The Y-axis presents the p-value ($-\log 10$) of the association based on quantitative-trait GWAS. The blue horizontal line represents $-\log 10 (0.05)$, while the red horizontal line represents $-\log 10 (5 \times 10^{-4})$.

*3.4. Conversion Analysis Based on Quantitative Traits and SNPs*

We used the baseline volumes of limbic region, basal ganglia region, and cerebellum region as quantitative traits and gene expression–determined cis–eQTL SNPs of longitudinal stably correlated genes in each region to perform a conversion analysis for the MCI samples. First, the MCI samples were clustered into two subgroups using quantitative traits or SNPs. Hierarchical clustering was applied based on the Euclidean distance in the *stats* R package (v4.0.4). Then, we compared the conversion times and performed Kaplan–Meier analyses between the two MCI subgroups. Figure 3 shows the Kaplan–Meier plots for the two groups using quantitative traits and SNPs. The volumes of the structures in the limbic region and cis–eQTL SNPs of longitudinally stable correlated genes in the limbic region showed effective predictive abilities (Figure 3A,B), while this was not true for basal ganglia and cerebellum (Figure 3C–F).

We calculated the percent of conversion and non–conversion of MCI samples in risk groups defined by quantitative traits and SNPs in the limbic region. Chi–square tests were used to determine between–group differences in the conversion and non–conversion of MCI samples. As shown in Figure 4, when using quantitative traits and SNPs, the high–risk groups and low–risk groups had significantly different proportions of conversion and non–

conversion, with the high–risk groups showing significantly higher percentages of conversion than the low–risk groups (quantitative traits, 66.7% vs. 38.2%; SNPs: 64.9% vs. 44.4%).

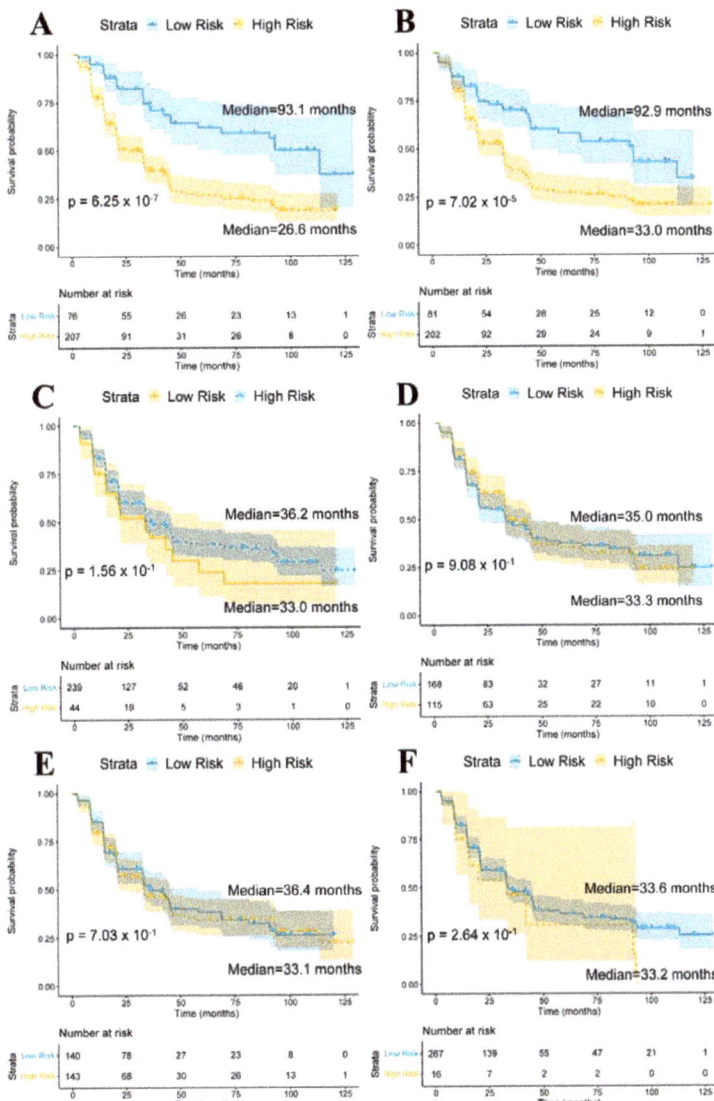

**Figure 3.** Survival curves of the two mild cognitive impairment (MCI) subgroups based on baseline volumes and cis-eQTL SNPs of limbic region (**A**,**B**), basal ganglia (**C**,**D**), cerebellum (**E**,**F**). Confidence intervals are indicated by shaded regions. The blue line represents the low-risk group, while the yellow line represents the-high risk group. Median means the median time (months) of conversion of MCI samples in the two subgroups.

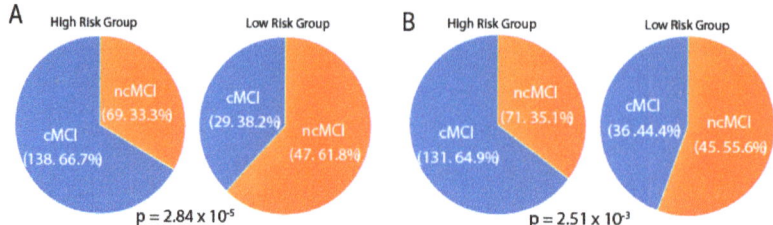

**Figure 4.** Percent of conversion mild cognitive impairment (MCI) (cMCI) and non-conversion MCI (ncMCI) samples in the high-risk group and low-risk group using quantitative traits (**A**) and SNPs derived from longitudinally stable correlated genes (**B**) in the limbic region. P, *p*-value of the chi-square test.

## 4. Discussion

In this study, we performed transcriptome–wide association analyses between gene expressions and longitudinal quantitative traits in specific brain subcortical structures to identify longitudinally stable correlated genes for MCI. Combining gene expression prediction models generated from GTEx data and quantitative traits extracted from T1–MRI data, we identified 9, 15, and 6 genes correlated with limbic region, basal ganglia region, and cerebellum region, of which 3, 8, and 6, respectively, have not been reported in previous studies. We also performed quantitative traits–based GWAS analysis using SNPs. Most SNPs derived from previously correlated genes were directly associated with the corresponding quantitative traits, indicating that those correlations between quantitative traits and predicted gene expressions were reasonable. Furthermore, quantitative traits and gene expression–determined cis–eQTL SNPs of longitudinally stable correlated genes were used for conversion analysis of the MCI samples. We found that limbic region structure volumes and cis–eQTL SNPs derived from longitudinally stable correlated genes in the limbic region showed effective conversion predictive ability.

Several studies performed transcriptome–wide association analyses using qualitative traits in Alzheimer's disease. To our knowledge, this is the first research using quantitative traits in transcriptome–wide association analyses. We found that genes associated with quantitative traits of different brain structures were specific. In the limbic region, we found nine longitudinally stable correlated genes, including four for amygdala volume and five for hippocampus volume. Within these nine genes, six genes have been reported to be associated with AD or MCI based on GeneCards. For example, we found that the expression of *EPHA4* was positively correlated with hippocampus volume in baseline and 12–month follow–up. Gene expression of *EPHA4* was predicted by rs149636195 in a hippocampal predictive model. Rs149636195 is located in the 5′–untranslated region of *EPHA4* and regulates *EPHA4* expression by modulating promoter activity and enhancer activity in the hippocampus [21]. A low level of EphA4 is likely to lead to synaptic dysfunction in early AD [27], EphA4 is responsible for amyloid β–protein production regulation, and *EPHA4* mRNA levels were significantly reduced in AD brains [28]. We speculate that rs149636195 is an eQTL of *EPHA4*, and the low expression of *EPHA4* results in a decrease in hippocampal volume, which may cause synaptic dysfunction in MCI. Additionally, we identified three genes in the limbic region which have not been reported in previous AD/MCI studies, including *NOXRED1*, *MYL6B*, and *FAM162B*. *NOXRED1* (NADP–Dependent Oxidoreductase Domain–Containing 1 protein) is a key gene in oxidoreductase activity (Gene Ontology: 0016491). Oxidative stress may play a role in neuron degeneration and, thus, in AD. We suspect that *NOXRED1* may influence the pathogenesis of AD/MCI through oxidative stress. *MYL6B* encodes myosin light–chain 6B protein and is a key component of myosin. *MYL6B* contributes to memory consolidation in the amygdala [29,30]. Myosin is essential for synapse remodeling [31]. We suspect that dysregulation of *MYL6B* may affect the integrity and function of myosin, leading to the impairment of synaptic function in the pathogenesis of early–stage AD. *FAM162B* (Family with Sequence Similarity 162 Member B) is a key gene in the membrane (Gene Ontology: 0016020) and an integral component of the membrane (Gene Ontology: 0016021). *FAM162B* plays an important role in endothelial cells in the blood–brain barrier (Lifemap discovery database). We propose that *FAM162B* is important to the maintenance of the blood–brain barrier, which is required for proper synaptic and neuronal functioning. Dysregulation of *FAM162B* may cause a breakdown of the blood–brain barrier, leading to increased susceptibility to AD [32].

We investigated the potential regulation patterns of gene expression–determined cis–eQTL SNPs affecting the expression of the corresponding genes. Due to the fact that gene expression prediction models are based on fine–mapped variants that may occasionally be absent in a typical GWAS and frequently absent in older GWAS [11], we explored the annotations of SNPs for longitudinally stable correlated genes using four databases, including SNPnexus, HaploReg, RegulomeDB, and VARAdb. First, these cis–eQTL SNPs appeared to be related to specific transcription factor binding sites. Transcription factors increase or decrease the transcription levels of genes by binding to super enhancers or promoters in specific DNA regions [33]. Second, we found more that than 57% and more than 44% cis–eQTL SNPs are in the promoters and enhancers of the corresponding genes, respectively. Promoters and enhancers are responsible for the initiation and reinforcement of transcription, respectively. SNPs within enhancers can alter transcription factor binding and alter enhancer–promoter interactions, leading to dysregulation of gene expression and diseases [34], such as AD [35,36]. Based on the above observations, we inferred that gene expression–determined cis–eQTL SNPs can affect the expression of corresponding genes by altering the binding ability of some transcription factors and/or by affecting promoter and enhancer activities. We also verified the possibility of SNPs affecting corresponding gene expression. We performed association analyses using these SNPs and all quantitative traits directly. We found that most SNPs in correlated genes were also correlated to corresponding quantitative traits, indicating that the correlations between quantitative traits and gene expressions were reasonable. SNPs appeared to be associated with quantitative traits by regulating the expression of their corresponding genes.

The identified longitudinally stable correlated genes could be drug candidates for AD or MCI. *EPHA4* encodes a tyrosine protein kinase receptor, and several studies have discussed the therapeutic potential to target EphA4 for AD [37,38]. *AHSA1* encodes an activator of heat shock protein 90 (Hsp90) ATPase. Small–molecule inhibitors of Hsp90 have been successful at ameliorating amyloid beta–protein and tau protein burden in AD [39]. *MYL6B* and *VAPA* have been reported to be related to synapse formation and remodeling [40,41]. The breakdown of synaptic connections can lead to a loss of cognitive ability, and synaptic repair is a disease–modifying strategy for neurodegenerative diseases, such as AD [42]. Mitochondrial dysfunction and oxidative stress are important pathogenetic mechanism of AD [43]. Antioxidants are often used in the clinical treatment of central nervous system diseases, such as AD. Antioxidants could improve mitochondrial energy metabolism, eliminate free radicals, reduce the damage of oxidative stress to the nervous system [44]. Targeted antioxidant drugs for the treatment of AD have been developed, such as idebenone [45]. We identified four genes related to mitochondrial dysfunction and oxidative stress in the limbic region, including *NDUFAF3*, *NOXRED1*, *ME3*, and *AGK*, and these genes may be used as drug targets in early–stage AD. Meanwhile, genes in the basal ganglia region and cerebellum region are related to the inflammatory response, signal transduction, and material transport, and could also be new targets for drug development.

We investigated and compared the potential of baseline quantitative traits and cis–eQTL of longitudinally stable correlated genes in each region in predicting conversion of MCI samples. Structure volumes in the limbic region, basal ganglia region, cerebellum region and corresponding cis–eQTL SNPs in each region were used for conversion analyses. Limbic region structure volumes and 12 SNPs in from longitudinally stable correlated genes in the limbic region showed effective predictive abilities. Our results support previous MRI studies of limbic region volumes in MCI progress prediction and found that SNPs obtained by gene–quantitative trait association also showed conversion prediction value [46–48]. We developed an SNP panel with 12 SNPs that can be used for conversion prediction for MCI patients. Based on conversion analyses using quantitative traits and SNPs, we estimated that about 65% of MCI patients in the high–risk group will convert to AD within the established follow–up in ADNI, compared with about 40% of those in the low–risk group.

## 5. Conclusions

In summary, our study revealed several genes which appeared to be stably correlated longitudinally with brain quantitative traits in the limbic region, basal ganglia region, and cerebellum region. These genes can be used as potential drug targets for the treatment of early–stage AD. Gene expression–determined cis–eQTL SNPs influence the expression of their corresponding genes by affecting transcription factor binding or the activities of promoters and enhancers. Quantitative traits and cis–eQTL SNPs in the limbic region can effectively predict the conversion risk of MCI patients.

**Supplementary Materials:** The following are available online at https://www.mdpi.com/article/10.3390/biomedicines9060658/s1, Table S1: Function Annotations of Selected Correlated Genes, Table S2: Genomic locations of cis-eQTL SNPs, Table S3: Annotations from HaploReg and RegulomeDB database, Table S4: Annotations of promoters of cis-eQTL SNPs, Table S5: Annotations of super enhancers of cis-eQTL SNPs, Figure S1: Bar plots of associations between 26 SNPs in the basal ganglia region and 6 subcortical structures, Figure S2: Bar plots of associations between 14 SNPs in the cerebellum region and 6 subcortical structures.

**Author Contributions:** Conceptualization, S.-X.Y.; methodology, S.-X.Y.; validation, S.-X.Y., H.-T.L. and X.S.; formal analysis, S.-X.Y. and X.S.; investigation, S.-X.Y.; writing—original draft preparation, S.-X.Y. and X.S.; writing—review and editing, S.-X.Y., Y.G. and X.S.; visualization, S.-X.Y.; supervision, X.S.; project administration, X.S.; funding acquisition, X.S. All authors have read and agreed to the published version of the manuscript.

**Funding:** This research was sponsored by the National Natural Science Foundation of China (81830053, 61972084) and the Key Research and Development Program of Jiangsu province (BE2016002-3).

**Institutional Review Board Statement:** This study did not involve patients. The data collection procedures were approved by the institutional review boards of all participating centers to the Alzheimer's Disease Neuroimaging Initiative.

**Informed Consent Statement:** Not applicable for this study. Participating centers to the Alzheimer's Disease Neuroimaging Initiative obtained written informed consent from all participants or their authorized representatives for data collection.

**Data Availability Statement:** Data used in this study are available through the Alzheimer's Disease Neuroimaging Initiative (ADNI) database (http://adni.loni.usc.edu) (accessed on 25 November 2019).

**Acknowledgments:** Data used in the preparation of this paper were obtained from the Alzheimer's Disease Neuroimaging Initiative (ADNI) database (http://www.loni.ucla.edu/ADNI) (accessed on 25 November 2019). As such, investigators within the ADNI contributed to the design and implementation of ADNI and/or provided data but did not participate in the analysis or writing of this report. A complete list of ADNI investigators is available at http://www.loni.ucla.edu/ADNI/Collaboration/ADNI_Auth-orship_list.pdf.

**Conflicts of Interest:** The authors declare no conflict of interest.

## References

1. Van Giau, V.; Bagyinszky, E.; An, S.S.A.; Kim, S. Clinical Genetic Strategies for Early Onset Neurodegenerative Diseases. *Mol. Cell. Toxicol.* **2018**, *14*, 123–142. [CrossRef]
2. Haines, J.L. Alzheimer Disease: Perspectives from Epidemiology and Genetics. *J. Law Med. Ethics* **2018**, *46*, 694–698. [CrossRef] [PubMed]
3. Hughes, T.F.; Snitz, B.E.; Ganguli, M. Should Mild Cognitive Impairment Be Subtyped? *Curr. Opin. Psychiatry* **2011**, *24*, 237–242. [CrossRef] [PubMed]
4. Lambert, J.-C.; Ibrahim-Verbaas, C.A.; Harold, D.; Naj, A.C.; Sims, R.; Bellenguez, C.; Jun, G.; DeStefano, A.L.; Bis, J.C.; Beecham, G.W.; et al. Meta-Analysis of 74,046 Individuals Identifies 11 New Susceptibility Loci for Alzheimer's Disease. *Nat. Genet.* **2013**, *45*, 1452–1458. [CrossRef] [PubMed]

5. Jansen, I.E.; Savage, J.E.; Watanabe, K.; Bryois, J.; Williams, D.M.; Steinberg, S.; Sealock, J.; Karlsson, I.K.; Hägg, S.; Athanasiu, L.; et al. Genome-Wide Meta-Analysis Identifies New Loci and Functional Pathways Influencing Alzheimer's Disease Risk. *Nat. Genet.* **2019**, *51*, 404–413. [CrossRef]
6. Schwartzentruber, J.; Cooper, S.; Liu, J.Z.; Barrio-Hernandez, I.; Bello, E.; Kumasaka, N.; Young, A.M.; Franklin, R.J.; Johnson, T.; Estrada, K.; et al. Genome-Wide Meta-Analysis, Fine-Mapping and Integrative Prioritization Implicate New Alzheimer's Disease Risk Genes. *Nat. Genet.* **2021**, *53*, 392–402. [CrossRef] [PubMed]
7. Shen, L.; Kim, S.; Risacher, S.L.; Nho, K.; Swaminathan, S.; West, J.D.; Foroud, T.; Pankratz, N.; Moore, J.H.; Sloan, C.D.; et al. Whole Genome Association Study of Brain-Wide Imaging Phenotypes for Identifying Quantitative Trait Loci in MCI and AD: A Study of the ADNI Cohort. *NeuroImage* **2010**, *53*, 1051–1063. [CrossRef]
8. Albert, F.W.; Kruglyak, L. The Role of Regulatory Variation in Complex Traits and Disease. *Nat. Rev. Genet.* **2015**, *16*, 197–212. [CrossRef]
9. Lappalainen, T.; Sammeth, M.; Friedländer, M.R.; AC't Hoen, P.; Monlong, J.; Rivas, M.A.; Gonzalez-Porta, M.; Kurbatova, N.; Griebel, T.; Ferreira, P.G.; et al. Transcriptome and Genome Sequencing Uncovers Functional Variation in Humans. *Nature* **2013**, *501*, 506–511. [CrossRef]
10. Gusev, A.; Ko, A.; Shi, H.; Bhatia, G.; Chung, W.; Penninx, B.W.; Jansen, R.; De Geus, E.J.; Boomsma, D.I.; Wright, F.A.; et al. Integrative Approaches for Large-Scale Transcriptome-Wide Association Studies. *Nat. Genet.* **2016**, *48*, 245–252. [CrossRef] [PubMed]
11. Gamazon, E.R.; Wheeler, H.E.; Shah, K.P.; Mozaffari, S.V.; Aquino-Michaels, K.; Carroll, R.J.; Eyler, A.E.; Denny, J.C.; Nicolae, D.L.; Cox, N.J.; et al. A Gene-Based Association Method for Mapping Traits Using Reference Transcriptome Data. *Nat. Genet.* **2015**, *47*, 1091–1098. [CrossRef] [PubMed]
12. Raj, T.; Li, Y.I.; Wong, G.; Humphrey, J.; Wang, M.; Ramdhani, S.; Wang, Y.-C.; Ng, B.; Gupta, I.; Haroutunian, V.; et al. Integrative Transcriptome Analyses of the Aging Brain Implicate Altered Splicing in Alzheimer's Disease Susceptibility. *Nat. Genet.* **2018**, *50*, 1584–1592. [CrossRef] [PubMed]
13. Hao, S.; Wang, R.; Zhang, Y.; Zhan, H. Prediction of Alzheimer's Disease-Associated Genes by Integration of GWAS Summary Data and Expression Data. *Front. Genet.* **2019**, *9*, 653. [CrossRef]
14. Jung, S.-H.; Nho, K.; Kim, D.; Won, H.-H.; Initiative, A.D.N. Genetic Risk Prediction of Late-Onset Alzheimer's Disease Based on Tissue-Specific Transcriptomic Analysis and Polygenic Risk Scores: Genetics/Genetic Factors of Alzheimer's Disease. *Alzheimer's Dement.* **2020**, *16*, e045184. [CrossRef]
15. Gerring, Z.F.; Lupton, M.K.; Edey, D.; Gamazon, E.R.; Derks, E.M. An Analysis of Genetically Regulated Gene Expression across Multiple Tissues Implicates Novel Gene Candidates in Alzheimer's Disease. *Alzheimer's Res. Ther.* **2020**, *12*, 1–10. [CrossRef]
16. GTEx Consortium. Genetic Effects on Gene Expression across Human Tissues. *Nature* **2017**, *550*, 204–213. [CrossRef] [PubMed]
17. Boyes, R.G.; Gunter, J.L.; Frost, C.; Janke, A.L.; Yeatman, T.; Hill, D.L.; Bernstein, M.A.; Thompson, P.M.; Weiner, M.W.; Schuff, N.; et al. Intensity Non-Uniformity Correction Using N3 on 3-T Scanners with Multichannel Phased Array Coils. *Neuroimage* **2008**, *39*, 1752–1762. [CrossRef] [PubMed]
18. Purcell, S.; Neale, B.; Todd-Brown, K.; Thomas, L.; Ferreira, M.A.; Bender, D.; Maller, J.; Sklar, P.; de Bakker, P.I.; Daly, M.J.; et al. PLINK: A Tool Set for Whole-Genome Association and Population-Based Linkage Analyses. *Am. J. Hum. Genet.* **2007**, *81*, 559–575. [CrossRef] [PubMed]
19. Howie, B.N.; Donnelly, P.; Marchini, J. A Flexible and Accurate Genotype Imputation Method for the next Generation of Genome-Wide Association Studies. *PLoS Genet.* **2009**, *5*, e1000529. [CrossRef] [PubMed]
20. Dayem Ullah, A.Z.; Lemoine, N.R.; Chelala, C. SNPnexus: A Web Server for Functional Annotation of Novel and Publicly Known Genetic Variants (2012 Update). *Nucleic Acids Res.* **2012**, *40*, W65–W70. [CrossRef]
21. Ward, L.D.; Kellis, M. HaploReg: A Resource for Exploring Chromatin States, Conservation, and Regulatory Motif Alterations within Sets of Genetically Linked Variants. *Nucleic Acids Res.* **2012**, *40*, D930–D934. [CrossRef]
22. Boyle, A.P.; Hong, E.L.; Hariharan, M.; Cheng, Y.; Schaub, M.A.; Kasowski, M.; Karczewski, K.J.; Park, J.; Hitz, B.C.; Weng, S.; et al. Annotation of Functional Variation in Personal Genomes Using RegulomeDB. *Genome Res.* **2012**, *22*, 1790–1797. [CrossRef]
23. Pan, Q.; Liu, Y.-J.; Bai, X.-F.; Han, X.-L.; Jiang, Y.; Ai, B.; Shi, S.-S.; Wang, F.; Xu, M.-C.; Wang, Y.-Z.; et al. VARAdb: A Comprehensive Variation Annotation Database for Human. *Nucleic Acids Res.* **2021**, *49*, D1431–D1444. [CrossRef]
24. Jiang, Y.; Qian, F.; Bai, X.; Liu, Y.; Wang, Q.; Ai, B.; Han, X.; Shi, S.; Zhang, J.; Li, X.; et al. SEdb: A Comprehensive Human Super-Enhancer Database. *Nucleic Acids Res.* **2019**, *47*, D235–D243. [CrossRef]
25. Barnes, D.E.; Cenzer, I.S.; Yaffe, K.; Ritchie, C.S.; Lee, S.J.; Alzheimer's Disease Neuroimaging Initiative. A Point-Based Tool to Predict Conversion from Mild Cognitive Impairment to Probable Alzheimer's Disease. *Alzheimer's Dement.* **2014**, *10*, 646–655. [CrossRef] [PubMed]
26. Liu, G.-M.; Zeng, H.-D.; Zhang, C.-Y.; Xu, J.-W. Identification of a Six-Gene Signature Predicting Overall Survival for Hepatocellular Carcinoma. *Cancer Cell Int.* **2019**, *19*, 1–13. [CrossRef] [PubMed]
27. Rosenberger, A.F.; Rozemuller, A.J.; van der Flier, W.M.; Scheltens, P.; van der Vies, S.M.; Hoozemans, J.J. Altered Distribution of the EphA4 Kinase in Hippocampal Brain Tissue of Patients with Alzheimer's Disease Correlates with Pathology. *Acta Neuropathol. Commun.* **2014**, *2*, 1–13. [CrossRef]
28. Tamura, K.; Chiu, Y.-W.; Shiohara, A.; Hori, Y.; Tomita, T. EphA4 Regulates Aβ Production via BACE1 Expression in Neurons. *FASEB J.* **2020**, *34*, 16383–16396. [CrossRef]

29. Gavin, C.F.; Rubio, M.D.; Young, E.; Miller, C.; Rumbaugh, G. Myosin II Motor Activity in the Lateral Amygdala Is Required for Fear Memory Consolidation. *Learn. Mem.* **2012**, *19*, 9–14. [CrossRef] [PubMed]
30. Lamprecht, R.; Margulies, D.; Farb, C.; Hou, M.; Johnson, L.; LeDoux, J. Myosin Light Chain Kinase Regulates Synaptic Plasticity and Fear Learning in the Lateral Amygdala. *Neuroscience* **2006**, *139*, 821–829. [CrossRef]
31. Kneussel, M.; Wagner, W. Myosin Motors at Neuronal Synapses: Drivers of Membrane Transport and Actin Dynamics. *Nat. Rev. Neurosci.* **2013**, *14*, 233–247. [CrossRef]
32. Ishii, M.; Iadecola, C. *Risk Factor for Alzheimer's Disease Breaks the Blood–Brain Barrier*; Nature Publishing Group: Berlin, Germany, 2020.
33. Gill, G. Regulation of the Initiation of Eukaryotic Transcription. *Essays Biochem.* **2001**, *37*, 33–44. [PubMed]
34. Khurana, E.; Fu, Y.; Chakravarty, D.; Demichelis, F.; Rubin, M.A.; Gerstein, M. Role of Non-Coding Sequence Variants in Cancer. *Nat. Rev. Genet.* **2016**, *17*, 93–108. [CrossRef]
35. Kikuchi, M.; Hara, N.; Hasegawa, M.; Miyashita, A.; Kuwano, R.; Ikeuchi, T.; Nakaya, A. Enhancer Variants Associated with Alzheimer's Disease Affect Gene Expression via Chromatin Looping. *BMC Med. Genom.* **2019**, *12*, 128. [CrossRef] [PubMed]
36. Choi, K.Y.; Lee, J.J.; Gunasekaran, T.I.; Kang, S.; Lee, W.; Jeong, J.; Lim, H.J.; Zhang, X.; Zhu, C.; Won, S.-Y.; et al. *APOE* Promoter Polymorphism-219T/G Is an Effect Modifier of the Influence of APOE E4 on Alzheimer's Disease Risk in a Multiracial Sample. *J. Clin. Med.* **2019**, *8*, 1236. [CrossRef] [PubMed]
37. Fu, A.K.; Hung, K.-W.; Huang, H.; Gu, S.; Shen, Y.; Cheng, E.Y.; Ip, F.C.; Huang, X.; Fu, W.-Y.; Ip, N.Y. Blockade of EphA4 Signaling Ameliorates Hippocampal Synaptic Dysfunctions in Mouse Models of Alzheimer's Disease. *Proc. Natl. Acad. Sci. USA* **2014**, *111*, 9959–9964. [CrossRef] [PubMed]
38. Vargas, L.; Cerpa, W.; Muñoz, F.; Zanlungo, S.; Alvarez, A. Amyloid-β Oligomers Synaptotoxicity: The Emerging Role of EphA4/c-Abl Signaling in Alzheimer's Disease. *Biochim. Biophys. Acta Mol. Basis Dis.* **2018**, *1864*, 1148–1159. [CrossRef]
39. Blair, L.J.; Sabbagh, J.J.; Dickey, C.A. Targeting Hsp90 and Its Co-Chaperones to Treat Alzheimer's Disease. *Expert Opin. Ther. Targets* **2014**, *18*, 1219–1232. [CrossRef]
40. Rudolf, R.; Bittins, C.M.; Gerdes, H.-H. The Role of Myosin V in Exocytosis and Synaptic Plasticity. *J. Neurochem.* **2011**, *116*, 177–191. [CrossRef]
41. Matteoli, M.; Coco, S.; Schenk, U.; Verderio, C. Vesicle Turnover in Developing Neurons: How to Build a Presynaptic Terminal. *Trends Cell Biol.* **2004**, *14*, 133–140. [CrossRef]
42. Lu, B.; Nagappan, G.; Guan, X.; Nathan, P.J.; Wren, P. BDNF-Based Synaptic Repair as a Disease-Modifying Strategy for Neurodegenerative Diseases. *Nat. Rev. Neurosci.* **2013**, *14*, 401–416. [CrossRef]
43. Butterfield, D.A.; Halliwell, B. Oxidative Stress, Dysfunctional Glucose Metabolism and Alzheimer Disease. *Nat. Rev. Neurosci.* **2019**, *20*, 148–160. [CrossRef]
44. Rottkamp, C.A.; Nunomura, A.; Raina, A.K.; Sayre, L.M.; Perry, G.; Smith, M.A. Oxidative Stress, Antioxidants, and Alzheimer Disease. *Alzheimer Dis. Assoc. Disord.* **2000**, *14*, S62–S66. [CrossRef]
45. Parkinson, M.H.; Schulz, J.B.; Giunti, P. Co-Enzyme Q10 and Idebenone Use in Friedreich's Ataxia. *J. Neurochem.* **2013**, *126*, 125–141. [CrossRef]
46. Qian, L.; Liu, R.; Qin, R.; Zhao, H.; Xu, Y. The Associated Volumes of Sub-Cortical Structures and Cognitive Domain in Patients of Mild Cognitive Impairment. *J. Clin. Neurosci.* **2018**, *56*, 56–62. [CrossRef] [PubMed]
47. Xu, L.; Wu, X.; Li, R.; Chen, K.; Long, Z.; Zhang, J.; Guo, X.; Yao, L. Prediction of Progressive Mild Cognitive Impairment by Multi-Modal Neuroimaging Biomarkers. *J. Alzheimer's Dis.* **2016**, *51*, 1045–1056. [CrossRef] [PubMed]
48. Yi, H.-A.; Möller, C.; Dieleman, N.; Bouwman, F.H.; Barkhof, F.; Scheltens, P.; van der Flier, W.M.; Vrenken, H. Relation between Subcortical Grey Matter Atrophy and Conversion from Mild Cognitive Impairment to Alzheimer's Disease. *J. Neurol. Neurosurg. Psychiatry* **2016**, *87*, 425–432. [CrossRef] [PubMed]

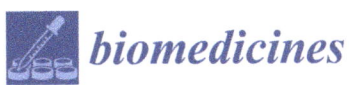 

Article

# Increased YKL-40 but Not C-Reactive Protein Levels in Patients with Alzheimer's Disease

Víctor Antonio Blanco-Palmero [1,2,3,†], Marcos Rubio-Fernández [1,2,†], Desireé Antequera [1,2], Alberto Villarejo-Galende [1,2,3], José Antonio Molina [1,2,3], Isidro Ferrer [1,4,5,6], Fernando Bartolome [1,2,*] and Eva Carro [1,2,*]

1. Network Center for Biomedical Research in Neurodegenerative Diseases (CIBERNED), 28031 Madrid, Spain; victorb1989@gmail.com (V.A.B.-P.); marcosrubio.imas12@h12o.es (M.R.-F.); eeara@yahoo.es (D.A.); avgalende@yahoo.es (A.V.-G.); cvillaiza@telefonica.net (J.A.M.); 8082ifa@gmail.com (I.F.)
2. Group of Neurodegenerative Diseases, Hospital 12 de Octubre Research Institute (imas12), 28041 Madrid, Spain
3. Neurology Service Hospital Universitario 12 de Octubre, 28041 Madrid, Spain
4. Bellvitge Biomedical Research Institute (IDIBELL), Hospitalet de Llobregat, E08907 Barcelona, Spain
5. Department of Pathology and Experimental Therapeutics, University of Barcelona, E08900 Barcelona, Spain
6. Institute of Neurosciences, University of Barcelona, E08000 Barcelona, Spain
* Correspondence: fbartolome.imas12@h12o.es (F.B.); carroeva@h12o.es (E.C.); Tel.: +34-913908765 (F.B. & E.C.); Fax: +34-913908544 (F.B. & E.C.)
† These authors contributed equally to this work.

**Abstract:** Neuroinflammation is a common feature in Alzheimer's (AD) and Parkinson's (PD) disease. In the last few decades, a testable hypothesis was proposed that protein-unfolding events might occur due to neuroinflammatory cascades involving alterations in the crosstalk between glial cells and neurons. Here, we tried to clarify the pattern of two of the most promising biomarkers of neuroinflammation in cerebrospinal fluid (CSF) in AD and PD. This study included cognitively unimpaired elderly patients, patients with mild cognitive impairment, patients with AD dementia, and patients with PD. CSF samples were analyzed for YKL-40 and C-reactive protein (CRP). We found that CSF YKL-40 levels were significantly increased only in dementia stages of AD. Additionally, increased YKL-40 levels were found in the cerebral orbitofrontal cortex from AD patients in agreement with augmented astrogliosis. Our study confirms that these biomarkers of neuroinflammation are differently detected in CSF from AD and PD patients.

**Keywords:** Alzheimer's disease; Parkinson's disease; YKL-40; C-reactive protein; CSF and plasma biomarkers; inflammation; astrogliosis

## 1. Introduction

Neuroinflammation is now widely accepted as a pathological hallmark of Alzheimer's (AD) [1,2] and Parkinson's (PD) [3–5] disease. Several damage signals appear to induce neuroinflammation, including β-amyloid (Aβ) oligomers, tau, and α-synuclein (α-syn), mediated by the progressive astrocyte and microglial cell activation with the consequent overproduction of proinflammatory agents that may leak toward cerebrospinal fluid (CSF) [6]. Despite the analysis of these agents in CSF being a tempting topic to study, levels of inflammatory markers in CSF from AD and PD patients have not been sufficiently investigated. A standard clinical application of inflammatory markers in the clinical diagnosis of these neurodegenerative disorders is lacking, likely owing to contradictory and heterogeneous findings of numerous studies [7,8].

Among these neuroinflammatory markers found in biological samples is YKL-40 (also named Chitinase 3-like I). This marker has been largely associated with the pathogenesis of a variety of human diseases, many of them sharing chronic inflammatory features and high cellular activity, including rheumatoid arthritis, hepatic fibrosis, and asthma,

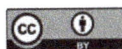

where YKL-40 levels were found elevated in patient peripheral blood [9–11]. YKL-40 is a secreted glycoprotein with functions including tissue remodeling during inflammation and angiogenic processes, which make YKL-40 a good marker of inflammation and endothelial dysfunction [12–14]. YKL-40 was found elevated in CSF from several acute and chronic neuroinflammatory conditions [15], as well as in preclinical and prodromal AD/mild cognitive impairment (MCI) [16–18]. This is consistent with the potential role of astrocytosis in early AD pathogenesis [19] and with the fact that YKL-40 expression and YKL-40 protein levels are abundant in reactive astrocytes and residual in microglial cells [15,20,21]. Additionally, YKL-40 was found close to amyloid plaques and neurofibrillary tangles in AD [16]. Contrarily, other works reported different results showing no significant differences in YKL-40 levels in CSF from MCI and AD patients compared with cognitively normal subjects [22]. Other works indicated increased CSF YKL-40 levels only in AD but not in MCI subjects compared with healthy controls [23,24]. Regarding PD, YKL-40 concentrations in CSF were found either decreased or unchanged [25,26].

Although YKL-40 can be considered one of the most promising neuroinflammatory biomarkers in AD, the abovementioned works indicate that brain YKL-40 levels patterns in different neurodegenerative diseases and the potential correlation between brain and CSF levels is largely unknown, indicating that more research regarding YKL-40 expression pattern is required.

On the other hand, C-reactive protein (CRP), a kind of acute-phase protein regulated by proinflammatory cytokines, is the most studied biomarker of systemic inflammation [27]. CRP was linked to chronic inflammatory and neurodegenerative diseases, such as AD and PD [28]. Elevated CRP peripheral blood levels have been frequently associated with increased risk of dementia and cognitive decline. Studies carried out investigating the association between markers of inflammation and risk of dementia showed conflicting results. A systematic review and meta-analysis found that elevation of peripheral CRP levels was associated with increased risk of developing dementia [29]. Nevertheless, another meta-analysis found no significant differences in serum CRP levels between patients with AD and healthy subjects [30]. Epidemiological studies have also explored the relationship between CRP levels and AD risk, describing lower CRP levels in CSF from AD patients [31,32]. Regarding PD and CRP levels, results in the literature are still contradictory. A significant increase in blood CRP levels was reported in subjects suffering from PD compared with healthy controls [33,34], while other works did not identify such a tendency, instead reporting no differences [35]. Furthermore, the CRP levels in CSF remained unchanged in PD patients when compared with healthy subjects [26,32]. Despite these differences, CRP is considered a prominent "risk factor" for PD [36].

Growing evidence indicates that blood-borne CRP can cross the blood–brain and blood–spinal cord barriers; thus, CRP can be found in the CSF and deposited in the diseased central nervous system (CNS). The source of CRP might also be local. However, CRP production may occur in multiple CNS-resident cells including neurons, microglia, and astrocytes [37–39]. Regardless of its origin (hepatic versus local), the presence of CRP in the CNS is associated with numerous diseases including AD [40]. CRP levels were also found increased in brain parenchyma tissue after intracerebral hemorrhage [41]. Additionally, large amounts of the protein were present in perihematomal regions and within neurons and glia of patients who died within 12 h of spontaneous intracerebral hemorrhage [41,42].

Despite these accumulative data supporting a role of neuroinflammation, particularly YKL-40 and CRP in AD and PD, there is no definitive evidence reflecting the peripheral (blood) and central (CSF) concentration changes of YKL-40 and CRP in AD and/or PD patients. We think that further research is needed to elucidate the variable pattern of these inflammatory biomarkers in the CSF and blood from AD and PD patients. In this work, we aimed at clarify YKL-40 and CRP concentrations measured in CSF and plasma and to determine their specificity in AD and PD. To address this issue, we analyzed YKL-40 and

CRP levels in CSF and plasma from a well-characterized cohort of patients with MCI, AD, and PD, using sensitive enzyme-linked immunosorbent assays (ELISAs).

## 2. Material and Methods

### 2.1. Human Donors

A total of 123 subjects were included in this study: (1) elderly nondemented subjects without any evidence of any neurodegenerative disease (healthy controls) classified as controls ($n = 37$); (2) MCI due to AD (MCI) patients ($n = 22$); (3) probable mild/moderate–severe sporadic AD patients ($n = 34$); (4) PD patients ($n = 30$). Study participants were enrolled from the Memory Clinic (controls, MCI and AD subjects) and Movement Disorders Unit (PD participants) of Hospital Universitario 12 de Octubre (Madrid, Spain). Subject demographic and clinical characteristics are listed in Table 1.

Table 1. Demographic and clinical data of participants.

|  | Control | PD | MCI | AD Dementia | p Value |
|---|---|---|---|---|---|
| n | 37 | 30 | 22 | 34 | NA |
| Sex (M/F) | 22/15 | 17/13 | 7/15 | 13/21 | ns |
| Age, mean (SD), y | 68.18 (11.2) | 66.39 (9.9) | 69.40 (6.4) | 73.53 (8.9) [a] | <0.05 |
| Age at onset, mean (SD), y | NA | 61.48 (10.7) | 66.53 (6.7) | 70.44 (8.9) [b] | <0.01 |
| Years since onset, mean (SD), y | NA | 3.89 (3.3) | 2.87 (1.3) | 3.09 (1.4) | ns |
| Hoehn & Yahr (1/2/3/4/5) | NA | 11/11/6/2/0 | NA | NA | NA |
| CDR (0.5/1/2/3) | NA | NA | 22/0/0/0 | 0/25/9/0 | NA |
| APOE ε4 carrier, No. (%) | 1 [c,d] | - | 54 | 32.4 | <0.0001 |

AD: Alzheimer's disease; MCI: mild cognitive impairment. PD: Parkinson's disease; n: number; F: female; ns: non-significant; y: year; M: male; SD: standard deviation; NA, not applicable; CDR: Clinical Dementia Rating. p value indicates statistical difference within the cohort1; -: not obtained data; [a] $p < 0.05$ vs PD; [b] $p < 0.01$ vs. PD; [c] $p < 0.0001$ vs. AD; [d] $p < 0.0001$ vs. PD.

All participants were classified using established diagnostic criteria into those with MCI or probable AD dementia [43–45]. Diagnosis was based on detailed clinical assessment, neuropsychological evaluation, and neuroimaging (MRI). Functional impairment was measured via the Clinical Dementia Rating (CDR) score [46]. PD patients were diagnosed following the Movement Disorder Society (MDS) clinical diagnostic criteria [47], and all fulfilled criteria for clinically established PD. PD patients did not refer cognitive complaints and did not exhibit symptoms of dementia. The control group was constituted by cognitively normal individuals aged 50 years or older, without clinical signs of cognitive impairment and without neurological or psychiatric disease history. Exclusion criteria for every participant were concomitant significant cerebrovascular disease and evidence of any neurological, psychiatric, medication, or non-neurological medical comorbidity that could affect cognition or motor function.

Approval of the study was obtained from the Research Ethics Committee of Hospital Universitario 12 de Octubre, and all participants provided written informed consent.

### 2.2. Fluid Sample Collection

CSF samples were collected from all subjects (including healthy patients and MCI, AD, and PD subjects) and processed according to standardized procedures by lumbar puncture in 15 mL sterile polypropylene tubes. Samples were then centrifuged at 3000 rpm at 4 °C for 10 min. Supernatant aliquots were stored at −80 °C into 0.5 mL polypropylene cryogenic tubes with Protease Inhibitor Cocktail (Roche, Basel, Switzerland).

Blood samples were obtained through antecubital vein puncture from patients and healthy subjects. Plasma was isolated from whole blood collected in 7 mL EDTA-2Na tubes. Whole blood was centrifuged at 2000 rpm for 10 min at room temperature. Supernatants were then collected and aliquoted in polypropylene cryogenic tubes with Protease Inhibitor Cocktail (Roche, Basel, Switzerland) and stored at −80 °C.

*2.3. Tissue Samples*

Postmortem cerebral orbitofrontal cortex tissue was obtained from brain donors diagnosed with AD and control individuals. Frozen samples were supplied by the Institute of Neuropathology Brain Bank IDIBELL-Hospital Universitari de Bellvitge (Hospitalet de Llobregat, Spain). Subject consent was obtained according to the Declaration of Helsinki, and approval came from the Research Ethics Committee of the responsible institution. For all cases, written informed consent was available. Subjects were selected on the basis of postmortem diagnosis of AD according to neurofibrillary tangle pathology and Aβ plaques [48]. AD cases showed high AD neuropathologic change (Braak stage V/VI and moderate to frequent neuritic plaque score). Control participants were considered those with/without neurological symptoms or a low grade of AD neuropathologic change. A total of 24 samples were categorized into AD and controls, as presented in Table 2.

**Table 2.** Demographic and clinical data of brain tissue donors.

|  | Control | AD |
| --- | --- | --- |
| n | 12 | 12 |
| Sex (M/F) | 6/6 | 6/6 |
| Age, mean (SD) | 73.25 (8.8) | 76.33 (10.3) |
| Braak stage (n) | None: 7<br>Braak I: 3<br>Braak II: 2 | Braak V: 9<br>Braak VI: 3 |

AD: Alzheimer's disease; n: number; F: female. M: male; SD: standard deviation.

*2.4. DNA Purification and Apolipoprotein E (APOE) Genotyping*

Genomic DNA was extracted from peripheral blood using QIAmp DNA Blood Mini Kit (Qiagen, Hilden, Germany), according to the manufacturer's instructions. Human APOE C112R and R158C polymorphisms were detected to identify the APOE ε2, ε3, and ε4 alleles, using the LightCycler 480 II Instruments Kit (Roche Diagnostics, Basel, Switzerland) following manufacturer instructions.

*2.5. Protein Analysis*

CSF and plasma concentrations of the neuroinflammatory biomarkers (YKL-40 and CRP) were analyzed using ELISA kits (Human Chitinase 3-like 1 Quantikine ELISA kit (DC3L10), R&D; Human CRP Quantikine ELISA kit (DCRP00), R&D) according to the manufacturer's instructions.

Brain YKL-40 and GFAP protein levels were also examined by Western blotting. Postmortem cerebral orbitofrontal cortex tissue was obtained from brain donors diagnosed with AD and control individuals. Briefly, human cerebral orbitofrontal cortex samples were incubated and homogenized in lysis buffer (50 mM Tris/HCl buffer, pH 7.4 containing 2 mM EDTA, 0.2% Nonidet P-40, 1 mM PMSF, Protease and Phosphatase Inhibitor Cocktails; Roche, Basel, Switzerland) and centrifuged for 10 min at 14,000 rpm at 4 °C. Supernatants were recovered and stored at −80 °C. Protein content was determined using the BCA method (Thermo Fisher Scientific, MA, USA). Equal amounts of protein (20 μg for YKL-40 and 5 μg for GFAP) were mixed with Laemmli sample buffer supplemented with β-mercaptoethanol, heated to 95 °C for 5 min, resolved by 10% NuPAGE Bis-Tris Gels (Thermo Fisher Scientific, MA, USA), and transferred onto polyvinylidene difluoride (PVDF) membranes (Millipore, MA, USA). Afterward, membranes were blocked and incubated overnight at 4 °C with primary antibodies: a recombinant rabbit monoclonal anti-YKL-40 antibody (ab255297, 1:500, Abcam) and a mouse monoclonal anti-GFAP antibody (G3893, 1:0000, Sigma Aldrich). Membranes were then incubated for 1 h with the appropriate horseradish peroxidase (HRP)-conjugated secondary antibodies (G-21234, 1:5000, Thermo Fisher Scientific, MA, USA; ab97023, 1:40000, Abcam). Protein loading was monitored using mouse monoclonal HRP-conjugated antibodies against α-tubulin (ab40742, 1:5000, Abcam) for YKL-40 or against β-actin (A1978, Sigma Aldrich) for GFAP detection. Immunocomplexes were revealed by an enhanced chemiluminescence reagent (ECL Clarity; Bio Rad, CA, USA). Densitometric quantification was carried out with Image Studio Lite 5.0 software (Li-COR Biosciences, NE, USA). Protein bands were normalized to loading controls and expressed as a percentage of the control group.

*2.6. Statistical Analysis*

Statistical analysis and graphs were performed using Stata/IC software (Stata 16.1, StataCorp LLC, College Station, TX, USA) and Prism (GraphPad Software version 8.00, La Jolla, CA, USA). After assessing the normality of the distribution, differences in CSF and plasma YKL-40 and CRP levels between groups were analyzed using the nonparametric Kruskal–Wallis rank test. The $p$-value for pairwise comparisons is displayed with Bonferroni correction. A descriptive multiple linear regression model was performed to account for confounding variables (age, sex, and APOE ε4) in CSF YKL-40 association analysis. Interactions of confounding variables with the clinical diagnosis were excluded from the model (significance for the whole set of interactions: $p > 0.10$). The regression coefficient is displayed as "b". Differences in sex distribution, age of participants, age at onset, and years since the onset of the disease between groups were evaluated with Pearson chi-squared and ANOVA tests, where appropriate. Associations between biomarkers and demographic characteristics were examined with Pearson correlation tests, Student $t$-tests and Mann–Whitney U tests, where appropriate. A nonparametric trend test (Jonckheere trend test) was performed to evaluate the existence of a trend when the exposition showed ordinal categories. ROC curves were constructed after modeling the presence or absence of a given clinical diagnosis with a regression logistic analysis. YKL-40 and GFAP Western blot expression levels were normalized to their respective loading controls (α-tubulin and β-actin) and compared with the mean of the control ratio with the nonparametric Mann–Whitney U test. In graphs, CSF and plasma YKL-40 and CRP levels are shown as median and interquartile range. The brain expression of YKL-40 is shown as the mean ± standard error of the mean (SEM). In all cases, statistical significance was set at $p < 0.05$.

## 3. Results

*3.1. Associations with Demographic Data*

Demographic and clinical data are shown in Table 1 for further characterization of the study cohort. A total of 34 subjects were clinically diagnosed with AD, 22 subjects were grouped as MCI, and 30 subjects were diagnosed with PD. Individuals diagnosed with AD were slightly older than the rest of the cohort, including PD, MCI, and healthy subjects. Female sex was overrepresented in the AD and MCI groups, while males represented around 60% of controls and PD subjects. APOE ε4 carriers were more prevalent in the MCI/AD group than in controls, according to previous publications [49]. Most AD patients had clinically mild dementia (74% scored 1 in CDR scale), and none of the PD patients reached the dementia stage. Furthermore, the majority of individuals diagnosed with PD exhibited mild motor impairment (73% of them were in Hoehn & Yahr stage 1 or 2).

*3.2. YKL-40 and CRP Levels in Different Diagnostic Groups*

YKL-40 and CRP levels across all clinical groups are illustrated in Figure 1. In CSF, YKL-40 levels were different among groups and were found to increase in AD dementia subjects compared with healthy controls (Figure 1A). No differences were found in YKL-40 levels between healthy controls and MCI or PD groups in CSF (Figure 1A). Nevertheless, a trend toward reduced levels was observed in PD patients, which were significantly lower compared to AD and MCI patient groups (Figure 1A). In plasma, YKL-40 levels remained unchanged across all clinical groups (Figure 1B).

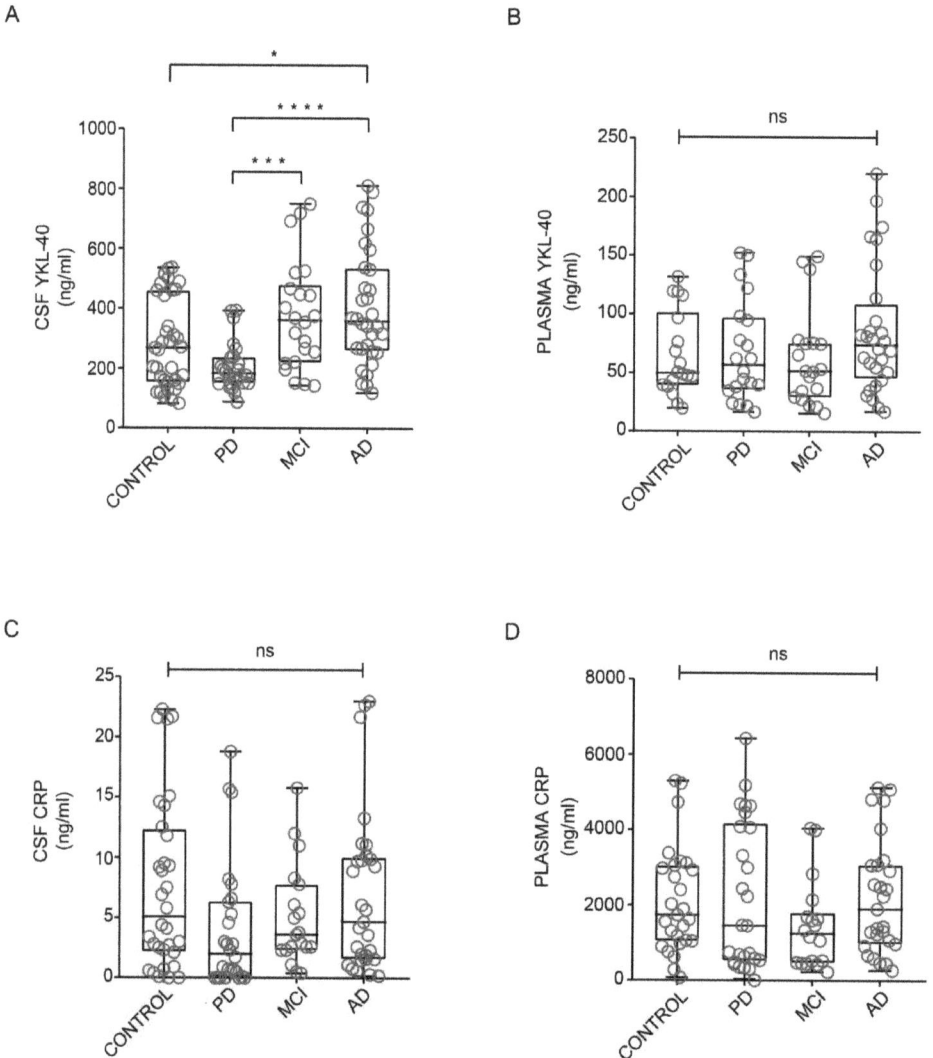

**Figure 1.** YKL-40 and CRP levels in CSF and plasma in different diagnostic groups. Box-and-whisker plots showing (**A,B**) YKL-40 and CRP levels (**C,D**) in CSF and plasma, respectively, across the diagnostic groups. Differences between groups were assessed using Kruskal–Wallis test followed by Bonferroni correction. * $p < 0.05$; *** $p < 0.001$; **** $p < 0.0001$. MCI, mild cognitive impairment; AD, Alzheimer's disease dementia; PD, Parkinson's disease. ns: non-significant.

A nonparametric trend test did not show any statistically significant rising tendency of CSF ($p = 0.48$) or plasma ($p = 0.053$) YKL-40 levels along with MCI or mild and moderate AD. When adjusting for age, sex, and APOE ε4 status, levels of CSF YKL-40 remained high in AD dementia patients when compared with controls (b = 125.5 ng/mL, 95% CI = 19.1 to 232.0 ng/mL, $p < 0.05$).

Regarding CRP levels in CSF and plasma, we did not find significant differences between healthy subjects and AD, MCI, and PD patients (Figure 1C,D). Our results are consistent with previous studies indicating no differences in CRP levels from CSF comparing healthy subjects and PD patients [26] or in serum CRP levels between patients with AD and healthy subjects [30].

In order to analyze the discriminative ability of both biomarkers for the diagnosis of PD and AD, we performed a logistic regression analysis and calculated the corresponding ROC curve for each CSF biomarker and diagnosis. CSF YKL-40 differentiated AD patients from the rest of the cohort, including PD, MCI, and healthy subjects, with 65.6% sensitivity and 66.3% specificity (AUC = 0.69, 95%CI = 0.58 to 0.80, cutoff point = 316.5 ng/mL) (Figure 2A). The combination with CSF CRP did not improve the performance. Nevertheless, for the diagnosis of PD, the combination of CSF YKL-40 and CRP yielded the best results, showing a moderate discriminative ability (AUC = 0.82, 95% CI =0.73 to 0.89, cutoff point of the model = 0.300), with 79.2% sensitivity and 82.1% specificity (Figure 2B).

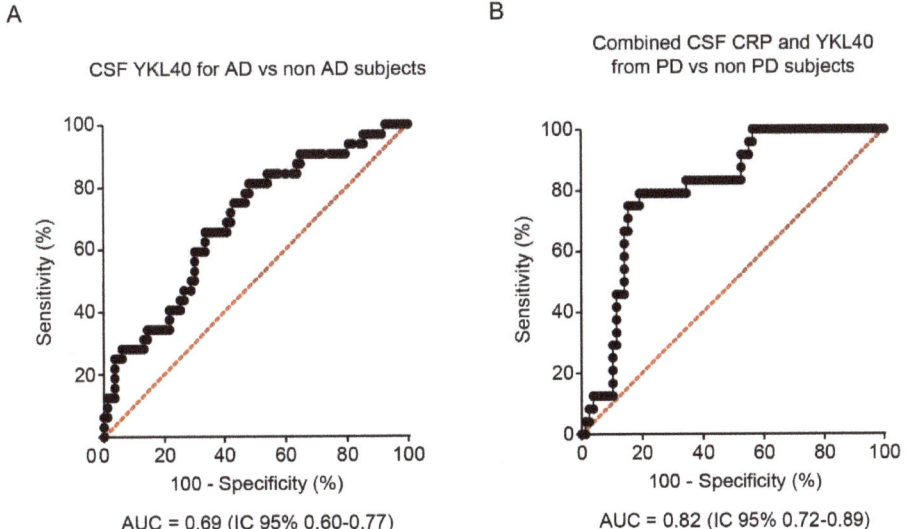

**Figure 2.** Receiver operating characteristic (ROC) analysis of YKL-40 and CRP levels in CSF. (**A**) ROC curve and its corresponding area under the curve (AUC) differentiating YKL-40 levels in CSF from AD patients and non-AD subjects including control subjects. (**B**) AUC differentiating the combination of YKL-40 and CRP levels in CSF from PD and non-PD patients. AUC, area under the curve; AD, Alzheimer's disease dementia; PD, Parkinson's disease.

*3.3. Correlations between YKL-40 and CRP Levels in Plasma and CSF*

Both CSF YKL-40 ($r = 0.39$, $p < 0.001$; Figure 3A) and CRP ($r = 0.56$, $p < 0.0001$; Figure 3B) correlated significantly with their respective plasma concentrations in the whole cohort. The stronger positive correlation was found in AD patients (YKL-40: $r = 0.69$, CRP: $r = 0.84$).

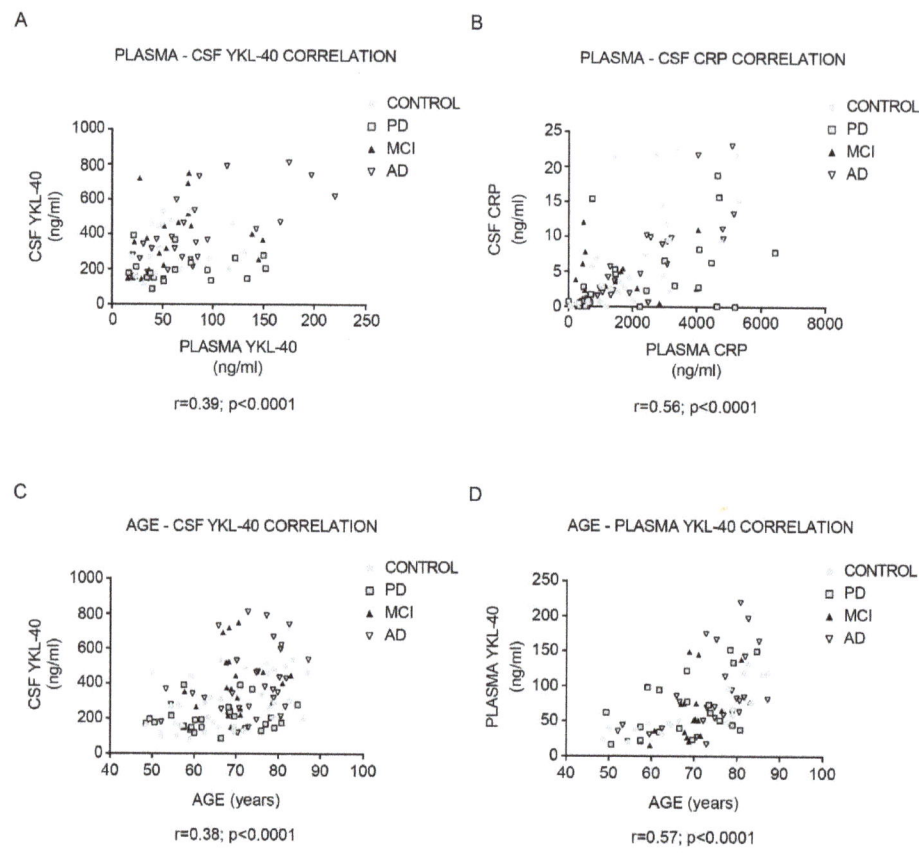

**Figure 3.** Correlation between YKL-40 and CRP levels in CSF and plasma, and between YKL-40 and age in the study cohort. Correlations between the expression levels of (**A**) YKL-40 and (**B**) CRP in CSF and plasma in the study cohort. Correlation between (**C**) CSF and (**D**) plasma YKL-40 and age within the diagnostic group. Correlations were examined with Pearson correlation test. MCI, mild cognitive impairment; AD, Alzheimer's disease dementia; PD, Parkinson's disease.

In the whole cohort, plasma and CSF YKL-40 levels positively correlated with age (CSF YKL-40: $r = 0.38$, $p < 0.0001$; Figure 3C; plasma YKL-40: $r = 0.57$, $p < 0.0001$; Figure 3D). This correlation was especially stronger for the control group (CSF YKL-40: $r = 0.46$, $p < 0.01$; plasma YKL-40: $r = 0.84$, $p < 0.0001$). No statistically significant correlation with age was found in the plasma and CSF CRP analysis. Furthermore, the time since symptom onset did not correlate with any biomarker level in any group. Plasma and CSF YKL-40 and CRP levels did not differ by sex or by the presence of an APOE ε4 allele.

### 3.4. YKL-40 Levels in AD Brain

Upon inflammation, YKL-40 is produced and secreted by many cells including vascular smooth muscle cells and macrophages [50]. In the brain, YKL-40 is mainly expressed in reactive astrocytes [20,25]. Thus, we investigated if the observed increase in YKL-40 levels in CSF from AD patients could be associated with higher YKL-40 levels in cerebral parenchyma. To explore this hypothesis, we examined the YKL-40 cellular levels in human brain tissue from AD patients and healthy subjects. Immunoblotting showed that YKL-40 levels in cerebral orbitofrontal cortex samples were significantly increased in AD patients compared with healthy subjects (Figure 4A). To determine if increased levels of YKL-40 in cerebral orbitofrontal cortex were associated with astrocyte reactivity, the levels of GFAP were also analyzed. Western blotting showed that GFAP levels were also higher in AD samples compared to those observed in control subjects (Figure 4B) in parallel with the observed rise in YKL-40 levels, proving that AD astrogliosis increases YKL-40 levels.

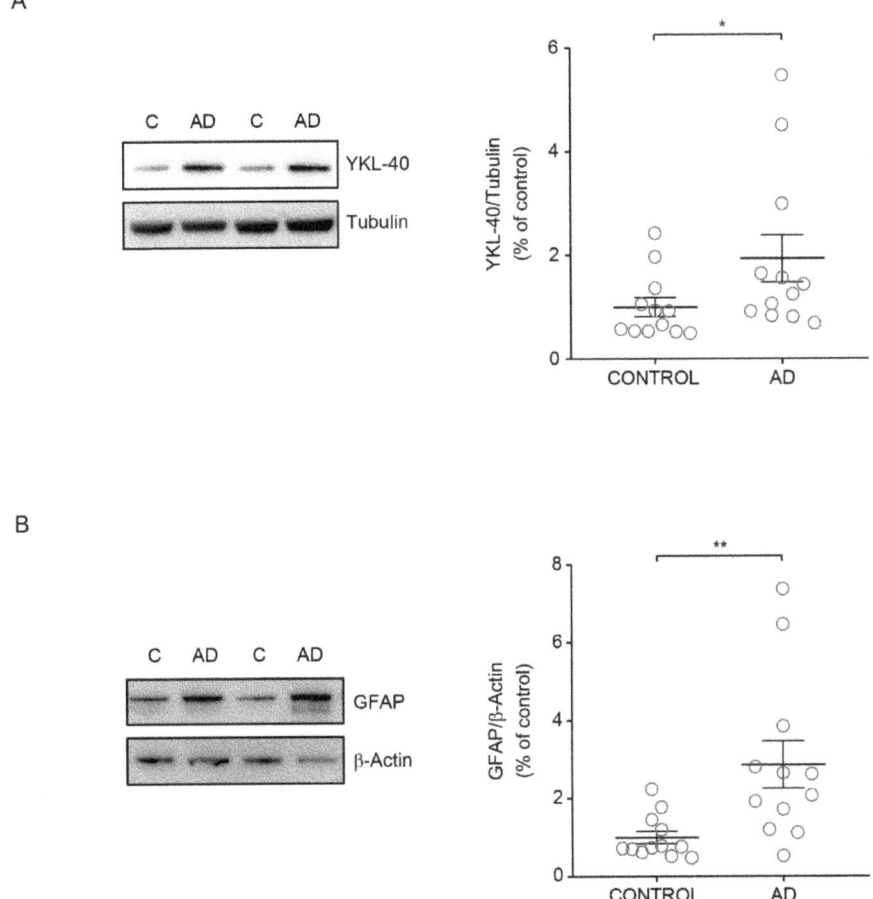

**Figure 4.** YKL-40 and GFAP levels in cerebral orbitofrontal cortex of AD patients and control group. Western blot analysis showing (**A**) YKL-40 and (**B**) GFAP in the cerebral orbitofrontal cortex of AD and control samples. Representative Western blots (left panels) and histograms with their densitometric analysis (right panels) are shown. Data are represented as the mean ± SEM. Differences between groups were assessed using Mann–Whitney test; * $p < 0.05$, ** $p < 0.01$.

## 4. Discussion

In this cross-sectional study, we showed a variable pattern of the inflammatory biomarkers YKL-40 and CRP in AD and PD patients. We confirmed that YKL-40 levels are significantly increased in CSF from AD patients compared to healthy controls, indicating an inflammatory response at the dementia stage. Such an increase was not seen in MCI or PD patients, where CSF YKL-40 levels remained unchanged. These results were also extended to the cerebral orbitofrontal cortex where we found that YKL-40 expression was augmented in AD patients, suggesting glial activation, thus corroborating our hypothesis. Another finding in this study was related to CRP levels in CSF and plasma. We found lower CRP levels in CSF from PD patients compared with other groups (AD, MCI, and healthy subjects), but this change did not reach statistical significance. Furthermore, we did not find evidence of significant alterations in plasma for YKL-40 or CRP.

Inflammation is increasingly recognized as part of the pathology of neurodegenerative conditions, including AD and PD. Evidence proposes that neurodegeneration occurs in part because the CNS environment is affected by a cascade of events collectively named neuroinflammation [51]. Despite biomarkers of neuroinflammation being useful for monitoring disease diagnosis, progression, and response to therapy, accurate and reliable biomarkers for many neurological diseases are scarce. In recent years, the interest in new neuroinflammatory biomarkers has grown at early and symptomatic stages of these diseases. Blood and CSF are commonly used to monitor biomarkers of neuroinflammation, with many of them being the consequence of the CNS pathology. Some examples are the levels of cytokines and chemokines, the loss of blood–brain barrier integrity, and neuronal damage indicators [52].

Only a few studies have shown the possibility of analyzing YKL-40 levels in CSF and blood from patients with AD and predementia stages. One of these studies found that YKL-40 concentration in CSF from AD patients was significantly elevated compared to cognitively normal subjects, with an AUC = 0.88 pointing to the potential value of YKL-40 levels in CSF for AD diagnosis [53]. Increased YKL-40 levels were observed not only in AD dementia, but also in the prodromal phase of AD when compared to cognitively normal controls [54]. Similar observations were found in patients with AD, where YKL-40 concentration in CSF was increased in very mild and mild dementia subjects in comparison with cognitively normal individuals [16]. In our study, we found a trend of increased YKL-40 levels in CSF from MCI subjects compared with healthy controls, and this increase was evident in AD patients. However, the resulting AUC in our study was lower; thus, we propose that YKL-40 might only be a modest AD biomarker candidate.

Significantly increased *chitinase-3 like 3* (*CHI3L3*) mRNA expression, a mouse homolog of YKL-40, was found in brains of AD mice models when compared to age-matched controls [55]. Similarly, in autopsied human brain samples from pathologically confirmed AD subjects, *YKL-40* mRNA levels were significantly increased in comparison with nondemented controls [55]. Although there is no clear explanation regarding which factors modulate YKL-40 levels in AD, it has been suggested that elevated *YKL-40* expression and protein levels might result from increased astrocytic reactivity and release in brain [21]. It was shown that astrocytes in the close vicinity of amyloid plaques were immunoreactive for YKL-40, which confirms the involvement of this protein in the neuroinflammatory response to Aβ deposition [16]. It is known that insoluble Aβ aggregates may induce inflammatory reactions and activation of microglia, resulting in increased proinflammatory mediator production. The relationship between YKL-40 and amyloid-related pathways in AD development was further discussed [17,25]. It seems that the YKL-40 concentration in CSF may be linked to AD pathology, particularly astrogliosis. Indeed, it has been shown that *YKL-40* is expressed by reactive astrocytes GFAP+ in AD [25]. Thus, increased expression of *YKL-40* and protein levels in reactive astrocytes may be reflected in the CSF, indicating that astrocyte-associated metabolites may be utilized as potential biomarkers. Although data regarding elevated YKL-40 levels in CSF from early stages of AD are contradictory [16,17,22–24,54], our results support the increase in YKL-40 levels in CSF from AD subjects, as well as the increased astrocytic YKL-40 levels associated with astrocytosis.

Interestingly, we found that YKL-40 levels in CSF from PD patients were significantly lower compared with those levels in AD subjects suggesting that YKL-40, a marker of astroglial activation, is downregulated in PD. It was reported that YKL-40 levels were decreased in synucleinopathies when compared with tauopathies, suggesting that glial activation may be lower in brains from PD patients and other synucleinopathies in comparison with patients who have tauopathies or healthy controls [26,56]. These data may suggest that CSF YKL-40, as a marker of astroglial activation, is downregulated in PD. Despite astrocytes exerting protection against the inflammatory response in PD [57,58], astroglial dysfunction due to α-syn inclusions may occur simultaneously. In vitro evidence showed that astrocytes are able to efficiently degrade the α-syn aggregates from the extracellular space [59]. More recently, it was shown that primary rat astrocytes receive α-syn aggregates from neurons in mixed cell culture and efficiently transfer them from astrocyte to astrocyte [60]. It is possible that the increase in α-syn levels in astrocytes is a consequence of an endocytic mechanism upon high α-syn levels from the extracellular space, leading to the typical α-syn astrocytic inclusions in PD brains [61]. This accumulation could then lead to the dysregulation of other astrocytic functions, including YKL-40 production/secretion.

Our study yielded no significant changes for CRP levels in CSF or in plasma from AD and PD subjects, although others have described contradictory results [30–32,34]. Pathological studies have demonstrated that CRP is present in the senile plaques and neurofibrillary tangles in AD brains, suggesting that this protein may play a role in the neuropathological processes in AD [62–64]. In PD, aggregated α-syn can promote microglial activation and stimulate the secretion of inflammatory molecules, including CRP [65], thus evoking neuroinflammation [66].

CRP is primarily produced in the liver but is also generated in neurons to a lesser extent [41]. Such residual production of CRP in the CNS does not appear to contribute significantly to CSF levels [39].

In summary, our present study revealed a different inflammatory biomarker profile in individuals with AD and PD. CSF YKL-40 levels were significantly elevated in the AD group, and this increment corroborated the analysis of the YKL-40 protein levels in the cerebral orbitofrontal cortex from pathologically confirmed AD subjects. In PD individuals, plasma and CSF CRP and YKL-40 levels remained unchanged. Notwithstanding, we identified a moderate discriminative ability by combining both biomarkers in CSF for PD diagnosis. Together, our data support the involvement of both inflammatory proteins in the pathogenesis of neurodegenerative diseases.

**Author Contributions:** F.B. and E.C. designed the study and wrote the manuscript; V.A.B.-P., M.R.-F., and D.A. carried out and analyzed experiments; A.V.-G., J.A.M. and I.F. provided CSF and blood samples from participants. All authors read and agreed to the published version of the manuscript.

**Funding:** This study was supported by grants from Instituto de Salud Carlos III (FIS18/00118), FEDER, Comunidad de Madrid (S2017/BMD-3700; NEUROMETAB-CM), and CIBERNED (CB07/502). V.A.B.-P. is supported by the Instituto de Salud Carlos III (ISCIII, Spanish Biomedical Research Institute) through a "Río Hortega" contract (CM 18/0095).

**Institutional Review Board Statement:** This study was conducted according to the guidelines of the Declaration of Helsinki and approved by the Research Ethics Committee of Hospital Universitario 12 de Octubre (18/459, 27 November 2018).

**Informed Consent Statement:** Informed consent to obtain their samples was obtained from all subjects involved in the study. Written informed consent was obtained from all subjects involved in this study to publish this paper using the results obtained with their biological samples.

**Data Availability Statement:** The data obtained and presented in this study are available upon reasoned request from the corresponding author.

**Acknowledgments:** We are grateful to the patients and donors without whom these studies would not have been possible.

**Conflicts of Interest:** The authors declare no conflict of interest.

## References

1. Heneka, M.T.; Carson, M.J.; El Khoury, J.; Landreth, G.E.; Brosseron, F.; Feinstein, D.L.; Jacobs, A.H.; Wyss-Coray, T.; Vitorica, J.; Ransohoff, R.M.; et al. Neuroinflammation in Alzheimer's disease. *Lancet Neurol.* **2015**, *14*, 388–405. [CrossRef]
2. Calsolaro, V.; Edison, P. Neuroinflammation in Alzheimer's disease: Current evidence and future directions. *Alzheimer's Dement.* **2016**, *12*, 719–732. [CrossRef] [PubMed]
3. McGeer, P.L.; McGeer, E.G. Inflammation and neurodegeneration in Parkinson's disease. *Park. Relat. Disord.* **2004**, *10*, S3–S7. [CrossRef]

4. Hirsch, E.C.; Hunot, S. Neuroinflammation in Parkinson's disease: A target for neuroprotection? *Lancet Neurol.* **2009**, *8*, 382–397. [CrossRef]
5. Tansey, M.G.; Goldberg, M.S. Neuroinflammation in Parkinson's disease: Its role in neuronal death and implications for therapeutic intervention. *Neurobiol. Dis.* **2010**, *37*, 510–518. [CrossRef]
6. Maccioni, R.B.; Rojo, L.; Fernández, J.A.; Kuljis, R. The Role of Neuroimmunomodulation in Alzheimer's Disease. *Ann. N. Y. Acad. Sci.* **2009**, *1153*, 240–246. [CrossRef] [PubMed]
7. Swardfager, W.; Lanctot, K.L.; Rothenburg, L.; Wong, A.; Cappell, J.; Herrmann, N. A Meta-Analysis of Cytokines in Alzheimer's Disease. *Biol. Psychiatry* **2010**, *68*, 930–941. [CrossRef] [PubMed]
8. Brosseron, F.; Krauthausen, M.; Kummer, M.; Heneka, M.T. Body Fluid Cytokine Levels in Mild Cognitive Impairment and Alzheimer's Disease: A Comparative Overview. *Mol. Neurobiol.* **2014**, *50*, 534–544. [CrossRef]
9. Létuvé, S.; Kozhich, A.; Arouche, N.; Grandsaigne, M.; Reed, J.; Dombret, M.-C.; Kiener, P.A.; Aubier, M.; Coyle, A.J.; Pretolani, M. YKL-40 Is Elevated in Patients with Chronic Obstructive Pulmonary Disease and Activates Alveolar Macrophages. *J. Immunol.* **2008**, *181*, 5167–5173. [CrossRef] [PubMed]
10. Sharif, M.; Granell, R.; Johansen, J.; Clarke, S.; Elson, C.; Kirwan, J.R. Serum cartilage oligomeric matrix protein and other biomarker profiles in tibiofemoral and patellofemoral osteoarthritis of the knee. *Rheumatol.* **2005**, *45*, 522–526. [CrossRef]
11. Johansen, J.S.; Christoffersen, P.; Møller, S.; A Price, P.; Henriksen, J.H.; Garbarsch, C.; Bendtsen, F. Serum YKL-40 is increased in patients with hepatic fibrosis. *J. Hepatol.* **2000**, *32*, 911–920. [CrossRef]
12. Shao, R.; Hamel, K.; Petersen, L.; Cao, Q.J.; Arenas, R.B.; Bigelow, C.; Bentley, B.; Yan, W. YKL-40, a secreted glycoprotein, promotes tumor angiogenesis. *Oncogene* **2009**, *28*, 4456–4468. [CrossRef]
13. Rathcke, C.N.; Vestergaard, H. YKL-40—An emerging biomarker in cardiovascular disease and diabetes. *Cardiovasc. Diabetol.* **2009**, *8*, 61. [CrossRef] [PubMed]
14. Rehli, M.; Niller, H.-H.; Ammon, C.; Langmann, S.; Schwarzfischer, L.; Andreesen, R.; Krause, S. Transcriptional Regulation of CHI3L1, a Marker Gene for Late Stages of Macrophage Differentiation. *J. Biol. Chem.* **2003**, *278*, 44058–44067. [CrossRef] [PubMed]
15. Bonneh-Barkay, D.; Wang, G.; Starkey, A.; Hamilton, R.L.; A Wiley, C. In vivo CHI3L1 (YKL-40) expression in astrocytes in acute and chronic neurological diseases. *J. Neuroinflamm.* **2010**, *7*, 34. [CrossRef] [PubMed]
16. Craig-Schapiro, R.; Perrin, R.J.; Roe, C.M.; Xiong, C.; Carter, D.; Cairns, N.J.; Mintun, M.A.; Peskind, E.R.; Li, G.; Galasko, D.R.; et al. YKL-40: A Novel Prognostic Fluid Biomarker for Preclinical Alzheimer's Disease. *Biol. Psychiatry* **2010**, *68*, 903–912. [CrossRef]
17. Alcolea, D.; Vilaplana, E.; Pegueroles, J.; Montal, V.; Sánchez-Juan, P.; González-Suárez, A.; Pozueta, A.; Rodriguez-Rodríguez, E.; Bartrés-Faz, D.; Vidal-Piñeiro, D.; et al. Relationship between cortical thickness and cerebrospinal fluid YKL-40 in predementia stages of Alzheimer's disease. *Neurobiol. Aging* **2015**, *36*, 2018–2023. [CrossRef]
18. Janelidze, S.; Mattsson, N.; Stomrud, E.; Lindberg, O.; Palmqvist, S.; Zetterberg, H.; Blennow, K.; Hansson, O. CSF biomarkers of neuroinflammation and cerebrovascular dysfunction in early Alzheimer disease. *Neurol.* **2018**, *91*, e867–e877. [CrossRef]
19. Verkhratsky, A.; Olabarria, M.; Noristani, H.; Yeh, C.-Y.; Rodriguez, J.J. Astrocytes in Alzheimer's disease. *Neurother.* **2010**, *7*, 399–412. [CrossRef]
20. Querol-Vilaseca, M.; Colom-Cadena, M.; Pegueroles, J.; Martín-Paniello, C.S.; Clarimon, J.; Belbin, O.; Fortea, J.; Lleó, A. YKL-40 (Chitinase 3-like I) is expressed in a subset of astrocytes in Alzheimer's disease and other tauopathies. *J. Neuroinflamm.* **2017**, *14*, 1–10. [CrossRef]
21. Bonneh-Barkay, D.; Bissel, S.J.; Kofler, J.; Starkey, A.; Wang, G.; Wiley, C.A. Astrocyte and Macrophage Regulation of YKL-40 Expression and Cellular Response in Neuroinflammation. *Brain Pathol.* **2011**, *22*, 530–546. [CrossRef]
22. Zhang, H.; Initiative, T.A.D.N.; Ng, K.P.; Therriault, J.; Kang, M.S.; Pascoal, T.A.; Rosa-Neto, P.; Gauthier, S. Cerebrospinal fluid phosphorylated tau, visinin-like protein-1, and chitinase-3-like protein 1 in mild cognitive impairment and Alzheimer's disease. *Transl. Neurodegener.* **2018**, *7*, 1–12. [CrossRef]
23. Nordengen, K.; Kirsebom, B.-E.; Henjum, K.; Selnes, P.; Gísladóttir, B.; Wettergreen, M.; Torsetnes, S.B.; Grøntvedt, G.R.; Waterloo, K.K.; Aarsland, D.; et al. Glial activation and inflammation along the Alzheimer's disease continuum. *J. Neuroinflamm.* **2019**, *16*, 1–13. [CrossRef]
24. Wang, L.; Gao, T.; Cai, T.; Li, K.; Zheng, P.; Liu, J. Cerebrospinal fluid levels of YKL-40 in prodromal Alzheimer's disease. *Neurosci. Lett.* **2020**, *715*, 134658. [CrossRef]
25. Llorens, F.; Thüne, K.; Tahir, W.; Kanata, E.; Diaz-Lucena, D.; Xanthopoulos, K.; Kovatsi, E.; Pleschka, C.; Garcia-Esparcia, P.; Schmitz, M.; et al. YKL-40 in the brain and cerebrospinal fluid of neurodegenerative dementias. *Mol. Neurodegener.* **2017**, *12*, 83. [CrossRef] [PubMed]
26. Hall, S.; Janelidze, S.; Surova, Y.; Widner, H.; Zetterberg, H.; Hansson, O. Cerebrospinal fluid concentrations of inflammatory markers in Parkinson's disease and atypical parkinsonian disorders. *Sci. Rep.* **2018**, *8*, 1–9. [CrossRef] [PubMed]
27. Gabay, C.; Kushner, I. Acute-Phase Proteins and Other Systemic Responses to Inflammation. *New Engl. J. Med.* **1999**, *340*, 448–454. [CrossRef]
28. Luan, Y.-Y.; Yao, Y.-M. The Clinical Significance and Potential Role of C-Reactive Protein in Chronic Inflammatory and Neurodegenerative Diseases. *Front. Immunol.* **2018**, *9*, 1302. [CrossRef] [PubMed]
29. Koyama, A.; O'Brien, J.; Weuve, J.; Blacker, D.; Metti, A.L.; Yaffe, K. The Role of Peripheral Inflammatory Markers in Dementia and Alzheimer's Disease: A Meta-Analysis. *J. Gerontol. Ser. A Boil. Sci. Med Sci.* **2012**, *68*, 433–440. [CrossRef]

30. Gong, C.; Wei, D.; Wang, Y.; Ma, J.; Yuan, C.; Zhang, W.; Yu, G.; Zhao, Y. A Meta-Analysis of C-Reactive Protein in Patients With Alzheimer's Disease. *Am. J. Alzheimer's Dis. Other Dementiasr* **2016**, *31*, 194–200. [CrossRef] [PubMed]
31. Schuitemaker, A.; Dik, M.G.; Veerhuis, R.; Scheltens, P.; Schoonenboom, N.S.; Hack, C.E.; Blankenstein, M.A.; Jonker, C. Inflammatory markers in AD and MCI patients with different biomarker profiles. *Neurobiol. Aging* **2009**, *30*, 1885–1889. [CrossRef] [PubMed]
32. Brosseron, F.; Traschütz, A.; Widmann, C.N.; Kummer, M.P.; Tacik, P.; Santarelli, F.; Jessen, F.; Heneka, M.T. Characterization and clinical use of inflammatory cerebrospinal fluid protein markers in Alzheimer's disease. *Alzheimer's Res. Ther.* **2018**, *10*, 1–14. [CrossRef] [PubMed]
33. Andican, G.; Konukoglu, D.; Bozluolcay, M.; Bayulkem, K.; Fırtına, S.; Burçak, G.; Konukoğlu, D. Plasma oxidative and inflammatory markers in patients with idiopathic Parkinson's disease. *Acta Neurol. Belg.* **2012**, *112*, 155–159. [CrossRef]
34. Song, I.-U.; Cho, H.-J.; Kim, J.-S.; Park, I.-S.; Lee, K.-S. Serum hs-CRP Levels are Increased in de Novo Parkinson's Disease Independently from Age of Onset. *Eur. Neurol.* **2014**, *72*, 285–289. [CrossRef]
35. Williams-Gray, C.; Wijeyekoon, R.; Yarnall, A.; Lawson, R.A.; Breen, D.P.; Evans, J.R.; Cummins, G.A.; Duncan, G.W.; Khoo, T.K.; Burn, D.; et al. Serum immune markers and disease progression in an incident Parkinson's disease cohort (ICICLE-PD). *Mov. Disord.* **2016**, *31*, 995–1003. [CrossRef]
36. Qiu, X.; Xiao, Y.; Wu, J.; Gan, L.; Huang, Y.; Wang, J. C-Reactive Protein and Risk of Parkinson's Disease: A Systematic Review and Meta-Analysis. *Front. Neurol.* **2019**, *10*, 384. [CrossRef]
37. Yasojima, K.; Schwab, C.; McGeer, E.G.; McGeer, P.L. Human neurons generate C-reactive protein and amyloid P: Upregulation in Alzheimer's disease. *Brain Res.* **2000**, *887*, 80–89. [CrossRef]
38. Wight, R.D.; Tull, C.A.; Deel, M.W.; Stroope, B.L.; Eubanks, A.G.; Chavis, J.A.; Drew, P.D.; Hensley, L.L. Resveratrol effects on astrocyte function: Relevance to neurodegenerative diseases. *Biochem. Biophys. Res. Commun.* **2012**, *426*, 112–115. [CrossRef]
39. Mulder, S.D.; Hack, C.E.; van der Flier, W.M.; Scheltens, P.; Blankenstein, M.A.; Veerhuis, R. Evaluation of Intrathecal Serum Amyloid P (SAP) and C-Reactive Protein (CRP) Synthesis in Alzheimer's Disease with the Use of Index Values. *J. Alzheimer's Dis.* **2011**, *22*, 1073–1079. [CrossRef] [PubMed]
40. McGeer, P.L.; Yasojima, K.; McGeer, E.G. Inflammation in Parkinson's disease. *Adv. Neurol.* **2001**, *86*, 83–89. [PubMed]
41. Di Napoli, M.; Godoy, D.A.; Campi, V.; Masotti, L.; Smith, C.; Jones, A.R.P.; Hopkins, S.; Slevin, M.; Papa, F.; Mogoanta, L.; et al. C-reactive protein in intracerebral hemorrhage: Time course, tissue localization, and prognosis. *Neurol.* **2012**, *79*, 690–699. [CrossRef]
42. Di Napoli, M.; Parry-Jones, A.R.; Smith, C.; Hopkins, S.; Slevin, M.; Masotti, L.; Campi, V.; Singh, P.; Papa, F.; Popa-Wagner, A.; et al. C-Reactive Protein Predicts Hematoma Growth in Intracerebral Hemorrhage. *Stroke* **2014**, *45*, 59–65. [CrossRef]
43. Albert, M.S.; DeKosky, S.; Dickson, D.W.; Dubois, B.; Feldman, H.; Fox, N.; Gamst, A.; Holtzman, D.M.; Jagust, W.J.; Petersen, R.C.; et al. The diagnosis of mild cognitive impairment due to Alzheimer's disease: Recommendations from the National Institute on Aging-Alzheimer's Association workgroups on diagnostic guidelines for Alzheimer's disease. *Alzheimer's Dement.* **2011**, *7*, 270–279. [CrossRef]
44. McKhann, G.M.; Knopman, D.S.; Chertkow, H.; Hyman, B.T.; Jack, C.R., Jr.; Kawas, C.H.; Klunk, W.E.; Koroshetz, W.J.; Manly, J.J.; Mayeux, R.; et al. The diagnosis of dementia due to Alzheimer's disease: Recommendations from the National Institute on Aging-Alzheimer's Association workgroups on diagnostic guidelines for Alzheimer's disease. *Alzheimer's Dement.* **2011**, *7*, 263–269. [CrossRef]
45. Winblad, B.; Palmer, K.; Kivipelto, M.; Jelic, V.; Fratiglioni, L.; Wahlund, L.-O.; Nordberg, A.; Backman, L.J.; Albert, M.S.; Almkvist, O.; et al. Mild cognitive impairment—Beyond controversies, towards a consensus: Report of the International Working Group on Mild Cognitive Impairment. *J. Intern. Med.* **2004**, *256*, 240–246. [CrossRef]
46. Morris, J.C. The Clinical Dementia Rating (CDR): Current version and scoring rules. *Neurology* **1993**, *43*, 2412–2414. [CrossRef]
47. Postuma, R.B.; Berg, D.; Stern, M.; Poewe, W.; Olanow, C.W.; Oertel, W.; Obeso, J.; Marek, K.; Litvan, I.; Lang, A.E.; et al. MDS clinical diagnostic criteria for Parkinson's disease. *Mov. Disord.* **2015**, *30*, 1591–1601. [CrossRef] [PubMed]
48. Hyman, B.T.; Phelps, C.H.; Beach, T.G.; Bigio, E.H.; Cairns, N.J.; Carrillo, M.C.; Dickson, D.W.; Duyckaerts, C.; Frosch, M.P.; Masliah, E.; et al. National Institute on Aging-Alzheimer's Association guidelines for the neuropathologic assessment of Alzheimer's disease. *Alzheimer's Dement.* **2012**, *8*, 1–13. [CrossRef] [PubMed]
49. Heffernan, A.; Chidgey, C.; Peng, P.; Masters, C.; Roberts, B.R. The Neurobiology and Age-Related Prevalence of the ε4 Allele of Apolipoprotein E in Alzheimer's Disease Cohorts. *J. Mol. Neurosci.* **2016**, *60*, 316–324. [CrossRef] [PubMed]
50. Rathcke, C.N.; Vestergaard, H. YKL-40, a new inflammatory marker with relation to insulin resistance and with a role in endothelial dysfunction and atherosclerosis. *Inflamm. Res.* **2006**, *55*, 221–227. [CrossRef] [PubMed]
51. Ransohoff, R.M. How neuroinflammation contributes to neurodegeneration. *Science* **2016**, *353*, 777–783. [CrossRef] [PubMed]
52. Kothur, K.; Wienholt, L.; Brilot, F.; Dale, R.C. CSF cytokines/chemokines as biomarkers in neuroinflammatory CNS disorders: A systematic review. *Cytokine* **2016**, *77*, 227–237. [CrossRef] [PubMed]
53. Andersson, C.-H.; Andreasson, U.; Bjerke, M.; Rami, L.; Blennow, K.; Zetterberg, H.; Rosén, C.; Molinuevo, J.L.; Lladó, A. Increased Levels of Chitotriosidase and YKL-40 in Cerebrospinal Fluid from Patients with Alzheimer's Disease. *Dement. Geriatr. Cogn. Disord. Extra* **2014**, *4*, 297–304. [CrossRef]
54. Antonell, A.; Mansilla, A.; Rami, L.; Lladó, A.; Iranzo, A.; Olives, J.; Balasa, M.; Sánchez-Valle, R.; Molinuevo, J.L. Cerebrospinal Fluid Level of YKL-40 Protein in Preclinical and Prodromal Alzheimer's Disease. *J. Alzheimer's Dis.* **2014**, *42*, 901–908. [CrossRef]

55. A Colton, C.; Mott, R.T.; Sharpe, H.; Xu, Q.; E Van Nostrand, W.; Vitek, M.P. Expression profiles for macrophage alternative activation genes in AD and in mouse models of AD. *J. Neuroinflamm.* **2006**, *3*, 27. [CrossRef] [PubMed]
56. Olsson, B.; Constantinescu, R.; Holmberg, B.; Andreasen, N.; Blennow, K.; Zetterberg, H. The glial marker YKL-40 is decreased in synucleinopathies. *Mov. Disord.* **2013**, *28*, 1882–1885. [CrossRef]
57. Sofroniew, M.V.; Vinters, H.V. Astrocytes: Biology and pathology. *Acta Neuropathol.* **2010**, *119*, 7–35. [CrossRef]
58. Gray, M.T.; Woulfe, J.M. Striatal Blood–Brain Barrier Permeability in Parkinson'S Disease. *Br. J. Pharmacol.* **2015**, *35*, 747–750. [CrossRef]
59. Li, J.-Y.; Englund, E.; Holton, J.L.; Soulet, D.; Hagell, P.; Lees, A.J.; Lashley, T.; Quinn, N.P.; Rehncrona, S.; Björklund, A.; et al. Lewy bodies in grafted neurons in subjects with Parkinson's disease suggest host-to-graft disease propagation. *Nat. Med.* **2008**, *14*, 501–503. [CrossRef]
60. Loria, F.; Vargas, J.Y.; Bousset, L.; Syan, S.; Salles, A.; Melki, R.; Zurzolo, C. α-Synuclein transfer between neurons and astrocytes indicates that astrocytes play a role in degradation rather than in spreading. *Acta Neuropathol.* **2017**, *134*, 789–808. [CrossRef]
61. Stevenson, T.; Murray, H.; Turner, C.; Faull, R.L.M.; Dieriks, B.V.; Curtis, M.A. α-synuclein inclusions are abundant in non-neuronal cells in the anterior olfactory nucleus of the Parkinson's disease olfactory bulb. *Sci. Rep.* **2020**, *10*, 1–10. [CrossRef] [PubMed]
62. McGeer, E. The pentraxins: Possible role in Alzheimer's disease and other innate inflammatory diseases. *Neurobiol. Aging* **2001**, *22*, 843–848. [CrossRef]
63. Duong, T.; Nikolaeva, M.; Acton, P.J. C-reactive protein-like immunoreactivity in the neurofibrillary tangles of Alzheimer's disease. *Brain Res.* **1997**, *749*, 152–156. [CrossRef]
64. Iwamoto, N.; Nishiyama, E.; Ohwada, J.; Arai, H. Demonstration of CRP immunoreactivity in brains of Alzheimer's disease: Immunohistochemical study using formic acid pretreatment of tissue sections. *Neurosci. Lett.* **1994**, *177*, 23–26. [CrossRef]
65. Sarkar, S.; Dammer, E.; Malovic, E.; Olsen, A.L.; Raza, S.A.; Gao, T.; Xiao, H.; Oliver, D.L.; Duong, D.; Joers, V.; et al. Molecular Signatures of Neuroinflammation Induced by αSynuclein Aggregates in Microglial Cells. *Front. Immunol.* **2020**, *11*, 33. [CrossRef]
66. Surendranathan, A.; Rowe, J.B.; O'Brien, J.T. Neuroinflammation in Lewy body dementia. *Park. Relat. Disord.* **2015**, *21*, 1398–1406. [CrossRef]

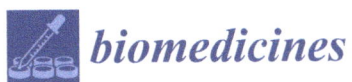 

*Review*

# Potential Roles of Sestrin2 in Alzheimer's Disease: Antioxidation, Autophagy Promotion, and Beyond

Shang-Der Chen [1,2,†], Jenq-Lin Yang [2,†], Yi-Heng Hsieh [3], Tsu-Kung Lin [1,4,5], Yi-Chun Lin [6], A-Ching Chao [7,8,*] and Ding-I Yang [3,9,*]

1. Department of Neurology, Kaohsiung Chang Gung Memorial Hospital, Kaohsiung City 83301, Taiwan; chensd@adm.cgmh.org.tw (S.-D.C.); tklin@adm.cgmh.org.tw (T.-K.L.)
2. Institute for Translation Research in Biomedicine, Kaohsiung Chang Gung Memorial Hospital, Kaohsiung City 83301, Taiwan; jyang@adm.cgmh.org.tw
3. Institute of Brain Science, National Yang Ming Chiao Tung University, Taipei City 11221, Taiwan; p400540226@gmail.com
4. College of Medicine, Chang Gung University, Taoyuan City 33302, Taiwan
5. Center for Mitochondrial Research and Medicine, Kaohsiung Chang Gung Memorial Hospital, Chang Gung University College of Medicine, Kaohsiung City 80708, Taiwan
6. Department of Neurology, Taipei City Hospital, Taipei City 10629, Taiwan; DAB16@tpech.gov.tw
7. Department of Neurology, College of Medicine, Kaohsiung Medical University, Kaohsiung City 80708, Taiwan
8. Department of Neurology, Kaohsiung Medical University Hospital, Kaohsiung City 80756, Taiwan
9. Brain Research Center, National Yang Ming Chiao Tung University, Taipei City 11221, Taiwan
* Correspondence: achch@cc.kmu.edu.tw (A.-C.C.); diyang@ym.edu.tw (D.-I.Y.); Tel.: +886-7-3121101 (A.-C.C.); Tel.: +886-2-28267386 (D.-I.Y.)
† Authors contributed equally to the work.

**Abstract:** Alzheimer's disease (AD) is the most common age-related neurodegenerative disease. It presents with progressive memory loss, worsens cognitive functions to the point of disability, and causes heavy socioeconomic burdens to patients, their families, and society as a whole. The underlying pathogenic mechanisms of AD are complex and may involve excitotoxicity, excessive generation of reactive oxygen species (ROS), aberrant cell cycle reentry, impaired mitochondrial function, and DNA damage. Up to now, there is no effective treatment available for AD, and it is therefore urgent to develop an effective therapeutic regimen for this devastating disease. Sestrin2, belonging to the sestrin family, can counteract oxidative stress, reduce activity of the mammalian/mechanistic target of rapamycin (mTOR), and improve cell survival. It may therefore play a crucial role in neurodegenerative diseases like AD. However, only limited studies of sestrin2 and AD have been conducted up to now. In this article, we discuss current experimental evidence to demonstrate the potential roles of sestrin2 in treating neurodegenerative diseases, focusing specifically on AD. Strategies for augmenting sestrin2 expression may strengthen neurons, adapting them to stressful conditions through counteracting oxidative stress, and may also adjust the autophagy process, these two effects together conferring neuronal resistance in cases of AD.

**Keywords:** Alzheimer's disease; autophagy; mTOR; oxidative stress; sestrin2

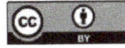

## 1. Introduction

Patients with age-related neurodegenerative diseases usually present with a relentlessly deteriorating clinical course. Worst of all, the lack of effective treatment results in heavy socioeconomic burdens to patients, family, and the whole of society [1–3]. Alzheimer's disease (AD), a type of dementia with progressive memory loss and declined cognitive functions, is the most common neurodegenerative disease in the elderly. Based on the information from the World Health Organization (WHO), approximately 50 million people suffer from dementia worldwide, and nearly 10 million new cases are added every year, making the disease one of the main causes of disability and dependence. AD may account for 60–70% of all dementia cases (https://www.who.int/news-room/fact-sheets/detail/dementia, accessed on 21 September 2020). According to "2021 Alzheimer's disease facts and figures", in the USA [4], approximately 6.2 million senior Americans over 65 years old have AD. By 2060, with a steep projected increase, the number of AD patients may rise to 13.8 million. Data revealed that, from 2000 to 2019, deaths resulting from human immunodeficiency virus (HIV), heart disease, and stroke declined, while deaths from AD increased more than 145% [4]. The total healthcare costs in 2020 are approximated at $305 billion and are expected to increase to more than $1 trillion as the population ages [5]. It is crucial to delay, reduce, or prevent the occurrence of disability from AD and lessen the heavy burden it places on society.

The major pathological hallmarks of AD brains are gross atrophy of the brain, as well microscopically observable senile plaques and neurofibrillary tangles (NFTs) [6–8]. Senile plaques are extracellular structures mainly composed of insoluble deposits of amyloid-beta peptide (A$\beta$), a peptide fragment of 39–43 amino acids derived from sequential cleavage of the transmembrane protein amyloid precursor protein (APP) by $\beta$- and $\gamma$-secretase [9–12]. Newly synthesized full-length APP is transported from the endoplasmic reticulum (ER) to the Golgi apparatus (GA)/*trans*-Golgi network (TGN) for further protein processing and maturation. The acidic environment (pH = 6.0–6.5) in the TGN or the late GA is optimal for the activity of many processing enzymes, including BACE1. The full-length APP delivered to the plasma membrane may be subjected to non-amyloidogenic cleavage by $\alpha$- and then $\gamma$-secretase to release the soluble APP-alpha (sAPP$\alpha$), the p3 fragment, and the APP intracellular domain (AICD). Alternatively, a portion of the full-length APP may also be endocytosed into early endosomes and possibly rerouted to the acidic recycling endosomes (REs), where BACE1 resides, to produce A$\beta$ [13]. In addition, extracellular A$\beta$ can also be taken up through receptor binding and subsequently internalized, thereby leading to its accumulation within various intracellular compartments, including endosomes, multivesicular bodies (MVBs), lysosomes, mitochondria, the ER, the TGN, and cytosol [14].

A$\beta$ can induce neurotoxicity through various mechanisms, such as excitotoxicity [15], excessive generation of reactive oxygen species (ROS) [16], aberrant cell cycle reentry [17,18], impaired mitochondrial function [19], and DNA damage [20], all of these mechanisms together contributing to neuronal damage or even death. Moreover, A$\beta$ can also alter gene transcription [19], and thereby affect protein expression, which may influence the survival or death of neuronal cells in AD-related pathophysiology.

Maintenance of neuronal functions depends on axonal transport of proteins, organelles, and vesicles from the soma to the nerve terminals [21]. Going the other way, neurotrophic factors, including the members of the neurotrophin family, secreted from postsynaptic targets must be transmitted retrogradely from nerve terminals via axonal transport back to the soma [22]. Thus, failure of axonal transport may contribute to neuronal death. As a microtubule-binding protein important for microtubule assembly and stabilization, hyperphosphorylation of tau compromises its biological functions and destabilizes the structures of microtubules, and is accompanied by disturbance to axonal transport [23]. Furthermore, increasing evidence suggests that A$\beta$ may also disrupt axonal transport and contribute to AD pathophysiology [21].

It was proposed two decades ago that fibrils may not be the only toxic form of A$\beta$; small oligomers of A$\beta$, or A$\beta$-derived diffusible ligand (ADDL), and A$\beta$ protofibrils may also have potent neurotoxicity [24]. Like A$\beta$ oligomers, tau oligomers formed during the early stages of aggregation are also pathologically relevant to the loss of neurons and behavioral impairments in several neurodegenerative disorders called tauopathies, the most common of which is AD [25]. In addition to the aggregation of extracellular amyloid plaques, emerging evidence has revealed the crucial role of intraneuronal amyloid species (iA$\beta$s) which can appear in the membrane or the lumen of late endosomes and precede further aggregation, eventually accumulating inside the endosome or endolysosome [26,27]. It was also noted that, besides the extracellular aggregation of homologous A$\beta$ species, cross-seeding of different amyloid proteins, or even between different misfolded proteins, such as Aβs and tau, may be biologically significant, and even critical in the progression of AD [28]. Apart from cross-seeding, crosstalk between Aβ and tau may also play a vital role contributing to AD pathogenesis. For example, Aβ has been shown to trigger alternative splicing of tau isoforms via glycogen synthase kinase-3beta (GSK-3β), making tau more susceptible to hyperphosphorylation [29,30]. Overall, these effects could further aggravate aberrant cellular signaling, induce excessive tau phosphorylation, worsen toxic tau accumulation, and lead to synapto/neurotoxic effects [26]. A simplified cartoon summarizing the pathogenic mechanisms of AD is shown in Figure 1, below.

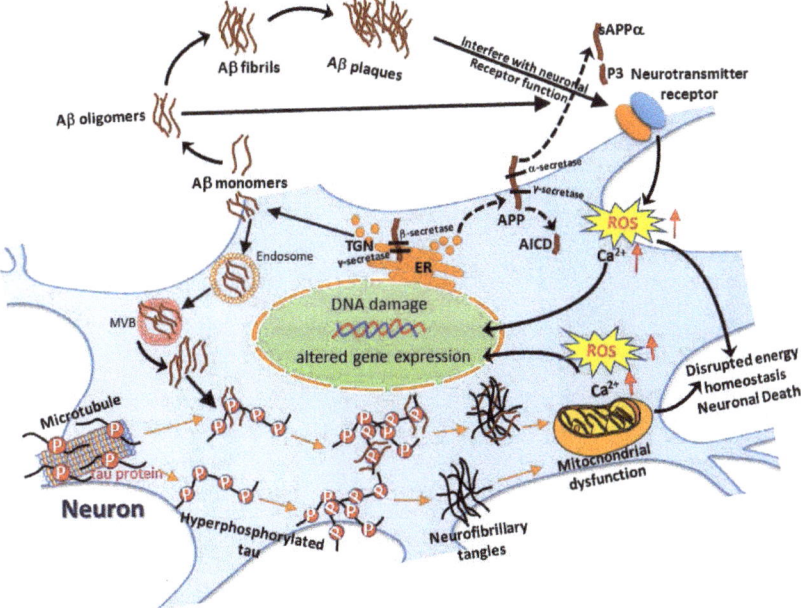

**Figure 1.** The cartoon diagram demonstrates the pathogenic processes of amyloid-beta peptide (Aβ) and tau protein. Through the amyloidogenic pathway, the full-length amyloid precursor protein (APP) is sequentially cleaved by β-secretase (encoded by beta-site amyloid precursor protein cleaving enzyme-1 or BACE1) and γ-secretase to generate Aβ. Newly synthesized APP is transported from the endoplasmic reticulum (ER) to the Golgi apparatus (GA) for protein maturation. The acidic pH in the trans-Golgi network (TGN) or the late GA is optimal for BACE1 activity, with production of secreted Aβ; the sequential amyloidogenic cleavages of full-length APP by β- and γ-secretase also generate soluble APP-beta (sAPPβ) and the APP intracellular domain (AICD), though these are not depicted in the diagram. A portion of the full-length APP reaching the plasma membrane may be subjected to the non-amyloidogenic cleavage by α- and then γ-secretase to release the soluble APP-alpha (sAPPα), the p3 fragment, and the AICD. Another portion of the full-length APP may also be endocytosed into early endosomes and possibly be rerouted to the acidic recycling endosomes (REs; not depicted), where BACE1 resides, for intracellular production of Aβ. Furthermore, extracellular Aβ can also be taken up through receptor binding and subsequent internalization, resulting in its accumulation within various intracellular compartments, including endosomes, multivesicular bodies (MVBs), and mitochondria (not depicted). The extracellular Aβ monomers aggregate into oligomers and then into fibrils, eventually forming senile plaques. Tau protein is a microtubule-binding protein, which is hyperphosphorylated in AD neurons. The phosphor-tau monomer may also aggregate into tau oligomers and, finally, into neurofibrillary tangles (NFTs). The intraneuronal Aβ species also oligomerize or even mix with tau proteins to form mixed aggregates. The extracellular senile plaques,

the extracellular and intraneuronal Aβ oligomers, as well as tau oligomers and NFTs, together lead to excessive production of reactive oxygen species (ROS), $Ca^{2+}$ overload, mitochondrial dysfunction, and disrupted energy homeostasis, ultimately causing neuronal death. In addition to those pictured above, other pathogenic mechanisms are not demonstrated in this figure due to limited space. For example, loss of tau binding destabilizes microtubules, thus compromising anterograde axonal transport of proteins, mitochondria, and vesicles from soma to the nerve terminals, which may negatively impact nerve transmission. Conversely, neurotrophic factors, especially neurotrophins, secreted from target cells also fail to be retrogradely transported from the nerve terminal back to the soma to nourish the neurons, also leading to neuronal demise. Please see the text for more details.

Sestrins, including sestrin1, sestrin2, and sestrin3, belong to a group of highly evolutionarily conserved proteins in mammalian cells, and may play a crucial role in stressful conditions, such as oxidative stress, hypoxia, and DNA damage [31–34]. While the structures of sestrin1 and sestrin3 await further elucidation, the essential characteristics of sestrin2 have been gradually revealed in recent years [35,36]. Three distinctive functional sites were identified, which are critical for inhibition of ROS production, modulation of the mammalian/mechanistic target of rapamycin (mTOR) complex 1 (mTORC1), and for leucine-binding [35,36]. Inhibiting either ROS for antioxidation or mTORC1 for autophagy promotion may attenuate degenerative processes associated with aging [35]. Therefore, sestrins may possess two beneficial effects that are pivotal for anti-aging [37,38].

Despite the potential effect of sestrins on age-related neurological disorders, only quite limited studies about AD have been reported. We have shown in a previous study that sestrin2 was induced by Aβ in primary rat cortical neurons and an increased expression of sestrin2 was also found in the cortices of 1-year-old AD transgenic mice [39]. We also showed that sestrin2 functions as an endogenous protective mediator against Aβ-induced neurotoxicity, in part through enhancement of autophagy activity [39]. In another recent study, we further demonstrated that Aβ-induced sestrin2 expression contributes to antioxidative activity in neurons; furthermore, Aβ induction of sestrin2 is at least partly mediated by the activation of transcription factors NF-κB and p53 [40]. In this review article, we discuss recent progress in revealing the underlying molecular mechanisms concerning the sestrin2-mediated protective effects against neuronal dysfunction in AD. Better understanding of the potential novel pathway in AD may guide further research into developing effective therapeutic regimens in the future. Finding the way to augmenting sestrin2 expression may have significant clinical implications, especially in treating many devastating neurodegenerative diseases, including AD.

## 2. The Biological Roles of Sestrin2

Sestrins, including sestrin1, sestrin2, and sestrin3, belong to a gene family and function as stress-inducible proteins that affect metabolism through perceiving nutrient status and redox level in living organisms. Sestrin1 (also known as PA26) was initially discovered in human Saos-2 osteosarcoma cells as one of the p53-induced transcripts and was mapped to chromosome 6q21 through a differential display screening [34,41]. Sestrin1 is ubiquitously expressed in most tissues, including lung, kidney, pancreas, skeletal muscle, and brain tissues [33], and it can be activated under oxidative stress and irradiation in a p53-dependent fashion [34,42]. Sestrin2 (also known as Hi95), located in chromosome 1p35.3, was first discovered in glioblastoma cells under prolonged hypoxia and its transcription was found to be increased following DNA damage [33]. Later, it was noted that sestrin1 and sestrin2, through activating the AMP-dependent kinase (AMPK) pathway, may affect tuberous sclerosis complex 2 (TSC2) expression to inhibit mTOR-mediated cell over-proliferation [43]. Sestrin3, located in chromosome 11q21, was identified from database mining of the PA26-related gene family [32,33]. mRNA expression of these sestrin genes is presented diffusely during mouse embryogenesis and also in adult tissues at various levels [32]. Sestrin1 is robustly expressed in the brain, heart, liver, and skeletal muscle; sestrin2 is expressed more in the kidney, leucocytes, lungs, and liver; sestrin3 is expressed at higher levels in the brain, kidney, small intestine, and skeletal muscle [32,34,44].

It has been revealed that the crystal structure of human sestrin2 (hSesn2) has distinct globular subdomains, each possessing separate functions [35]. As shown below in Figure 2A, the N-terminal domain (Sesn-A) diminishes alkyl hydroperoxide radicals through the helix-turn-helix oxidoreductase motif. Mutations of Cys125, His132, and Tyr127, which are, respectively, the catalytic cysteine, the residue critical for the conserved proton relay system, and the residue potentially involved in the catalytic process, reduce this redox activity. The C-terminal domain (Sesn-C) of hSesn2, whose sequence is highly conserved across the sestrin family, has lost its antioxidant activity but acquired another important function in mTORC1 inhibition via physical association with GTPase-activating protein activity toward the Rags-2 (GATOR2) complex, in which process Asp406 and Asp407 (the DD motif) are vital. Furthermore, the DD motif is involved in activation of AMP-dependent protein kinase (AMPK), which is also important for mTORC1 inhibition. Besides GATOR2 binding and AMPK activation for mTOR inhibition, sestrin2 may also carry the guanosine nucleotide dissociation inhibition (GDI) function. However, mutation studies of Arg419/Lys422/Lys426 in Sesn-C suggested that whether these amino acid residues are truly critical for GDI functions is still in question [35].

The availability of amino acids is critical for the regulation of protein synthesis in living organisms. Leucine, one of the essential amino acids, is indispensable for this process and, more importantly, leucine was found to be crucial for mTORC1 activation in cells [45]. Located in the Sesn-C of hSesn2 (Figure 2A), charged residues Glu451 and Arg390, from two sides of a single binding pocket, anchor leucine in place through salt bridges with the free amine and carboxyl groups, respectively, whereas the isopropyl side chain of the bound leucine forms extensive hydrophobic interactions with residues Leu389, Trp444, and Phe447 in the pocket. In addition to contacting the charged sides and hydrophobic base of the pocket, three threonine residues (Thr374, Thr377, and Thr386) are positioned directly above the leucine to form a "lid" that encloses the top of the leucine, thereby locking the ligand in place [36]. As a leucine sensor, sestrin2 inhibits mTORC1 activity through the Rag guanosine triphosphatases (GTPase) and its regulators-GATOR1 and GATOR2. Thus, the binding of leucine with sestrin2 disrupts the connection of sestrin2 with GATOR2, allowing GATOR2 to enhance mTORC1 activity [36]. It has previously been demonstrated that adult sestrin2 gene knockout mice subject to a fasting/refeeding regimen or maintained with a high-fat diet suffered from various metabolic derangements, such as hepatosteatosis, insulin resistance, and glucose intolerance, with increased ROS extent and mTORC1 activity [38,46].

Despite the availability of the crystal structure of hSesn2, the detailed molecular information for sestrin1 and sestrin3 remains to be fully elucidated. However, sequence alignment of the three human sestrins revealed an overall 44.8% amino acid sequence identity [47]. Furthermore, the amino acid residues critical for alkyl hydroperoxidase activity (Cys125, His132, and Tyr127), GATOR2-binding and AMPK activation for mTORC1 inhibition (Asp406 and Asp407), and leucine-binding (Glu451 and Arg390; Leu389, Trp444, and Phe447; Thr374, Thr377, and Thr386) are all evolutionarily conserved in the three human sestrins. It is therefore reasonable to speculate that hSesn1 and hSesn3 may share most, if not all, of the functional roles of hSesn2. However, as compared with sestrin2, the potential involvement of sestrin1 and sestrin3 in nervous systems has been studied much less well. Below, in Figure 2B, is the list of known biological functions of all three sestrins.

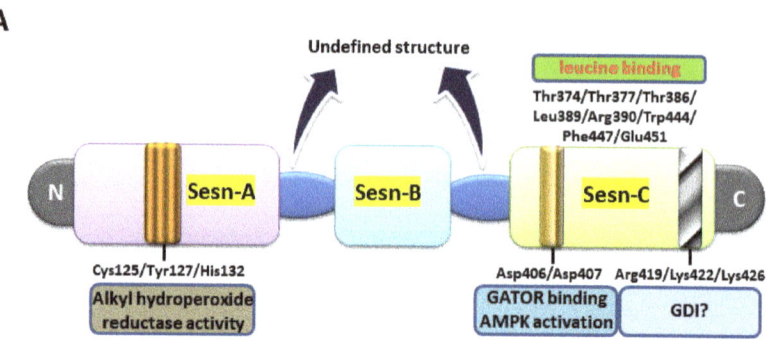

Figure 2. The structural and functional domains as well as the biological functions of three sestrin members. (**A**) The strip diagram illustrates the three major structural domains (Sesn-A, Sesn-B, and Sesn-C). Cys125/Tyr127/His132, located within the Sesn-A domain, is critical for alkyl hydroperoxidase activity. The Asp406/Asp407 residues, the so-called "DD motif", located within Sesn-C are vital for GATOR2 binding and AMPK activation, both contributing to mTORC1 suppression. The leucine binding pocket spanning from Thr374 to Glu451 in the Sesn-C is also important for amino acid sensing and mTOR regulation. The guanosine nucleotide dissociation inhibition (GDI) domain containing Arg419/Lys422/Lys426 is also shown in Sesn-C. Based on the crystal structure, however, whether these amino acid residues are critical for GDI functions remains questionable. All the information was based on Kim et al., 2015 [35] and Saxton et al., 2016 [36]. (**B**) Potential biological functions of three sestrins are listed. Information was derived from UniProt (https://www.uniprot.org) for human sestrin1 [UniProtKB-Q9Y6P5 (SESN1_HUMAN)], human sestrin2 [UniProtKB-P58004 (SESN2_HUMAN), human sestrin3 [UniProtKB-P58005 (SESN3_HUMAN)], and mouse sestrin3 [UniProtKB- Q9CYP7 (SESN3_MOUSE)].

Expression of the sestrin2 genes is regulated by several critical transcription factors, enabling the cells to cope with various stressful insults. Initially the crucial role of the p53 tumor suppressor in regulating the expression of sestrin2 under hypoxic and genotoxic stress was revealed [33]. Later, additional studies revealed further transcription factors that are critical for the expression of sestrin2 under a variety of stressful conditions. Oxidative stress can activate the nuclear factor erythroid 2-related factor-2 (Nrf2) to regulate sestrin2 expression [48,49]. Hypoxia may induce sestrin2 expression where hypoxia-inducible factor-1 (HIF-1) may play a certain role [33,50–52], although the detailed mechanism is not well understood. In our earlier study [53], we found that brain-derived neurotrophic factor (BDNF) induced sestrin2 expression, which required dimerization of nuclear factor-κB (NF-κB) subunits p65 and p50. Further, BDNF also enhanced production of nitric oxide (NO), formation of 3′,5′-cyclic guanosine monophosphate (cGMP), and activation of cGMP-dependent protein kinase (PKG). Indeed, BDNF induced nuclear translocation of PKG-1 and its direct interaction with p65/p50 to form a ternary complex, thereby leading to heightened NF-κB binding to the sestrin2 gene promoter with resultant upregulation of its mRNA and proteins [53]. Apart from PKG/NF-κB, BDNF has also been shown to induce sestrin2 in neurons by activating transcription factor-4 (ATF4) [54]. In another recent study [40], we also found that NF-κB and p53 are involved in Aβ-induced sestrin2 expression in primary cortical neurons. Additional regulatory mechanisms responsible for sestrin2 induction under various stressful or physiological conditions may emerge in the near future.

Nutrients including amino acids, lipids, and glucose are crucial for the biosynthetic processes in the cell. An inadequate supply of nutrients can seriously modify cellular metabolism. Sestrin2 activation may serve as one of the metabolic accommodations to nutrient deficiency in cells [38]. Glucose starvation, inhibition of glycolysis, and impairment of mitochondrial respiration can disrupt energy production, leading to the activation of two transcription factors, ATF4 and Nrf2, that can bind directly to the consensus sequences within the promoter to induce sestrin2 gene transcription [49,55–57]. ATF4 is also involved in the induction of sestrin2 as a result of a deficiency in amino acid supply in mouse embryonic fibroblasts [58]. The inadequacy of growth factors may result in the expression of sestrin2. It has been demonstrated in cancer cells that serum deprivation can activate the c-Jun N-terminal kinase (JNK) pathway and upregulate sestrin2 expression, which could be abolished by specific siRNAs against JNK1/2 or c-Jun [59]. Various physiological and pathological conditions, such as excessive ROS generation, ischemia, $Ca^{2+}$ dyshomeostasis, and inflammatory response can all cause an accumulation of misfolded proteins in the endoplasmic reticulum (ER), with resultant ER stress [60]. ER stress may lead to cellular dysfunction and/or cell death and contributes to the progression of many diseases. Modulation of ER stress pathways may represent a potential therapeutic strategy. It was reported that activating transcription factor-6 (ATF6)-dependent sestrin2 induction can lessen the severity of ER stress-mediated liver injury [61]. In another study, it was shown that the hepatoprotective role of sestrin2 against chronic ER stress depends on the regulation of CCAAT-enhancer-binding protein-beta (c/EBPβ) [62]. Together, these previous reports identify the crucial roles played by sestrin2 in dealing with various cellular stresses under diverse physiological and pathological conditions. A simplified diagram (Figure 3) demonstrates that distinct transcription factors are activated under a variety of stressful conditions, thereby leading to induction of sestrin2 expression, which can regulate autophagy and contribute to antioxidation.

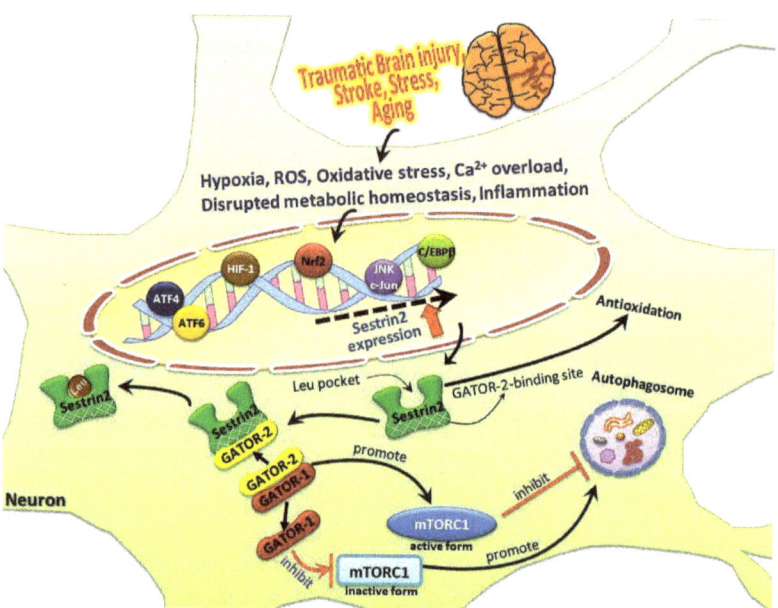

**Figure 3.** Brain trauma, stroke, neurological disorders, and aging induce hypoxia, the production of reactive oxygen species (ROS), $Ca^{2+}$ overload, metabolic dyshomeostasis, and neuronal inflammation. Subsequently, the injury-induced signaling pathways promote sestrin2 expression via the activation of various transcription factors (which particular factors depending on which stressors), such as transcription factor-4 (ATF4), ATF6, hypoxia-inducible factor-1 (HIF-1), nuclear factor erythroid 2-related factor-2 (Nrf2), c-Jun N-terminal kinase (JNK)/c-Jun, and CCAAT-enhancer-binding protein-beta (C/EBPβ). Sestrin2, as a sensor for essential amino acids with a leucine-binding pocket, also has a binding site for the GTPase-activating protein activity toward Rags-2 (GATOR2). In the presence of sufficient amino acids available for protein synthesis, sestrin2 may bind to leucine and release the bound GATOR2. The freed GATOR2 can then physically associate with GATOR1, which can no longer bind to, and hence inhibit, mTORC1, thereby promoting protein synthesis while inhibiting autophagy. Under the stressful condition in which amino acids are insufficient, binding of GATOR2 to sestrin2 allows GATOR1 to inhibit mTORC1, thereby promoting autophagy while inhibiting protein synthesis. In addition to regulating autophagy and protein synthesis via binding with leucine or GATOR2, the endogenous alkyl hydroperoxidase activity of sestrin2 also exerts direct antioxidative actions.

## 3. Sestrin2 in Age-Related Clinical Conditions

Persuasive evidence supports the notion that aging is related to various harmful mechanisms, such as escalation of oxidative stress, instability of genetic materials, declined protein homeostasis, impaired mitochondrial function, increased cellular senescence, and stem cell exhaustion [63]. The accumulation of various cellular damages among tissues in aging organisms leads eventually to functional breakdown, causing disability or death. Therefore, aging is believed to be a risk factor for various disorders, such as cardiovascular diseases, stroke, type II diabetes, cancers, and neurodegenerative diseases [63–65]. Inhibition of either ROS production or mTORC1 activation may counteract aging [35], and as sestrin2 is characterized by both these functions, it may exert such beneficial effects [66,67]. In fact, enhancement of sestrin2 expression reduces aging markers. Conversely, lessening sestrin2 expression accelerates aging processes [68].

Aging is a predetermined time-related deterioration in various physiological conditions, and is a critical risk factor for cancer development. Cancer and aging involve similar processes of progressive time-dependent cellular damage. As sestrin2 is critically involved in aging [38,67], it may play a pivotal role in cancer progression, and is regarded as a potential tumor suppressor. In non-small cell lung cancer patients, higher sestrin2 expression was a favorable prognostic factor, while lower sestrin2 expression was accompanied by poor tumor cell differentiation, as well as more advanced staging in terms of tumor, node, and metastasis (TNM) [69]. It was shown that colorectal cancer patients with lower expression of sestrin2 showed poor prognostic outcomes [70]. Docosahexaenoic acid (DHA) can increase oxaliplatin-induced autophagic cell death through the ER stress/sestrin2 pathway in colorectal cancer [71], whereas downregulation of sestrin2 can accelerate colon carcinogenesis [72].

Hypernutrition, causing obesity, hepatosteatosis, and insulin resistance, is related to chronic activation of p70S6 kinase and mTORC1 [73]. Activation of sestrin2 can lower the extents of fatty liver and insulin resistance [73]. Sestrin2 can activate AMPK, inhibit mTORC1 activity, and maintain a high AKT level to suppress the extent of gluconeogenesis in the liver, thereby reducing the level of blood sugar. Sestrin2-deficient obese mice were found to present an evident decline of AKT activity, leading to insulin resistance and a higher level of glucose production [73]. In a recent study, serum levels of sestrins are significantly decreased in patients with diabetes and dyslipidemia. It appears that sestrin2 levels are robustly associated with diabetes, dyslipidemia, atherosclerosis, and the atherogenic index [74]. Declined serum sestrin2 levels were also observed in diabetic patients with nephropathy, particularly in those with macroalbuminuria [75].

It was demonstrated previously that loss of dSestrin (the only one sestrin homologue in Drosophila) results in age-associated pathologies, including cardiac dysfunction, muscle degeneration, and triglyceride accumulation. The cardiac dysfunction showed reduced heart rate and compromised heart function. The detrimental effects induced by dSestrin deficiency were generally inhibited by AICAR and rapamycin, the AMPK activator and the mTORC1 inhibitor, respectively [67]. These results indicate that the sestrin family may play crucial roles in the pathophysiology of cardiac regulation [76]. In a recent review article, sestrin2 is considered a rising star among antioxidants, with future therapeutic potential for reducing heart injury induced by oxidative stress, promoting cell survival through the activation of Nrf2/AMPK, and inhibiting mTORC1 to combat various cardiovascular diseases, such as cardiomyopathy, heart failure, and myocardial infarction [77]. Despite these promises, however, the occurrence of major adverse cardiac events is predicted in patients with chronic heart failure who have higher plasma sestrin2 concentrations [78]. The conflicting results as far as the beneficial or detrimental effects of sestrin2 in heart failure are concerned await further clarification.

Stroke is the most common age-related cerebral vascular disease and the chief cause of physical and intellectual disability in adults, as well as the leading cause of mortality in developed countries [79]. Several studies have investigated the roles of sestrin2 in cerebral ischemia [80–83]. It was demonstrated that sestrin2 can activate the Nrf2/heme oxygenase-1 (HO-1) pathway, leading to augmentation of angiogenesis following focal cerebral ischemia [82]. Another study also showed the critical role of sestrin2 in promoting angiogenesis in focal cerebral ischemia by activating the Nrf2/p62 pathway [81]. In contrast, silencing sestrin2 expression may reduce mitochondrial activity, suppress mitochondrial biogenesis, and ultimately exacerbate cerebral ischemia/reperfusion injury by preventing the AMPK/PGC-1α pathway [83]. Although sestrin2 seems to have pro-survival characteristics in the context of ischemic brain injury, the anti-inflammatory role of sestrin2 is unknown. In a recent study, it was demonstrated that sestrin2 exerts neuroprotective effects by changing microglial polarization and mitigating the extent of inflammation in the ischemic mouse brain, which may be due to the inhibition of the mTOR pathway and the restoration of autophagic flux [80]. It is to be expected that knowledge of the mechanisms underlying additional protective effects of sestrin2 may emerge in the not too distant future.

## 4. Potential Roles of Sestrin2 in Age-Related Neurodegenerative Diseases: Focusing on AD

As mentioned above, the sequences of the critical amino acid residues important for known biological activities of hSesn2, including alkyl hydroperoxide reductase, mTORC1 inhibition, and leucine binding, are also conserved in hSesn1 and hSesn3. However, the crystal structures of sestrin1 and sestrin3 are still not available. Nevertheless, there are a few studies implicating sestrin1 and sestrin3 in nervous system disorders. For example, sestrin1 may exert protective effects in oxygen-glucose deprivation/reoxygenation (OGD/R)-induced neuronal injury, a cellular model for mimicking cerebral ischemia/reperfusion injury in vitro [84]. Furthermore, sestrin3 has been identified as a pro-convulsant gene network in the human epileptic hippocampus [85]. Results derived from sestrin3 knockout rats also suggested that sestrin3 may increase the occurrence and/or severity of seizures [86]. Conversely, silencing rno-miR-155-5p in vivo mitigated the pathophysiological features associated with the status epilepticus, which was accompanied by attenuation of apoptosis in the hippocampus, by enhancing expression of sestrin3 in rats, implying that sestrin3 plays a beneficial role in offsetting temporal lobe epilepsy [87]. Further dissection of the pathophysiological roles of sestrin1 and sestrin3 will require a greater understanding of their molecular structures, as well as the upstream regulatory mechanisms involved in their expression in nervous systems.

Among age-related disorders, chronic neurodegenerative diseases are particularly concerning due to the lack of efficacious treatments, their irremediable clinical course, and their association with substantial social-economic burdens [1–3]. The potential roles of sestrin2 in combatting neurodegenerative diseases, including AD, Parkinson's disease (PD), and Huntington's disease (HD), while still awaiting further evidence, have gradually been recognized in recent years.

It is widely accepted that maintaining proper levels of reactive nitrogen species and ROS are crucial for ensuring regular neuronal function [88]. Yet, excessive ROS generation with heightened levels of oxidation in lipids, proteins, and DNA, or inherent lower antioxidant competence in the brain, may have detrimental effects on the organism and play a role in the pathophysiology of various chronic neurodegenerative diseases, including AD, PD, and HD [89,90]. Numerous mechanisms underlie oxidative stress-mediated neurodegeneration; these include calcium overload, glutamate excitotoxicity, inflammation, functional impairment of mitochondria, and apoptotic processes [88]. The ability to lessen these harmful effects may be the key to developing effective treatments for neurodegenerative diseases.

As mentioned above, sestrin2, with its dual functions, can directly reduce oxidative stress through restoring overoxidized peroxiredoxins, and indirectly lessen oxidative stress through regulating mTOR to augment the activity of autophagy, or specifically, mitophagy, to remove the worn-out or damaged mitochondria with higher levels of electron leakage and hence free radical production. The N-terminal domain of sestrin2 decreases oxidative stress by its helix-turn-helix motif, while the C-terminal domain of sestrin2 may physically associate with GATOR2, thereby causing the inhibition of mTORC1 [35]. Apart from the effect of oxidative stress, one more common pathogenic mechanism in chronic neurodegeneration is the deposition of aberrant and/or misfolded proteins, such as $A\beta$ and tau protein in AD, Lewy body (LB) in PD, and mutant huntingtin in HD. Enhancing the activity of autophagy may help to eradicate neuronal dysfunction induced by misfolded proteins, thereby opening an opportunity towards developing a new therapeutic strategy for treating neurodegenerative diseases [91]. The dual biological functions of sestrin2, with increasing antioxidative ability and autophagy-promoting activity to eliminate aggregated proteins and damaged mitochondria, give this molecule a unique position in protecting neurons against degeneration.

PD is the second most common aging-related neurodegenerative disease that mainly presents syndromes with slow movements, tremors, and rigidity. The underlying cause of PD is not well understood but may involve various genetic and environmental factors [92]. The main pathological feature of PD is LB, which is composed of ubiquitin-bound, misfolded α-synuclein protein in the dopamine neurons in the substantia nigra of the midbrain [93,94]. In an in vitro PD model with 1-methyl-4-phenylpyridinium (MPP$^+$), it was revealed that MPP$^+$ neurotoxicity increases sestrin2 expression, whereas downregulation of sestrin2 with small interference RNA augments MPP$^+$-related neurotoxicity in SH-SY5Y cells [95]. In another in vivo PD model induced by rotenone, sestrin2 exerts a protective effect over dopaminergic neurons against rotenone-induced neurotoxicity by activating an AMPK-dependent autophagy pathway [96]. In a clinical study, serum sestrin2 levels were found to be elevated in PD patients compared to controls [97]. In postmortem human samples, it was found that PD patients had higher expression levels of sestrin2 in the midbrain [95].

No report was available concerning HD and sestrin2 either in the clinical or pre-clinical studies. 3-Nitropropionic acid (3-NP) can inhibit the function of the mitochondrial respiratory complex II (also named succinate dehydrogenase), decrease ATP production, impair cellular energy metabolism, aggravate the extent of oxidative stress, cause mitochondrial DNA damage, and thus impair the function of mitochondria [98,99]. Although genetic models of HD are more popular due to their similarity to the phenotypes observed in HD, 3-NP is still a useful model to study neurotoxic phenomena, mitochondrial alterations, and neuroprotective effects for HD patients [100]. Therefore, 3-NP has been used as a pharmacological model to study neurodegeneration and neuronal death involving mitochondrial dysfunction in HD [101]. Despite the indirect relationship, we have shown that BDNF protects 3-NP-induced oxidative stress through augmenting sestrin2 expression. Furthermore, BDNF induction of sestrin2 implicates the NO/PKG/NF-κB pathway [53]. This study thus highlights the probable beneficial role of sestrin2 in this devastating hereditary neurodegenerative disease. Understanding the potential role of sestrin2 in impeding HD pathogenesis may require further investigation into the genetic models of HD, such as R6/2 or other knock-in mice.

AD is the most common age-related neurodegenerative disease involving various pathogenic mechanisms such as excitotoxicity, excessive generation of ROS, aberrant cell cycle reentry, impaired mitochondrial function, and DNA damage [15–19]. Although emerging roles of sestrin2 in various neurological diseases have been suggested before [102], limited studies concerning sestrin2 and AD have been reported [39,40,103–107]. In a 2003 study, in which human neuroblastoma CHP134 cells were analyzed with cDNA microarray technology with confirmation by semi-quantitative RT-PCR, it was revealed that sestrin2 is overexpressed under treatment of Aβ [107]. Furthermore, in human neuroblastoma SH-SY5Y cells, Aβ1-42 dose-dependently enhanced sestrin2 expression, whereas cotreatment with atorvastatin reversed sestrin2 back to the control level [103]. We have also demonstrated, in primary cortical neurons, that both Aβ25-35 and Aβ1-42 triggered the expression of sestrin2 [39,40], as is discussed in more detail below. In addition to these pre-clinical studies, the first human study reported in 2012 using postmortem brain tissues from advanced AD patients with immunohistochemistry findings showed intense sestrin2 expression in the neuropil, which may suggest a diffuse expression in various components among neurons, glia, and vascular cells. Using double-labeling immunofluorescence microscopy, co-localization between phosphorylated tau and sestrin2 is observed in the neurons and the neurites in neurofibrillary lesions [106]. These findings together implied that sestrin2 is expressed at least in the neurons of AD patients. Another clinical study demonstrated significant overexpression of sestrin2 protein and mRNA in the serum of AD patients as compared to the mild cognitive impairment (MCI) and the age-matched control groups. A difference in serum sestrin2 concentration between MCI and the control groups was also evident. However, no significant difference in sestrin1 levels was observed among the study groups. These results therefore suggested the potential role of sestrin2 as a biomarker in the analysis of peripheral blood in AD patients, and highlighted the importance of sestrin2, as opposed to sestrin1, in the progression of AD [104]. Despite these arguments supporting the important roles of sestrin2 in AD, it should be noted that, with similar biological functions and significantly conserved amino acid sequences identified across the different members of the sestrin family, although potential involvements of sestrin1 and sestrin3 in AD have not been reported, they certainly cannot be overlooked. Overall, this review has only focused on discussing the potential roles of sestrin2 in neurodegenerative disorders, AD in particular.

We have explored the potential link between sestrin2 and Aβ-induced neurotoxicity [39,40]. In an in vitro study, we demonstrated that sestrin2 was induced by Aβs, including both Aβ25-35 and Aβ1-42, in primary culture of fetal rat cortical neurons. We further showed an in vivo result of increased sestrin2 expression in the aged APPswe/PSEN1dE9 transgenic mice. More importantly, sestrin2 functions as an endogenous protective moderator, through the adjustment of autophagy, against Aβ-induced neurotoxicity [39]. It is well known that sestrin2 has an antioxidant character and plays a critical role in age-related diseases [66]. In our recent report [40], Aβ-induced sestrin2 expression in primary cortical neurons was found to have an antioxidant effect, resulting in the suppression of Aβ-mediated ROS production, enhancement of lipid peroxidation, and formation of 8-hydroxy-2-deoxyguanosine (8-OH-dG) as an index of oxidative DNA damage. Interestingly, we found that lentivirus-mediated overexpression of the N-terminal domain of sestrin2 in primary cortical neurons completely blocked Aβ25-35-induced ROS production, whereas overexpression of the C-terminal domain partially, but statistically significantly, suppressed ROS formation. Although the sestrin2 C-terminal domain is known to have the capability of inhibiting mTORC1 to promote autophagy [35], we speculated that augmentation of autophagy with enhanced removal of damaged mitochondria, or mitophagy, may also contribute to the antioxidant function of sestrin2. Upstream of sestrin2, we found that the observed Aβ effect on sestrin2 expression is at least partially mediated by p53 and NF-κB. Indeed, apart from regulating sestrin2 induction, p53 and NF-κB subunits p65/p50 also affect the expression of each other [40]. Furthermore, upstream of p53 and NF-κB, we identified at least two signaling pathways, namely nitric oxide synthase/cGMP-dependent protein kinase (NOS/PKG) and phosphatidylinositol 3-kinase (PI3K)/Akt, that may have contributed to the observed Aβ induction of sestrin2 in cortical neurons [40]. A diagram summarizing our findings is shown in Figure 4, below.

The synaptic activity of neurons can affect the homeostasis of Aβ and tau. Both are aggregated and accumulated during the progression of AD and are critical for neuronal function. Furthermore, impairment of synaptic activity is linked with AD [108]. Physiologic synaptic activity, through NMDA receptor signaling, can enhance antioxidant activity and increase sestrin2 expression to exert a protective effect through transcription factor C/EBPbeta [109]. Presenilin proteins are catalytic components of γ-secretase involved in various functions such as proteolytic cleavage of the Notch and APP, adjustment of neurotransmitter release, and are vital for the survival of neurons in aging [110]. Mutations of the presenilin genes are one of the main causes of familial AD [111]. Impairment of presenilin activity may compromise synaptic functions, resulting in neurodegeneration and ultimately dementia [112]. It was demonstrated that cells deficient in presenilin have lower levels of sestrin2 and are accompanied with mTORC1 dysregulation. These findings show that sestrin2, through attenuation of oxidative stress and its nutrient-sensing ability via mTOR, plays a critical role in AD-related conditions [105].

Emerging evidence suggested the potential benefit of sestrin2 in AD. Medications with the capability to alter sestrin2 expression may therefore have the potential to prevent or delay the clinical deterioration of this neurodegenerative disease. It was previously shown that atorvastatin reduces Aβ-induced synaptotoxicity and memory impairment through a p38MAP kinase pathway [113]. Atorvastatin could also activate autophagy through AMPK/mTOR signaling [113,114]. In a recent study, it was demonstrated that sestrin2 and the autophagy marker LC3II were increased with Aβ treatment in human neuroblastoma cells; co-treatment of atorvastatin and Aβ reduced oxidative stress and decreased sestrin2 expression [103]. We have shown before that BDNF can induce sestrin2 expression in rat primary cortical neurons and exert a protective effect against 3-NP neurotoxicity by reducing the production of free radicals [53]. BDNF is known to protect against Aβ-induced neurotoxicity in vitro as well as in rodent and primate models [115,116]. However, whether sestrin2 induction by BDNF contributes to this neuroprotective effect has not been tested. The possibility certainly cannot, however, be excluded.

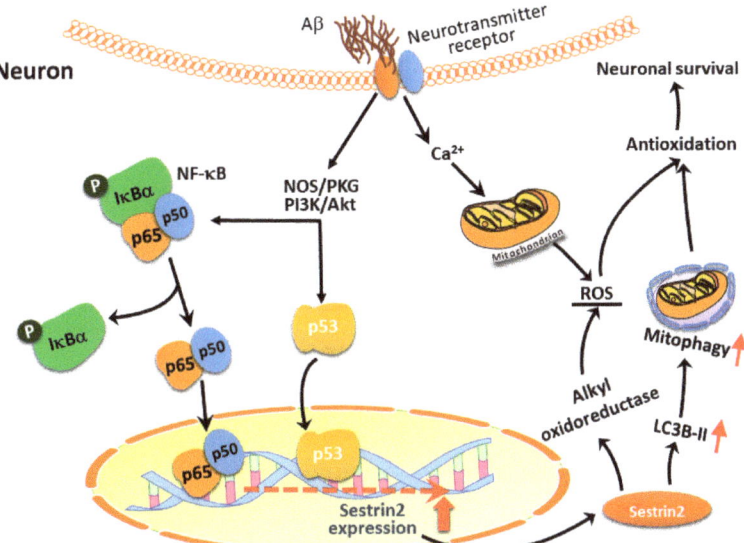

**Figure 4.** Amyloid-beta peptide (Aβ) enhances calcium dyshomeostasis and the generation of reactive oxygen species (ROS), thereby leading to oxidative stress with damaged mitochondria. Meanwhile, Aβ also induces p53, as well as nuclear factor-kappaB (NF-κB) subunits p65 and p50 via activation of nitric oxide synthase (NOS)/cGMP-dependent protein kinase (PKG) and phosphatidylinositol 3-kinase (PI3K)/Akt. The transcription factors, p50, p65, and p53 translocate into the nucleus of the neuron to promote expression of sestrin2 mRNA, as indicated by the red dashed arrow. The alkyl hydroperoxidase activity of sestrin2 may neutralize excessive ROS generated by Aβ with antioxidative functions. In addition, sestrin2 may trigger autophagy, as is indicated by the conversion of the microtubule-associated protein-1 light-chain 3B-I (LC3B-I) into LC3B-II, and possibly also mitophagy, in order to remove Aβ-damaged mitochondria known to produce more ROS. Sestrin2 thus may function as an endogenous protective mediator inducible by Aβ that contributes to neuronal survival against Aβ neurotoxicity.

In addition to alkyl hydroperoxidase activity and enhanced autophagy to alleviate oxidative stress, sestrin2 may also trigger the Nrf2/ARE pathway to augment antioxidant responses. For example, following photochemical cerebral ischemia in rats, expression of sestrin2, Nrf2, HO-1, and VEGF were significantly increased. Overexpression of sestrin2 by AAV injection further enhanced their expression [82]. In another study of photothrombotic ischemia in rats, sestrin2 may promote angiogenesis by activating Nrf2 via upregulation of p62 with enhanced interaction between p62 and Keap1, thereby improving the neurological function, reducing brain infarction, and alleviating brain edema [81]. Sestrin2 was also a direct target of microRNA miR-148b-3p in the HT22 hippocampal neurons challenged with OGD/R. Furthermore, Nrf2/ARE was a downstream antioxidant signal contributing to the observed protective effects through miR-148b-3p inhibition, and hence sestrin2 induction, in response to OGD/R injury [117]. In the $H_2O_2$-stimulated retinal ganglion cells (RGCs), sestrin2 overexpression increased the nuclear translocation of Nrf2, thereby upregulating the Nrf2/ARE target genes, including HO-1 and NAD(P)H quinone oxidoreductase-1 [118]. As mentioned above, sestrin2 itself may be a downstream target of Nrf2 [48,49]. Although these studies were conducted in non-neuronal cells like mammary epithelial cells and hepatocytes, the possibility that Nrf2 activation may induce sestrin2 expression in the nervous system cannot be excluded. Whether sestrin2 may trigger its own expression, thereby forming a positive feedforward loop, via Nrf2/ARE in neurons, also requires further investigation. The potential role of sestrin2 in age-related neurodegenerative diseases is demonstrated in Figure 5.

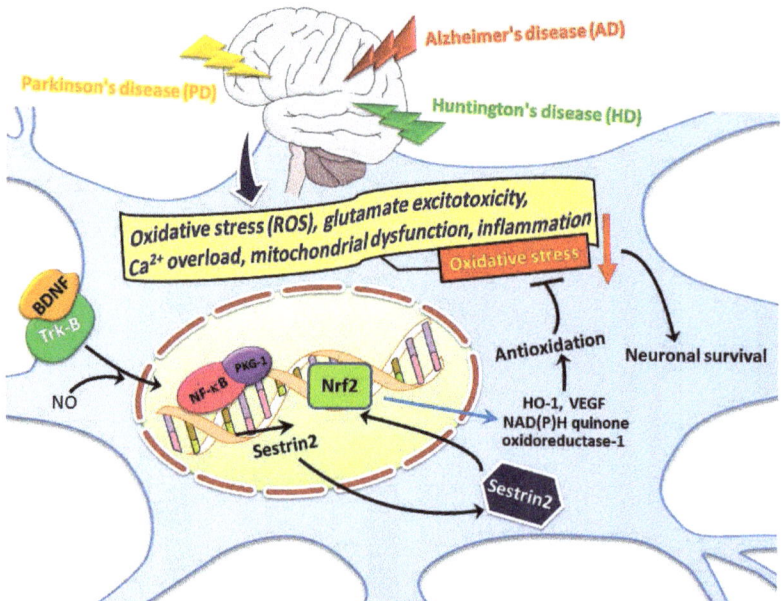

**Figure 5.** Multiple pathogenic mechanisms including oxidative stress, with excessive production of reactive oxygen species (ROS), glutamate-induced excitotoxicity, calcium overload, mitochondrial dysfunction, and inflammation contribute to neuronal death in various neurodegenerative disorders like Alzheimer's disease (AD), Parkinson's disease (PD), and Huntington's disease (HD). Brain-derived neurotrophic factor (BDNF) enhances sestrin2 expression via signaling pathways involving nitric oxide (NO)/3′,5′-cyclic guanosine monophosphate (cGMP)-dependent protein kinase-1 (PKG-1)/nuclear factor-kappaB (NF-κB). In addition to the alkyl hydroperoxidase activity and autophagy promotion, sestrin2 may also have antioxidant properties by activating nuclear factor erythroid 2-related factor-2 (Nrf2) with enhanced expression of antioxidant proteins like heme oxygenase-1 (HO-1), vascular endothelial growth factor (VEGF), and NAD(P)H quinone oxidoreductase-1. These antioxidant proteins then mitigate oxidative stress, as indicated by the red arrow, that is commonly observed in various neurodegenerative diseases. The possibility that BDNF may exert its neuroprotective effects, in addition to its well-known neurotrophic actions, via induction of sestrin2 in various neurodegenerative disorders, requires further investigation.

## 5. Medications or Chemical Compounds Capable of Altering Sestrin2 Expression

The outcomes of clinical trials using drugs to target amyloid and tau have been unsatisfactory up to now, thereby leading to enthusiasm in targeting alternative mechanisms in AD studies [119,120]. Drug repurposing involves taking the research into an existing, ready-to-use drug and assessing its therapeutic potential with respect to another disease [121,122]. Several well-known success stories include aspirin, sildenafil, and thalidomide [123]. This approach may provide a less expensive and quicker method of drug discovery. Several recent review articles emphasize the clinical potential of drug repurposing in the context of AD [120,124–126]. It would be worthwhile to search among medications with neuroprotective effects, as these are likely to have a better chance of achieving clinically meaningful results with neurodegenerative diseases [127]. The potential of certain medications to activate sestrin2 expression requires further investigation.

Several studies revealed that certain drugs capable of activating sestrin2 expression in various disease models may be worth testing in AD as well. It was shown that empagliflozin, which is a sodium-glucose cotransporter 2 (SGLT2) inhibitor useful for treating diabetes mellitus (DM) patients, can regulate sestrin2, the AMPK-mTOR pathway, and ROS homeostasis to improve obesity-related cardiac dysfunction in mice [128]. Another study demonstrated that liraglutide, a glucagon-like peptide 1 (GLP-1) agonist for DM patients, may lessen obesity-related fatty liver disease through regulating the sestrin2-mediated Nrf2/HO-1 pathway [129].

5-Fluorouracil is an antimetabolite widely used for chemotherapeutic treatment of cancers [130,131]. It was shown that 5-fluorouracil increases sestrin2 levels in a p53-dependent pathway and inhibits cancer cell migration in an in vitro colon cancer study [132]. Nelfinavir, an ER stress-inducing agent, and bortezomib, a proteasome inhibitor, can both enhance sestrin2 expression, which may be useful to treat cancers [133]. Interestingly, nelfinavir inhibited endogenous Aβ1-40 production from primary cultured human cortical neurons [134]. Whether these reagents may also carry therapeutic potential for AD requires further investigation.

Other chemical compounds such as resveratrol and melatonin possessing pleiotropic effects like antioxidancy or anti-inflammation were studied based on their capability of upregulating sestrin2 in various disease models [135–137]. Resveratrol is a naturally occurring polyphenol that is abundant in grape seeds and skin [138,139]. It can offer protective effects against various age-related diseases like AD through diverse mechanisms [138,140]. These molecular mechanisms include modulation of NF-κB, regulation of inflammatory cytokines, production of antioxidant enzymes, angiogenesis, apoptosis, lipid metabolism, and mitochondrial biogenesis-all critical for its potential clinical application [141,142]. It was demonstrated before that resveratrol affects sestrin2 gene induction and inhibits liver X receptor-alpha (LXRα)-mediated hepatic lipogenesis [137]. Methylglyoxal is implicated in the formation of advanced glycation end-products associated with diabetes and age-related neurodegenerative diseases [143]. In a previous study using methylglyoxal to induce cell death in HepG2, a human liver cancer cell line, it was found that resveratrol reduces methylglyoxal-induced mitochondrial impairment and apoptosis through sestrin2 induction [136]. Other flavonoid polyphenols or flavone derivatives, such as eupatilin [144,145], pentamethylquercetin [146], and isorhamentin [147], also possess the capability to alter sestrin2 expression and are worth studying further in AD models.

Melatonin, a molecule widely distributed in living organisms, is involved in various physiological and biological functions among diverse tissues and organs. It possesses prominent antioxidant effects, functions as a free radical scavenger, augments antioxidant enzymes, lessens mitochondrial electron leakage, and reduces pro-inflammatory signaling pathways [148]. These properties of melatonin underline the possibility for future clinical use in numerous disorders, including neurodegeneration [149]. It was shown that melatonin can inhibit proliferation and apoptosis in the vascular smooth muscle through upregulation of sestrin2, which may be important in preventing atherosclerosis and restenosis of vessel lumen [135]. It would be interesting to know the effect of sestrin2 expression under melatonin treatment in a stressful condition, such as in Aβ-induced neurotoxicity.

It is believed that a long list of medications, natural products, chemical compounds, or small molecules capable of altering sestrin2 expression may exert beneficial effects over AD-related mechanisms. This awaits further investigation and may lead to more opportunities for treating such devastating neurodegenerative diseases as AD.

## 6. Conclusions and Future Perspectives

Being a member of the sestrin family, sestrin2 acts as a crucial intracellular detector capable of regulating various biological processes to maintain the homeostasis of living organisms. Emerging evidence reveals that sestrin2 may have beneficial effects for vulnerable cells, such that they may adapt to numerous pathological situations under diverse stressful conditions, including DNA injury, hypoxic state, metabolic dyshomeostasis, and oxidative stress. In age-related neurodegenerative disorders, excessive generation of ROS and dysfunction of autophagy may play pivotal roles in the pathogenesis among these diseases. Sestrin2, with distinctive dual-functional sites to counteract excessive ROS generation and inhibit mTOR activity for autophagy promotion, is presumed to play a crucial role in AD, although at present only limited information is available to firmly establish this notion. Certain medicinal compounds or natural products, such as flavonoid-related products, can alter the expression levels of sestrin2. It is believed that any means of increasing sestrin2 expression may possess significant clinical implications for the abatement of AD-related neurodegeneration. The possibility awaits further investigation. It is uncertain, however, whether the overactivation of sestrin2 may result in detrimental effects due to autophagic dysfunction. It may be difficult to determine the pros and cons of excessive activation or inhibition of autophagy in terms of neurodegenerative diseases, including AD. This concern further reveals the crucial need for a thorough understanding of both the downstream targets, as well as the upstream regulators, of sestrin2. Fuller elucidation of the signaling pathways of sestrin2 would accelerate the discovery of novel therapies for disease treatment, especially for those diseases with a devastating clinical course, such as AD.

**Funding:** This study was supported by the Ministry of Science and Technology (MOST) in Taiwan (MOST 104-2314-B-010-014-MY2, MOST 107-2314-B-010-020-MY3, and MOST 109-2314-B-010-038-MY3 to Ding-I Yang; MOST 108-2314-B-037-038-MY3 to A-Ching Chao; MOST 109-2314-B-182A-078-MY3 to Shang-Der Chen; MOST 108-2320-B-182A-005-MY3 to Jenq-Lin Yang), Department of Health in Taipei City Government (11001-62-038 to Ding-I Yang), and Chang Gung Medical Foundation (CMRPG8I0051, CMRPG8I0052, and CMRPG8I0053 to Shang-Der Chen; CMRPG8K0652 to Jenq-Lin Yang). This study was also financially supported by Kaohsiung Medical University Hospital (KMUH109-9R72 to A-Ching Chao) and Brain Research Center, National Yang Ming Chiao Tung University, from The Featured Areas Research Center Program within the framework of the Higher Education Sprout Project by the Ministry of Education (MOE) in Taiwan (110BRC-B407 to Ding-I Yang).

**Conflicts of Interest:** The authors declare no conflict of interest.

## References

1. Dugger, B.N.; Dickson, D.W. Pathology of Neurodegenerative Diseases. *Cold Spring Harb. Perspect. Biol.* **2017**, *9*, a028035. [CrossRef]
2. Takizawa, C.; Thompson, P.L.; van Walsem, A.; Faure, C.; Maier, W.C. Epidemiological and Economic Burden of Alzheimer's Disease: A Systematic Literature Review of Data across Europe and the United States of America. *J. Alzheimer's Dis.* **2014**, *43*, 1271–1284. [CrossRef]
3. Hung, C.-W.; Chen, Y.-C.; Hsieh, W.-L.; Chiou, S.-H.; Kao, C.-L. Ageing and neurodegenerative diseases. *Ageing Res. Rev.* **2010**, *9*, S36–S46. [CrossRef]
4. 2021 Alzheimer's disease facts and figures. *Alzheimer's Dement.* **2021**, *17*, 327–406. [CrossRef] [PubMed]
5. Economic burden of Alzheimer disease and managed care considerations. *Am. J. Manag. Care* **2020**, *26*, S177–S183. [PubMed]
6. DeTure, M.A.; Dickson, D.W. The neuropathological diagnosis of Alzheimer's disease. *Mol. Neurodegener.* **2019**, *14*, 32. [CrossRef]
7. Jack, C.R., Jr.; Bennett, D.A.; Blennow, K.; Carrillo, M.C.; Dunn, B.; Haeberlein, S.B.; Holtzman, D.M.; Jagust, W.; Jessen, F.; Karlawish, J.; et al. NIA-AA Research Framework: Toward a biological definition of Alzheimer's disease. *Alzheimer's Dement.* **2018**, *14*, 535–562. [CrossRef] [PubMed]
8. Murphy, M.P.; LeVine, H., III. Alzheimer's Disease and the Amyloid-β Peptide. *J. Alzheimer's Dis.* **2010**, *19*, 311–323. [CrossRef] [PubMed]
9. O'Brien, R.J.; Wong, P.C. Amyloid Precursor Protein Processing and Alzheimer's Disease. *Annu. Rev. Neurosci.* **2011**, *34*, 185–204. [CrossRef]
10. Octave, J.N. The amyloid peptide precursor in Alzheimer's disease. *Acta Neurol. Belg.* **1995**, *95*, 197–209. [CrossRef]

11. Seubert, P.; Oltersdorf, T.; Lee, M.G.; Barbour, R.; Blomquist, C.; Davis, D.L.; Bryant, K.; Fritz, L.C.; Galasko, D.; Thal, L.J.; et al. Secretion of β-amyloid precursor protein cleaved at the amino terminus of the β-amyloid peptide. *Nat. Cell Biol.* **1993**, *361*, 260–263. [CrossRef]
12. Haass, C.; Schlossmacher, M.G.; Hung, A.Y.; Vigo-Pelfrey, C.; Mellon, A.; Ostaszewski, B.L.; Lieberburg, I.; Koo, E.H.; Schenk, D.; Teplow, D.B.; et al. Amyloid β-peptide is produced by cultured cells during normal metabolism. *Nat. Cell Biol.* **1992**, *359*, 322–325. [CrossRef] [PubMed]
13. Lin, T.; Tjernberg, L.; Schedin-Weiss, S. Neuronal Trafficking of the Amyloid Precursor Protein—What Do We Really Know? *BioMed* **2021**, *9*, 801. [CrossRef]
14. LaFerla, F.M.; Green, K.N.; Oddo, S. Intracellular amyloid-beta in Alzheimer's disease. *Nat. Rev. Neurosci.* **2007**, *8*, 499–509. [CrossRef] [PubMed]
15. Esposito, Z.; Belli, L.; Toniolo, S.; Sancesario, G.; Bianconi, C.; Martorana, A. Amyloid beta, glutamate, excitotoxicity in Alzheimer's disease: Are we on the right track? *CNS Neurosci. Ther.* **2013**, *19*, 549–555. [CrossRef] [PubMed]
16. Ju, T.C.; Chen, S.D.; Liu, C.C.; Yang, D.I. Protective effects of S-nitrosoglutathione against amyloid beta-peptide neurotoxicity. *Free Radic. Biol. Med.* **2005**, *38*, 938–949. [CrossRef] [PubMed]
17. Chao, A.C.; Chen, C.H.; Wu, M.H.; Hou, B.Y.; Yang, D.I. Roles of Id1/HIF-1 and CDK5/HIF-1 in cell cycle reentry induced by amyloid-beta peptide in post-mitotic cortical neuron. *Biochim. Biophys. Acta-Mol. Cell Res.* **2020**, *1867*, 118628. [CrossRef] [PubMed]
18. Chao, A.-C.; Chen, C.-H.; Chang, S.-H.; Huang, C.-T.; Hwang, W.-C.; Yang, D.-I. Id1 and Sonic Hedgehog Mediate Cell Cycle Reentry and Apoptosis Induced by Amyloid Beta-Peptide in Post-mitotic Cortical Neurons. *Mol. Neurobiol.* **2018**, *56*, 465–489. [CrossRef]
19. Caldeira, G.L.; Ferreira, I.L.; Rego, A.C. Impaired Transcription in Alzheimer's Disease: Key Role in Mitochondrial Dysfunction and Oxidative Stress. *J. Alzheimer's Dis.* **2013**, *34*, 115–131. [CrossRef]
20. Wu, M.-F.; Yin, J.-H.; Hwang, C.-S.; Tang, C.-M.; Yang, D.-I. NAD attenuates oxidative DNA damages induced by amyloid beta-peptide in primary rat cortical neurons. *Free Radic. Res.* **2014**, *48*, 794–805. [CrossRef]
21. Vicario-Orri, E.; Opazo, C.M.; Muñoz, F.J. The Pathophysiology of Axonal Transport in Alzheimer's Disease. *J. Alzheimer's Dis.* **2014**, *43*, 1097–1113. [CrossRef]
22. Chen, X.-Q.; Sawa, M.; Mobley, W.C. Dysregulation of neurotrophin signaling in the pathogenesis of Alzheimer disease and of Alzheimer disease in Down syndrome. *Free Radic. Biol. Med.* **2018**, *114*, 52–61. [CrossRef]
23. Lauretti, E.; Praticò, D. Alzheimer's disease: Phenotypic approaches using disease models and the targeting of tau protein. *Expert Opin. Ther. Targets* **2020**, *24*, 319–330. [CrossRef] [PubMed]
24. Klein, W.L.; Krafft, G.A.; Finch, C.E. Targeting small Abeta oligomers: The solution to an Alzheimer's disease conundrum? *Trends Neurosci.* **2001**, *24*, 219–224. [CrossRef]
25. Niewiadomska, G.; Niewiadomski, W.; Steczkowska, M.; Gasiorowska, A. Tau Oligomers Neurotoxicity. *Life* **2021**, *11*, 28. [CrossRef] [PubMed]
26. Perić, A.; Annaert, W. Early etiology of Alzheimer's disease: Tipping the balance toward autophagy or endosomal dysfunction? *Acta Neuropathol.* **2015**, *129*, 363–381. [CrossRef]
27. Brewer, G.J.; Herrera, R.A.; Philipp, S.; Sosna, J.; Reyes-Ruiz, J.M.; Glabe, C.G. Age-related intraneuronal aggregation of amyloid-beta in endosomes, mitochondria, autophagosomes, and lysosomes. *J. Alzheimers Dis.* **2020**, *73*, 229–246. [CrossRef]
28. Ren, B.; Zhang, Y.; Zhang, M.; Liu, Y.; Zhang, D.; Gong, X.; Feng, Z.; Tang, J.; Chang, Y.; Zheng, J. Fundamentals of cross-seeding of amyloid proteins: An introduction. *J. Mater. Chem. B* **2019**, *7*, 7267–7282. [CrossRef] [PubMed]
29. Chen, K.L.; Yuan, R.Y.; Hu, C.J.; Hsu, C.Y. Amyloid-beta peptide alteration of tau exon-10 splicing via the GSK3beta-SC35 pathway. *Neurobiol. Dis.* **2010**, *40*, 378–385. [CrossRef]
30. Sayas, C.; Ávila, J. GSK-3 and Tau: A Key Duet in Alzheimer's Disease. *Cells* **2021**, *10*, 721. [CrossRef]
31. Budanov, A.V.; Sablina, A.A.; Feinstein, E.; Koonin, E.V.; Chumakov, P. Regeneration of Peroxiredoxins by p53-Regulated Sestrins, Homologs of Bacterial AhpD. *Science* **2004**, *304*, 596–600. [CrossRef] [PubMed]
32. Peeters, H.; Debeer, P.; Bairoch, A.; Wilquet, V.; Huysmans, C.; Parthoens, E.; Fryns, J.P.; Gewillig, M.; Nakamura, Y.; Niikawa, N.; et al. PA26 is a candidate gene for heterotaxia in humans: Identification of a novel PA26-related gene family in human and mouse. *Qual. Life Res.* **2003**, *112*, 573–580. [CrossRef]
33. Budanov, A.V.; Shoshani, T.; Faerman, A.; Zelin, E.; Kamer, I.; Kalinski, H.; Gorodin, S.; Fishman, A.; Chajut, A.; Einat, P.; et al. Identification of a novel stress-responsive gene Hi95 involved in regulation of cell viability. *Oncogene* **2002**, *21*, 6017–6031. [CrossRef] [PubMed]
34. Velasco-Miguel, S.; Buckbinder, L.; Jean, P.; Gelbert, L.; Talbott, R.; Laidlaw, J.; Seizinger, B.; Kley, N. PA26, a novel target of the p53 tumor suppressor and member of the GADD family of DNA damage and growth arrest inducible genes. *Oncogene* **1999**, *18*, 127–137. [CrossRef] [PubMed]
35. Kim, H.; An, S.; Ro, S.-H.; Teixeira, F.; Park, G.J.; Kim, C.; Cho, C.-S.; Kim, J.-S.; Jakob, U.; Lee, J.H.; et al. Janus-faced Sestrin2 controls ROS and mTOR signalling through two separate functional domains. *Nat. Commun.* **2015**, *6*, 10025. [CrossRef]
36. Saxton, R.A.; Knockenhauer, K.E.; Wolfson, R.L.; Chantranupong, L.; Pacold, M.E.; Wang, T.; Schwartz, T.U.; Sabatini, D.M. Structural basis for leucine sensing by the Sestrin2-mTORC1 pathway. *Science* **2015**, *351*, 53–58. [CrossRef]

37. Haidurov, A.; Budanov, A.V. Sestrin family—The stem controlling healthy ageing. *Mech. Ageing Dev.* **2020**, *192*, 111379. [CrossRef] [PubMed]
38. Lee, J.H.; Budanov, A.V.; Karin, M. Sestrins Orchestrate Cellular Metabolism to Attenuate Aging. *Cell Metab.* **2013**, *18*, 792–801. [CrossRef]
39. Chen, Y.-S.; Chen, S.-D.; Wu, C.-L.; Huang, S.-S.; Yang, D.-I. Induction of sestrin2 as an endogenous protective mechanism against amyloid beta-peptide neurotoxicity in primary cortical culture. *Exp. Neurol.* **2014**, *253*, 63–71. [CrossRef]
40. Hsieh, Y.H.; Chao, A.C.; Lin, Y.C.; Chen, S.D.; Yang, D.I. The p53/NF-kappaB-dependent induction of sestrin2 by amyloid-beta peptides exerts antioxidative actions in neurons. *Free Radic. Biol. Med.* **2021**, *169*, 36–61. [CrossRef]
41. Buckbinder, L.; Talbott, R.; Seizinger, B.R.; Kley, N. Gene regulation by temperature-sensitive p53 mutants: Identification of p53 response genes. *Proc. Natl. Acad. Sci. USA* **1994**, *91*, 10640–10644. [CrossRef] [PubMed]
42. A Sablina, A.; Budanov, A.V.; Ilyinskaya, G.V.; Agapova, L.S.; E Kravchenko, J.; Chumakov, P. The antioxidant function of the p53 tumor suppressor. *Nat. Med.* **2005**, *11*, 1306–1313. [CrossRef] [PubMed]
43. Budanov, A.V.; Karin, M. p53 Target Genes Sestrin1 and Sestrin2 Connect Genotoxic Stress and mTOR Signaling. *Cell* **2008**, *134*, 451–460. [CrossRef] [PubMed]
44. Parmigiani, A.; Budanov, A. Sensing the Environment Through Sestrins: Implications for Cellular Metabolism. *Pancreat. ß-Cell Biol. Health Dis.* **2016**, *327*, 1–42. [CrossRef]
45. Wolfson, R.L.; Chantranupong, L.; Saxton, R.A.; Shen, K.; Scaria, S.M.; Cantor, J.R.; Sabatini, D.M. Sestrin2 is a leucine sensor for the mTORC1 pathway. *Science* **2015**, *351*, 43–48. [CrossRef]
46. Bae, S.H.; Sung, S.H.; Oh, S.Y.; Lim, J.M.; Lee, S.K.; Park, Y.N.; Lee, H.E.; Kang, D.; Rhee, S.G. Sestrins Activate Nrf2 by Promoting p62-Dependent Autophagic Degradation of Keap1 and Prevent Oxidative Liver Damage. *Cell Metab.* **2013**, *17*, 73–84. [CrossRef]
47. The UniProt Consortium. UniProt: A worldwide hub of protein knowledge. *Nucleic Acids Res.* **2019**, *47*, D506–D515. [CrossRef]
48. Chen, M.; Xi, Y.; Chen, K.; Xiao, P.; Li, S.; Sun, X.; Han, Z. Upregulation Sestrin2 protects against hydrogen peroxide-induced oxidative damage bovine mammary epithelial cells via a Keap1-Nrf2/ARE pathway. *J. Cell. Physiol.* **2021**, *236*, 392–404. [CrossRef]
49. Shin, B.Y.; Jin, S.H.; Cho, I.J.; Ki, S.H. Nrf2-ARE pathway regulates induction of Sestrin-2 expression. *Free Radic. Biol. Med.* **2012**, *53*, 834–841. [CrossRef]
50. Olson, N.; Hristova, M.; Heintz, N.H.; Lounsbury, K.M.; Van Der Vliet, A. Activation of hypoxia-inducible factor-1 protects airway epithelium against oxidant-induced barrier dysfunction. *Am. J. Physiol. Cell. Mol. Physiol.* **2011**, *301*, L993–L1002. [CrossRef]
51. Essler, S.; Dehne, N.; Brüne, B. Role of sestrin2 in peroxide signaling in macrophages. *FEBS Lett.* **2009**, *583*, 3531–3535. [CrossRef] [PubMed]
52. Shoshani, T.; Faerman, A.; Mett, I.; Zelin, E.; Tenne, T.; Gorodin, S.; Moshel, Y.; Elbaz, S.; Budanov, A.; Chajut, A.; et al. Identification of a Novel Hypoxia-Inducible Factor 1-Responsive Gene, RTP801, Involved in Apoptosis. *Mol. Cell. Biol.* **2002**, *22*, 2283–2293. [CrossRef] [PubMed]
53. Wu, C.L.; Chen, S.D.; Yin, J.H.; Hwang, C.S.; Yang, D.I. Nuclear factor-kappaB-dependent Sestrin2 induction mediates the antioxidant effects of BDNF against mitochondrial inhibition in rat cortical neurons. *Mol. Neurobiol.* **2016**, *53*, 4126–4142. [CrossRef]
54. Liu, J.; Amar, F.; Corona, C.; So, R.; Andrews, S.J.; Nagy, P.L.; Shelanski, M.L.; Greene, L.A. Brain-Derived Neurotrophic Factor Elevates Activating Transcription Factor 4 (ATF4) in Neurons and Promotes ATF4-Dependent Induction of Sesn2. *Front. Mol. Neurosci.* **2018**, *11*, 62. [CrossRef] [PubMed]
55. Ding, B.; Parmigiani, A.; Divakaruni, A.S.; Archer, K.; Murphy, A.N.; Budanov, A.V. Sestrin2 is induced by glucose starvation via the unfolded protein response and protects cells from non-canonical necroptotic cell death. *Sci. Rep.* **2016**, *6*, 22538. [CrossRef] [PubMed]
56. Garaeva, A.; Kovaleva, I.E.; Chumakov, P.M.; Evstafieva, A.G. Mitochondrial dysfunction induces SESN2 gene expression through Activating Transcription Factor 4. *Cell Cycle* **2016**, *15*, 64–71. [CrossRef] [PubMed]
57. Wang, S.; Chen, X.A.; Hu, J.; Jiang, J.-K.; Li, Y.; Chan-Salis, K.Y.; Gu, Y.; Chen, G.; Thomas, C.; Pugh, B.F.; et al. ATF4 Gene Network Mediates Cellular Response to the Anticancer PAD Inhibitor YW3-56 in Triple-Negative Breast Cancer Cells. *Mol. Cancer Ther.* **2015**, *14*, 877–888. [CrossRef]
58. Ye, J.; Palm, W.; Peng, M.; King, B.; Lindsten, T.; Li, M.; Koumenis, C.; Thompson, C.B. GCN2 sustains mTORC1 suppression upon amino acid deprivation by inducing Sestrin2. *Genes Dev.* **2015**, *29*, 2331–2336. [CrossRef]
59. Zhang, X.-Y.; Wu, X.-Q.; Deng, R.; Sun, T.; Feng, G.-K.; Zhu, X.-F. Upregulation of sestrin 2 expression via JNK pathway activation contributes to autophagy induction in cancer cells. *Cell. Signal.* **2013**, *25*, 150–158. [CrossRef]
60. Hotamisligil, G.S. Endoplasmic Reticulum Stress and the Inflammatory Basis of Metabolic Disease. *Cell* **2010**, *140*, 900–917. [CrossRef]
61. Jegal, K.H.; Park, S.M.; Cho, S.S.; Byun, S.H.; Ku, S.K.; Kim, S.C.; Ki, S.H.; Cho, I.J. Activating transcription factor 6-dependent sestrin 2 induction ameliorates ER stress-mediated liver injury. *Biochim. Biophys. Acta (BBA) Bioenerget.* **2017**, *1864*, 1295–1307. [CrossRef] [PubMed]
62. Park, H.-W.; Park, H.; Ro, S.-H.; Jang, I.; Semple, I.A.; Kim, D.N.; Kim, M.; Nam, M.; Zhang, D.; Yin, L.; et al. Hepatoprotective role of Sestrin2 against chronic ER stress. *Nat. Commun.* **2014**, *5*, 1–11. [CrossRef] [PubMed]
63. Lopez-Otin, C.; Blasco, M.A.; Partridge, L.; Serrano, M.; Kroemer, G. The hallmarks of aging. *Cell* **2013**, *153*, 1194–1217. [CrossRef] [PubMed]

64. Hou, Y.; Dan, X.; Babbar, M.; Wei, Y.; Hasselbalch, S.G.; Croteau, D.L.; Bohr, V.A. Ageing as a risk factor for neurodegenerative disease. *Nat. Rev. Neurol.* **2019**, *15*, 565–581. [CrossRef]
65. Niccoli, T.; Partridge, L. Ageing as a Risk Factor for Disease. *Curr. Biol.* **2012**, *22*, R741–R752. [CrossRef]
66. Lee, J.H.; Bodmer, R.; Bier, E.; Karin, M. Sestrins at the crossroad between stress and aging. *Aging* **2010**, *2*, 369–374. [CrossRef]
67. Lee, J.H.; Budanov, A.V.; Park, E.J.; Birse, R.; Kim, T.E.; Perkins, G.A.; Ocorr, K.; Ellisman, M.H.; Bodmer, R.; Bier, E.; et al. Sestrin as a Feedback Inhibitor of TOR That Prevents Age-Related Pathologies. *Science* **2010**, *327*, 1223–1228. [CrossRef]
68. Budanov, A.V.; Lee, J.H.; Karin, M. Stressin' Sestrins take an aging fight. *EMBO Mol. Med.* **2010**, *2*, 388–400. [CrossRef] [PubMed]
69. Chen, K.-B.; Xuan, Y.; Shi, W.-J.; Chi, F.; Xing, R.; Zeng, Y.-C. Sestrin2 expression is a favorable prognostic factor in patients with non-small cell lung cancer. *Am. J. Transl. Res.* **2016**, *8*, 1903–1909.
70. Wei, J.-L.; Fu, Z.-X.; Fang, M.; Guo, J.-B.; Zhao, Q.-N.; Lu, W.-D.; Zhou, Q.-Y. Decreased expression of sestrin 2 predicts unfavorable outcome in colorectal cancer. *Oncol. Rep.* **2014**, *33*, 1349–1357. [CrossRef] [PubMed]
71. Jeong, S.; Kim, D.Y.; Kang, S.H.; Yun, H.K.; Kim, J.L.; Kim, B.R.; Park, S.H.; Na, Y.J.; Jo, M.J.; Jeong, Y.A.; et al. Docosahexaenoic Acid Enhances Oxaliplatin-Induced Autophagic Cell Death via the ER Stress/Sesn2 Pathway in Colorectal Cancer. *Cancers* **2019**, *11*, 982. [CrossRef]
72. Ro, S.-H.; Xue, X.; Ramakrishnan, S.K.; Cho, C.-S.; Namkoong, S.; Jang, I.; A Semple, I.; Ho, A.; Park, H.-W.; Shah, Y.M.; et al. Tumor suppressive role of sestrin2 during colitis and colon carcinogenesis. *eLife* **2016**, *5*, e12204. [CrossRef]
73. Lee, J.H.; Budanov, A.V.; Talukdar, S.; Park, E.J.; Park, H.L.; Park, H.-W.; Bandyopadhyay, G.; Li, N.; Aghajan, M.; Jang, I.; et al. Maintenance of Metabolic Homeostasis by Sestrin2 and Sestrin3. *Cell Metab.* **2012**, *16*, 311–321. [CrossRef] [PubMed]
74. Sundararajan, S.; Jayachandran, I.; Subramanian, S.C.; Anjana, R.M.; Balasubramanyam, M.; Mohan, V.; Venkatesan, B.; Manickam, N. Decreased Sestrin levels in patients with type 2 diabetes and dyslipidemia and their association with the severity of atherogenic index. *J. Endocrinol. Investig.* **2021**, *44*, 1395–1405. [CrossRef]
75. Mohany, K.M.; Al Rugaie, O. Association of serum sestrin 2 and betatrophin with serum neutrophil gelatinase associated lipocalin levels in type 2 diabetic patients with diabetic nephropathy. *J. Diabetes Metab. Disord.* **2020**, *19*, 249–256. [CrossRef]
76. Liao, H.-H.; Ruan, J.-Y.; Liu, H.-J.; Liu, Y.; Feng, H.; Tang, Q.-Z. Sestrin family may play important roles in the regulation of cardiac pathophysiology. *Int. J. Cardiol.* **2016**, *202*, 183–184. [CrossRef] [PubMed]
77. Liu, Y.; Li, M.; Du, X.; Huang, Z.; Quan, N. Sestrin 2, a potential star of antioxidant stress in cardiovascular diseases. *Free. Radic. Biol. Med.* **2021**, *163*, 56–68. [CrossRef] [PubMed]
78. Wang, H.; Li, N.; Shao, X.; Li, J.; Guo, L.; Yu, X.; Sun, Y.; Hao, J.; Niu, H.; Xiang, J.; et al. Increased plasma sestrin2 concentrations in patients with chronic heart failure and predicted the occurrence of major adverse cardiac events: A 36-month follow-up cohort study. *Clin. Chim. Acta* **2019**, *495*, 338–344. [CrossRef] [PubMed]
79. Boehme, A.K.; Esenwa, C.; Elkind, M.S.V. Stroke Risk Factors, Genetics, and Prevention. *Circ. Res.* **2017**, *120*, 472–495. [CrossRef] [PubMed]
80. He, T.; Li, W.; Song, Y.; Li, Z.; Tang, Y.; Zhang, Z.; Yang, G.Y. Sestrin2 regulates microglia polarization through mTOR-mediated autophagic flux to attenuate inflammation during experimental brain ischemia. *J. Neuroinflamm.* **2020**, *17*, 329. [CrossRef]
81. Li, Y.; Wu, J.; Yu, S.; Zhu, J.; Zhou, Y.; Wang, P.; Li, L.; Zhao, Y. Sestrin2 promotes angiogenesis to alleviate brain injury by activating Nrf2 through regulating the interaction between p62 and Keap1 following photothrombotic stroke in rats. *Brain Res.* **2020**, *1745*, 146948. [CrossRef] [PubMed]
82. Wang, P.; Zhao, Y.; Li, Y.; Wu, J.; Yu, S.; Zhu, J.; Li, L.; Zhao, Y. Sestrin2 overexpression attenuates focal cerebral ischemic injury in rat by increasing Nrf2/HO-1 pathway-mediated angiogenesis. *Neuroscience* **2019**, *410*, 140–149. [CrossRef] [PubMed]
83. Li, L.; Xiao, L.; Hou, Y.; He, Q.; Zhu, J.; Li, Y.; Wu, J.; Zhao, J.; Yu, S.; Zhao, Y. Sestrin2 Silencing Exacerbates Cerebral Ischemia/Reperfusion Injury by Decreasing Mitochondrial Biogenesis through the AMPK/PGC-1α Pathway in Rats. *Sci. Rep.* **2016**, *6*, 30272. [CrossRef]
84. Yang, F.; Chen, R. Sestrin1 exerts a cytoprotective role against oxygen-glucose deprivation/reoxygenation-induced neuronal injury by potentiating Nrf2 activation via the modulation of Keap1. *Brain Res.* **2021**, *1750*, 147165. [CrossRef] [PubMed]
85. Johnson, M.R.; Behmoaras, J.; Bottolo, L.; Krishnan, M.L.; Pernhorst, K.; Santoscoy, P.L.M.; Rossetti, T.; Speed, D.; Srivastava, P.K.; Chadeau-Hyam, M.; et al. Systems genetics identifies Sestrin 3 as a regulator of a proconvulsant gene network in human epileptic hippocampus. *Nat. Commun.* **2015**, *6*, 1–11. [CrossRef] [PubMed]
86. Lovisari, F.; Roncon, P.; Soukoupova, M.; Paolone, G.; Labasque, M.; Ingusci, S.; Falcicchia, C.; Marino, P.; Johnson, M.; Rossetti, T.; et al. Implication of sestrin3 in epilepsy and its comorbidities. *Brain Commun.* **2021**, *3*, fcaa130. [CrossRef] [PubMed]
87. Huang, L.G.; Zou, J.; Lu, Q.C. Silencing rno-miR-155-5p in rat temporal lobe epilepsy model reduces pathophysiological features and cell apoptosis by activating Sestrin-3. *Brain Res.* **2018**, *1689*, 109–122. [CrossRef]
88. Numakawa, T.; Matsumoto, T.; Numakawa, Y.; Richards, M.; Yamawaki, S.; Kunugi, H. Protective Action of Neurotrophic Factors and Estrogen against Oxidative Stress-Mediated Neurodegeneration. *J. Toxicol.* **2011**, *2011*, 1–12. [CrossRef]
89. Niedzielska, E.; Smaga, I.; Gawlik, M.; Moniczewski, A.; Stankowicz, P.; Pera, J.; Filip, M. Oxidative Stress in Neurodegenerative Diseases. *Mol. Neurobiol.* **2016**, *53*, 4094–4125. [CrossRef]
90. Andersen, J.K. Oxidative stress in neurodegeneration: Cause or consequence? *Nat. Med.* **2004**, *10*, S18–S25. [CrossRef]
91. Thellung, S.; Corsaro, A.; Nizzari, M.; Barbieri, F.; Florio, T. Autophagy Activator Drugs: A New Opportunity in Neuroprotection from Misfolded Protein Toxicity. *Int. J. Mol. Sci.* **2019**, *20*, 901. [CrossRef]
92. Kalia, L.V.; Lang, A.E. Parkinson's disease. *Lancet* **2015**, *386*, 896–912. [CrossRef]

93. Rocha, E.; De Miranda, B.; Sanders, L.H. Alpha-synuclein: Pathology, mitochondrial dysfunction and neuroinflammation in Parkinson's disease. *Neurobiol. Dis.* **2018**, *109*, 249–257. [CrossRef] [PubMed]
94. Del Tredici, K.; Braak, H. Review: Sporadic Parkinson's disease: Development and distribution of α-synuclein pathology. *Neuropathol. Appl. Neurobiol.* **2016**, *42*, 33–50. [CrossRef] [PubMed]
95. Zhou, D.; Zhan, C.; Zhong, Q.; Li, S. Upregulation of sestrin-2 expression via P53 protects against 1-methyl-4-phenylpyridinium (MPP+) neurotoxicity. *J. Mol. Neurosci.* **2013**, *51*, 967–975. [CrossRef] [PubMed]
96. Hou, Y.-S.; Guan, J.-J.; Xu, H.-D.; Wu, F.; Sheng, R.; Qin, Z.-H. Sestrin2 Protects Dopaminergic Cells against Rotenone Toxicity through AMPK-Dependent Autophagy Activation. *Mol. Cell. Biol.* **2015**, *35*, 2740–2751. [CrossRef] [PubMed]
97. Rai, N.; Upadhyay, A.D.; Goyal, V.; Dwivedi, S.; Dey, A.B.; Dey, S. Sestrin2 as Serum Protein Marker and Potential Therapeutic Target for Parkinson's Disease. *J. Gerontol. Ser. A: Boil. Sci. Med. Sci.* **2019**, *75*, 690–695. [CrossRef]
98. Chen, S.-D.; Wu, C.-L.; Hwang, W.-C.; Yang, D.-I. More Insight into BDNF against Neurodegeneration: Anti-Apoptosis, Anti-Oxidation, and Suppression of Autophagy. *Int. J. Mol. Sci.* **2017**, *18*, 545. [CrossRef]
99. Johri, A.; Chandra, A.; Beal, M.F. PGC-1α, mitochondrial dysfunction, and Huntington's disease. *Free Radic. Biol. Med.* **2013**, *62*, 37–46. [CrossRef] [PubMed]
100. Tunez, I.; Tasset, I.; Perez-De La Cruz, V.; Santamaria, A. 3-Nitropropionic acid as a tool to study the mechanisms involved in Huntington's disease: Past, present and future. *Molecules* **2010**, *15*, 878–916. [CrossRef] [PubMed]
101. Wu, C.-L.; Hwang, C.-S.; Chen, S.-D.; Yin, J.; Yang, D.-I. Neuroprotective mechanisms of brain-derived neurotrophic factor against 3-nitropropionic acid toxicity: Therapeutic implications for Huntington's disease. *Ann. N. Y. Acad. Sci.* **2010**, *1201*, 8–12. [CrossRef] [PubMed]
102. Chen, S.-D.; Yang, J.-L.; Lin, T.-K.; Yang, D.-I. Emerging Roles of Sestrins in Neurodegenerative Diseases: Counteracting Oxidative Stress and Beyond. *J. Clin. Med.* **2019**, *8*, 1001. [CrossRef]
103. Celik, H.; Karahan, H.; Kelicen-Ugur, P. Effect of atorvastatin on Abeta1-42-induced alteration of SESN2, SIRT1, LC3II and TPP1 protein expressions in neuronal cell cultures. *J. Pharm. Pharmacol.* **2020**, *72*, 424–436. [CrossRef] [PubMed]
104. Rai, N.; Kumar, R.; Desai, G.R.; Venugopalan, G.; Shekhar, S.; Chatterjee, P.; Tripathi, M.; Upadhyay, A.D.; Dwivedi, S.; Dey, A.B.; et al. Relative Alterations in Blood-Based Levels of Sestrin in Alzheimer's Disease and Mild Cognitive Impairment Patients. *J. Alzheimer's Dis.* **2016**, *54*, 1147–1155. [CrossRef]
105. Reddy, K.; Cusack, C.L.; Nnah, I.C.; Khayati, K.; Saqcena, C.; Huynh, T.B.; Noggle, S.; Ballabio, A.; Dobrowolski, R. Dysregulation of Nutrient Sensing and CLEARance in Presenilin Deficiency. *Cell Rep.* **2016**, *14*, 2166–2179. [CrossRef] [PubMed]
106. Soontornniyomkij, V.; Soontornniyomkij, B.; Moore, D.J.; Gouaux, B.; Masliah, E.; Tung, S.; Vinters, H.V.; Grant, I.; Achim, C.L. Antioxidant Sestrin-2 Redistribution to Neuronal Soma in Human Immunodeficiency Virus-Associated Neurocognitive Disorders. *J. Neuroimmune Pharmacol.* **2012**, *7*, 579–590. [CrossRef]
107. Kim, J.R.; Lee, S.R.; Chung, H.J.; Kim, S.; Baek, S.H.; Kim, J.H.; Kim, Y.S. Identification of amyloid beta-peptide responsive genes by cDNA microarray technology: Involvement of RTP801 in amyloid beta-peptide toxicity. *Exp. Mol. Med.* **2003**, *35*, 403–411. [CrossRef]
108. Tampellini, D. Synaptic activity and Alzheimer's disease: A critical update. *Front. Neurosci.* **2015**, *9*, 423. [CrossRef] [PubMed]
109. Papadia, S.; Soriano, F.; Léveillé, F.; Martel, M.-A.; A Dakin, K.; Hansen, H.H.; Kaindl, A.; Sifringer, M.; Fowler, J.; Stefovska, V.; et al. Synaptic NMDA receptor activity boosts intrinsic antioxidant defenses. *Nat. Neurosci.* **2008**, *11*, 476–487. [CrossRef] [PubMed]
110. Shen, J. Function and dysfunction of presenilin. *Neurodegener. Dis.* **2013**, *13*, 61–63. [CrossRef]
111. Sherrington, R.; Rogaev, E.I.; Liang, Y.; Rogaeva, E.A.; Levesque, G.; Ikeda, M.; Chi, H.; Lin, C.; Li, G.; Holman, K.; et al. Cloning of a gene bearing missense mutations in early-onset familial Alzheimer's disease. *Nature* **1995**, *375*, 754–760. [CrossRef]
112. Zhang, C.; Wu, B.; Beglopoulos, V.; Wines-Samuelson, M.; Zhang, D.; Dragatsis, I.; Südhof, T.C.; Shen, J. Presenilins are essential for regulating neurotransmitter release. *Nat. Cell Biol.* **2009**, *460*, 632–636. [CrossRef]
113. Zhang, L.L.; Sui, H.J.; Liang, B.; Wang, H.M.; Qu, W.H.; Yu, S.X.; Jin, Y. Atorvastatin prevents amyloid-beta peptide oligomer-induced synaptotoxicity and memory dysfunction in rats through a p38 MAPK-dependent pathway. *Acta Pharmacol. Sin.* **2014**, *35*, 716–726. [CrossRef]
114. Zhang, Q.; Yang, Y.-J.; Wang, H.; Dong, Q.-T.; Wang, T.-J.; Qian, H.-Y.; Xu, H. Autophagy Activation: A Novel Mechanism of Atorvastatin to Protect Mesenchymal Stem Cells from Hypoxia and Serum Deprivation via AMP-Activated Protein Kinase/Mammalian Target of Rapamycin Pathway. *Stem Cells Dev.* **2012**, *21*, 1321–1332. [CrossRef] [PubMed]
115. Arancibia, S.; Silhol, M.; Mouliere, F.; Meffre, J.; Höllinger, I.; Maurice, T.; Tapia-Arancibia, L. Protective effect of BDNF against beta-amyloid induced neurotoxicity in vitro and in vivo in rats. *Neurobiol. Dis.* **2008**, *31*, 316–326. [CrossRef]
116. Nagahara, A.H.; Merrill, D.; Coppola, G.; Tsukada, S.; E Schroeder, B.; Shaked, G.M.; Wang, L.; Blesch, A.; Kim, A.; Conner, J.M.; et al. Neuroprotective effects of brain-derived neurotrophic factor in rodent and primate models of Alzheimer's disease. *Nat. Med.* **2009**, *15*, 331–337. [CrossRef]
117. Du, Y.; Ma, X.; Ma, L.; Li, S.; Zheng, J.; Lv, J.; Cui, L.; Lv, J. Inhibition of microRNA-148b-3p alleviates oxygen-glucose deprivation/reoxygenation-induced apoptosis and oxidative stress in HT22 hippocampal neuron via reinforcing Sestrin2/Nrf2 signalling. *Clin. Exp. Pharmacol. Physiol.* **2020**, *47*, 561–570. [CrossRef] [PubMed]

118. Fan, Y.; Xing, Y.; Xiong, L.; Wang, J. Sestrin2 overexpression alleviates hydrogen peroxide-induced apoptosis and oxidative stress in retinal ganglion cells by enhancing Nrf2 activation via Keap1 downregulation. *Chem. Interact.* **2020**, *324*, 109086. [CrossRef] [PubMed]
119. Huang, L.-K.; Chao, S.-P.; Hu, C.-J. Clinical trials of new drugs for Alzheimer disease. *J. Biomed. Sci.* **2020**, *27*, 1–13. [CrossRef] [PubMed]
120. Khan, A.; Corbett, A.; Ballard, C. Emerging treatments for Alzheimer's disease for non-amyloid and non-tau targets. *Expert Rev. Neurother.* **2017**, *17*, 683–695. [CrossRef]
121. Nabirotchkin, S.; E Peluffo, A.; Rinaudo, P.; Yu, J.; Hajj, R.; Cohen, D. Next-generation drug repurposing using human genetics and network biology. *Curr. Opin. Pharmacol.* **2020**, *51*, 78–92. [CrossRef] [PubMed]
122. Ashburn, T.T.; Thor, K.B. Drug repositioning: Identifying and developing new uses for existing drugs. *Nat. Rev. Drug Discov.* **2004**, *3*, 673–683. [CrossRef]
123. Yang, J.-L.; Yang, Y.-R.; Chen, S.-D. The potential of drug repurposing combined with reperfusion therapy in cerebral ischemic stroke: A supplementary strategy to endovascular thrombectomy. *Life Sci.* **2019**, *236*, 116889. [CrossRef]
124. Ballard, C.; Aarsland, D.; Cummings, J.; O'Brien, J.; Mills, R.; Molinuevo, J.L.; Fladby, T.; Williams, G.; Doherty, P.; Corbett, A.; et al. Drug repositioning and repurposing for Alzheimer disease. *Nat. Rev. Neurol.* **2020**, *16*, 661–673. [CrossRef]
125. Ihara, M.; Saito, S. Drug Repositioning for Alzheimer's Disease: Finding Hidden Clues in Old Drugs. *J. Alzheimer's Dis.* **2020**, *74*, 1013–1028. [CrossRef]
126. Singh, R.K. Recent Trends in the Management of Alzheimer's Disease: Current Therapeutic Options and Drug Repurposing Approaches. *Curr. Neuropharmacol.* **2020**, *18*, 868–882. [CrossRef] [PubMed]
127. Dunkel, P.; Chai, C.; Sperlágh, B.; Huleatt, P.B.; Mátyus, P. Clinical utility of neuroprotective agents in neurodegenerative diseases: Current status of drug development for Alzheimer's, Parkinson's and Huntington's diseases, and amyotrophic lateral sclerosis. *Expert Opin. Investig. Drugs* **2012**, *21*, 1267–1308. [CrossRef]
128. Sun, X.; Han, F.; Lu, Q.; Li, X.; Ren, D.; Zhang, J.; Han, Y.; Xiang, Y.K. Empagliflozin ameliorates obesity-related cardiac dysfunction by regulating Sestrin2-mediated AMPK-mTOR signaling and redox homeostasis in high-fat diet-induced obese mice. *Diabetes* **2020**, *69*, 1292–1305. [CrossRef] [PubMed]
129. Han, X.; Ding, C.; Zhang, G.; Pan, R.; Liu, Y.; Huang, N.; Hou, N.; Han, F.; Xu, W.; Sun, X. Liraglutide ameliorates obesity-related nonalcoholic fatty liver disease by regulating Sestrin2-mediated Nrf2/HO-1 pathway. *Biochem. Biophys. Res. Commun.* **2020**, *525*, 895–901. [CrossRef] [PubMed]
130. Entezar-Almahdi, E.; Mohammadi-Samani, S.; Tayebi, L.; Farjadian, F. Recent Advances in Designing 5-Fluorouracil Delivery Systems: A Stepping Stone in the Safe Treatment of Colorectal Cancer. *Int. J. Nanomed.* **2020**, *15*, 5445–5458. [CrossRef]
131. Vodenkova, S.; Buchler, T.; Cervena, K.; Veskrnova, V.; Vodicka, P.; Vymetalkova, V. 5-fluorouracil and other fluoropyrimidines in colorectal cancer: Past, present and future. *Pharmacol. Ther.* **2020**, *206*, 107447. [CrossRef]
132. Seo, K.; Ki, S.H.; Park, E.Y.; Shin, S.M. 5-Fluorouracil inhibits cell migration by induction of Sestrin2 in colon cancer cells. *Arch. Pharmacal Res.* **2016**, *40*, 231–239. [CrossRef]
133. Brüning, A.; Rahmeh, M.; Friese, K. Nelfinavir and bortezomib inhibit mTOR activity via ATF4-mediated sestrin-2 regulation. *Mol. Oncol.* **2013**, *7*, 1012–1018. [CrossRef]
134. Lan, X.; Kiyota, T.; Hanamsagar, R.; Huang, Y.; Andrews, S.; Peng, H.; Zheng, J.C.; Swindells, S. The effect of HIV protease inhibitors on amyloid-beta peptide degradation and synthesis in human cells and Alzheimer's disease animal model. *J. Neuroimmune Pharmacol.* **2012**, *7*, 412–423. [CrossRef] [PubMed]
135. Lee, S.; Byun, J.; Park, M.; Kim, S.W.; Lee, S.; Kim, J.; Lee, I.; Choi, Y.; Park, K. Melatonin inhibits vascular smooth muscle cell proliferation and apoptosis through upregulation of Sestrin2. *Exp. Ther. Med.* **2020**, *19*, 3454–3460. [CrossRef] [PubMed]
136. Seo, K.; Seo, S.; Han, J.Y.; Ki, S.H.; Shin, S.M. Resveratrol attenuates methylglyoxal-induced mitochondrial dysfunction and apoptosis by Sestrin2 induction. *Toxicol. Appl. Pharmacol.* **2014**, *280*, 314–322. [CrossRef] [PubMed]
137. Jin, S.H.; Yang, J.H.; Shin, B.Y.; Seo, K.; Shin, S.M.; Cho, I.J.; Ki, S.H. Resveratrol inhibits LXRalpha-dependent hepatic lipogenesis through novel antioxidant Sestrin2 gene induction. *Toxicol. Appl. Pharmacol.* **2013**, *271*, 95–105. [CrossRef]
138. Galiniak, S.; Aebisher, D.; Bartusik-Aebisher, D. Health benefits of resveratrol administration. *Acta Biochim. Pol.* **2019**, *66*, 13–21. [CrossRef]
139. Del Rio, D.; Rodriguez-Mateos, A.; Spencer, J.P.E.; Tognolini, M.; Borges, G.; Crozier, A. Dietary (Poly)phenolics in Human Health: Structures, Bioavailability, and Evidence of Protective Effects Against Chronic Diseases. *Antioxid. Redox Signal.* **2013**, *18*, 1818–1892. [CrossRef]
140. Sun, A.Y.; Wang, Q.; Simonyi, A.; Sun, G.Y. Resveratrol as a Therapeutic Agent for Neurodegenerative Diseases. *Mol. Neurobiol.* **2010**, *41*, 375–383. [CrossRef]
141. Malaguarnera, L. Influence of Resveratrol on the Immune Response. *Nutrients* **2019**, *11*, 946. [CrossRef]
142. Singh, A.P.; Singh, R.; Verma, S.S.; Rai, V.; Kaschula, C.H.; Maiti, P.; Gupta, S.C. Health benefits of resveratrol: Evidence from clinical studies. *Med. Res. Rev.* **2019**, *39*, 1851–1891. [CrossRef]
143. Allaman, I.; Belanger, M.; Magistretti, P.J. Methylglyoxal, the dark side of glycolysis. *Front. Neurosci.* **2015**, *9*, 23. [CrossRef] [PubMed]
144. Lou, Y.; Wu, J.; Liang, J.; Yang, C.; Wang, K.; Wang, J.; Guo, X. Eupatilin protects chondrocytes from apoptosis via activating sestrin2-dependent autophagy. *Int. Immunopharmacol.* **2019**, *75*, 105748. [CrossRef]

145. Jegal, K.H.; Ko, H.L.; Park, S.M.; Byun, S.H.; Kang, K.W.; Cho, I.J.; Kim, S.C. Eupatilin induces Sestrin2-dependent autophagy to prevent oxidative stress. *Apoptosis* **2016**, *21*, 642–656. [CrossRef] [PubMed]
146. Du, J.-X.; Wu, J.-Z.; Li, Z.; Zhang, C.; Shi, M.-T.; Zhao, J.; Jin, M.-W.; Liu, H. Pentamethylquercetin protects against cardiac remodeling via activation of Sestrin2. *Biochem. Biophys. Res. Commun.* **2019**, *512*, 412–420. [CrossRef] [PubMed]
147. Yang, J.H.; Shin, B.Y.; Han, J.Y.; Kim, M.G.; Wi, J.E.; Kim, Y.W.; Cho, I.J.; Kim, S.C.; Shin, S.M.; Ki, S.H. Isorhamnetin protects against oxidative stress by activating Nrf2 and inducing the expression of its target genes. *Toxicol. Appl. Pharmacol.* **2014**, *274*, 293–301. [CrossRef] [PubMed]
148. Salehi, B.; Sharopov, F.; Fokou, P.V.T.; Kobylinska, A.; De Jonge, L.; Tadio, K.; Sharifi-Rad, J.; Posmyk, M.M.; Martorell, M.; Martins, N.; et al. Melatonin in Medicinal and Food Plants: Occurrence, Bioavailability, and Health Potential for Humans. *Cells* **2019**, *8*, 681. [CrossRef] [PubMed]
149. Tordjman, S.; Chokron, S.; Delorme, R.; Charrier, A.; Bellissant, E.; Jaafari, N.; Fougerou, C. Melatonin: Pharmacology, Functions and Therapeutic Benefits. *Curr. Neuropharmacol.* **2017**, *15*, 434–443. [CrossRef]

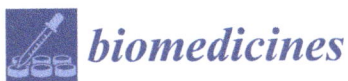 

*Case Report*

# From Cerebrospinal Fluid Neurochemistry to Clinical Diagnosis of Alzheimer's Disease in the Era of Anti-Amyloid Treatments. Report of Four Patients

Ioanna Tsantzali [1,†], Fotini Boufidou [2,†], Eleni Sideri [1], Antonis Mavromatos [1], Myrto G. Papaioannou [2], Aikaterini Foska [1], Ioannis Tollos [1], Sotirios G. Paraskevas [2], Anastasios Bonakis [1], Konstantinos I. Voumvourakis [1], Georgios Tsivgoulis [1], Elisabeth Kapaki [2] and George P. Paraskevas [1,2,*]

1. 2nd Department of Neurology, School of Medicine, National and Kapodistrian University of Athens, "Attikon" General University Hospital, 12462 Athens, Greece; docjo1989@gmail.com (I.T.); elenisideri1985@gmail.com (E.S.); amavro01@hotmail.com (A.M.); dkfoska@gmail.com (A.F.); iw_toll@yahoo.gr (I.T.); bonakistasos@med.uoa.gr (A.B.); cvoumvou@otenet.gr (K.I.V.); tsivgoulisgiorg@yahoo.gr (G.T.)
2. Neurochemistry and Biological Markers Unit, 1st Department of Neurology, School of Medicine, National and Kapodistrian University of Athens, "Eginition" Hospital, 11528 Athens, Greece; fboufidou@med.uoa.gr (F.B.); myrtop@yahoo.com (M.G.P.); sotirispar5@gmail.com (S.G.P.); ekapaki@med.uoa.gr (E.K.)
* Correspondence: geoprskvs44@gmail.com; Tel.: +30-2105832466
† These authors contributed equally to this work.

**Abstract:** Analysis of classical cerebrospinal fluid biomarkers, especially when incorporated in a classification/diagnostic system such as the AT(N), may offer a significant diagnostic tool allowing correct identification of Alzheimer's disease during life. We describe four patients with more or less atypical or mixed clinical presentation, in which the classical cerebrospinal fluid biomarkers amyloid peptide with 42 and 40 amino acids ($A\beta_{42}$ and $A\beta_{40}$, respectively), phospho-tau ($\tau_{P-181}$) and total tau ($\tau_T$) were measured. Despite the unusual clinical presentation, the biomarker profile was compatible with Alzheimer's disease in all four patients. The measurement of classical biomarkers in the cerebrospinal fluid may be a useful tool in identifying the biochemical fingerprints of Alzheimer's disease, especially currently, due to the recent approval of the first disease-modifying treatment, allowing not only typical but also atypical cases to be enrolled in trials of such treatments.

**Keywords:** Alzheimer's disease; beta amyloid; tau protein; phospho-tau; cerebrospinal fluid; biomarkers; anti-amyloid antibodies; aducanumab

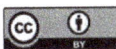

## 1. Introduction

Alzheimer's disease (AD), the most common cause of dementia, is a neurodegenerative disorder characterized by neuronal and synaptic loss and eventually brain atrophy, due to extracellular polymerization and the accumulation of amyloid peptide with 40 and especially 42 amino acids ($A\beta_{40}$ and $A\beta_{42}$, respectively) in the form of amyloid plaques and intracellular polymerization of hyper-phosphorylated tau protein in the form of paired helical filaments, viewed microscopically as neurofibrillary tangles [1]. This pathophysiological/pathobiochemical process of AD starts many years before, and likely, one to three decades prior to symptom onset [2,3]. Following this long asymptomatic or "preclinical" phase of the disease [4], the symptomatic phase starts [5] initially with mild cognitive impairment (MCI) [6] and finally dementia [7]. At the symptomatic phase, the typical presentation of AD is usually of the "hippocampal amnestic-type", characterized by a deficit in episodic memory with difficulty in both free and cued recall [8]. However, in approximately 10–15% of AD patients, atypical (non-amnestic) presentations have been described [5] and this percentage may rise to 22–64% in early-onset (pre-senile) cases [9]. Such atypical presentations include primary progressive aphasia (PPA) [10], frontal dementia which may mimic frontotemporal degeneration [11], corticobasal syndrome (CBS) [12], and posterior cortical atrophy [13]. Furthermore, cases of AD mixed with cerebrovascular disease [14], Lewy body pathology [15], and even normal pressure hydrocephalus (NPH) [16] are not uncommon, especially in the elderly. Thus, AD is no longer viewed as synonymous with amnestic dementia [17]. It may be viewed as a biological process, irrespective of the presence (or absence) and the type and severity of symptoms at a certain time point during disease evolution and progression [18]. Then, how can we diagnose AD?

As in any aspect of medicine, the initial approach is always clinical and, clinical criteria formulated more than 35 years ago [19], may show a diagnostic accuracy > 90% when typical patients are examined in specialized centers [20]. However, in the community, in early disease, in atypical or mixed cases, and the presence of comorbidities, diagnostic accuracy may decrease substantially [21]. Thus, it has been estimated that up to 30% of patients with a clinical diagnosis of AD during life will prove to have non-AD pathology at autopsy [22] and, vice versa, for patients with a clinical presentation suggestive of a non-AD disorder, there is a 39% chance that an autopsy will prove the (co)occurrence of AD pathology [23]. The gold standard for verification of the AD diagnosis is a *postmortem* neuropathological examination. However, correct diagnosis during life is needed, since it allows a more accurate estimation of prognosis and better therapeutic decisions [24,25].

Until now, the pharmaceutical treatment of Alzheimer's disease was dependent on drugs introduced 20–25 years ago. However, on 7 June 2021, the Food and Drug Administration (FDA) in the USA, approved the anti-amyloid monoclonal antibody aducanumab, as the first disease-modifying treatment for AD in the early clinical stages (MCI, mild dementia) [26]. Aducanumab was approved under the accelerated approval pathway, which requires a long (nine years) post-marketing phase IV study to confirm the drug's cognitive benefits. Despite the intense discussion, the arguments and debates triggered, all agree that, if such a specific disease-modifying treatment is to be used the diagnosis of AD should be verified with the maximum accuracy as possible.

For in vivo diagnosis, various biomarkers have been studied during the last 25 years, including cerebrospinal fluid (CSF) biomarkers [27]. Among these, three are considered as classical or "core" biomarkers for AD [28]: $A\beta_{42}$, which is decreased in AD and is inversely related to amyloid plaque burden [29]; tau protein phosphorylated to a threonine residue at position 181 ($\tau_{P-181}$) which is increased in AD and it is considered as a marker of tangle formation [30]; total tau protein ($\tau_T$) which is increased in AD and it is a nonspecific marker of neuronal and/or axonal loss [31]. The $A\beta_{42}/A\beta_{40}$ ratio may be used instead of $A\beta_{42}$ and seems to perform diagnostically better than the latter [32]. With sensitivities and specificities approaching or exceeding 90%, CSF biomarkers offer added diagnostic value compared to clinically-based diagnosis alone [5] and they have been incorporated in newer diagnostic criteria and guidelines [5–7]. A combination of decreased $A\beta_{42}$ with increased $\tau_{P-181}$ and $\tau_T$ is highly specific for the presence of AD, while normal levels of all three biomarkers are highly specific for the absence of AD [33]. Increased levels of the $\tau_{P-181}/A\beta_{42}$ ratio have also been observed to provide high specificity for the differential diagnosis of AD from other dementias [34]. More recently, the AT(N) classification system has been introduced for diagnostic classification of AD (and possibly other dementia disorders), based on biomarkers [35]. The letter A stands for markers of amyloid pathology, T for markers of tau pathology (tangle formation), and N for markers of neurodegeneration (neuronal/axonal loss). Each letter is followed by either $^+$ or $^-$, representing the positive (abnormal) or negative (normal) result of testing, respectively. The profile ("fingerprint") of AD is either $A^+T^+(N)^+$ or $A^+T^+(N)^-$ [18]. Profiles such as $A^+T^-(N)^-$ or $A^+T^-(N)^+$ are compatible with Alzheimer's *pathological change* (change from normal with the acquisition of amyloid biochemistry/pathology, without or with additional non-AD pathologies), but not Alzheimer's disease (which requires *both* amyloid plaques and neurofibrillary tangles [1]) [18]. Although the AT(N) system was designed mainly for research purposes, it can be used in clinical practice, even with clinically relevant prognostic value [36] and it may be suitable for in vivo AD verification in patients suitable for aducanumab treatment, especially during the long phase IV trial of aducanumab.

## 2. Patients and Methods

### 2.1. Patients

The four patients presented here were examined at the 2nd Department of Neurology. They had cognitive impairment with an atypical presentation, creating clinical diagnostic uncertainty, with CSF biomarkers resolving the problem by revealing the CSF "neurochemical fingerprint" of AD (otherwise, there were no specific selection criteria).

Initially, history, neurological and complete physical examination were recorded routinely. Secondary causes including thyroid disease, B12 deficiency, neurosyphilis, brain tumor, or subdural hematoma (but not normal pressure hydrocephalus) were excluded. Written informed consent was obtained for all cases. The study had the approval of the Scientific Board and Ethics Committee of "Attikon" Hospital (project identification codes of approval: A13, 7 April 2021 and 157, 16 March 2021 respectively) and was conducted according to the ethical guidelines of the 1964 Declaration of Helsinki.

### 2.2. Neuropsychological Approach

Following history and clinical examination, a battery of neuropsychological tests was performed. Global tests for the assessment of cognition and activities of daily living included the Addenbrooke's Cognitive Examination-Revised version (ACE-R), the Mini Mental State Examination (MMSE), and the Instrumental Activities of Daily Living (IADL), all of which have been validated in Greece [37–39]. Brief bed-side tests for memory (free and cued recall), frontal function, visuospatial skills, and possible depression included the 5-words memory test [40], the Frontal Assessment Battery (FAB) [41], the CLOX (1 and 2) [42], and the short version of the Geriatric Depression Scale (GDS) [43], respectively. Finally, as a tool for the concomitant assessment of cognitive and functional status, the Clinical Dementia Rating (CDR, both sum of boxes and overall score) was used [44].

### 2.3. Neuroimaging

A routine 1.5 or 3T brain magnetic resonance imaging (MRI) scan was the preferred method of neuroimaging, including 3D T1W sequences, suitable for assessing cortical and central atrophy, including medial temporal atrophy, according to a visual scale [45]. The Evans index and callosal angle were also calculated as appropriate [46]. Alternatively, a brain computerized (CT) scan was obtained in cases with MRI contraindication (orthopedic prostheses).

### 2.4. Lumbar Puncture and CSF Biomarker Measurements

A lumbar puncture was performed using a standard, 21–22G, Quincke-type needle, at the L4–L5 interspace, at 9–12 a.m. according to widely accepted recommendations on standardized operative procedures for CSF biomarkers [47]. In brief, CSF was collected in six polypropylene tubes. The first and second tubes (1 mL each) were used for routine CSF cytology and biochemistry, respectively. The third tube (2 mL) was used for oligoclonal bands and IgG index determinations. The following two tubes (5 mL each) were used for biomarker determinations. The last tube (~2 mL) was used for syphilis serology or other tests according to clinical indications. All CSF samples had <500 red blood cells/µL.

The two tubes intended for CSF biomarker analysis were immediately centrifuged ($2000\times g$ 15 min), aliquoted in polypropylene tubes (1 mL each), and finally stored at $-80\ °C$. Aliquots were thawed only once, just before analysis, which was performed within three months of storage.

Classical CSF biomarkers ($A\beta_{42}$, $A\beta_{40}$, $\tau_{P-181}$, and $\tau_T$) were measured in a Euroimmun Analyzer I (Euroimmun, Lübeck, Germany), in duplicate, with a double sandwich enzyme-linked immunosorbent assay (ELISA) by commercially available kits (EUROIMMUN Beta-Amyloid (1-42) ELISA, EUROIMMUN Beta-Amyloid (1-40) ELISA, EUROIMMUN pTau(181) ELISA, and EUROIMMUN Total-Tau ELISA, respectively), according to the manufacturer's instructions and by the use of 4-parameter logistic curves as described elsewhere [48]. All procedures were performed under a stable temperature (21 ± 2 °C) and quality control samples (both in-house and provided by the manufacturer) were used in each run. The inter- and intra-assay coefficients of variation were both <7% for all biomarkers. CSF biomarkers were considered normal according to cut-off values of the Neurochemistry and Biological Markers Unit ($A\beta_{42}$ > 480–500 pg/mL, $A\beta_{42}/A\beta_{40}$ > 0.09, $\tau_{P-181}$ < 60 pg/mL, $\tau_T$ < 400 pg/mL).

The CSF AD profile ("fingerprint") was defined as decreased $A\beta_{42}$ or decreased $A\beta_{42}/A\beta_{40}$ and increased $\tau_{P-181}$, and thus, compatible with the $A^+T^+(N)^+$ or $A^+T^+(N)^-$ profiles of the AT(N) classification system [18], according to Figure 1.

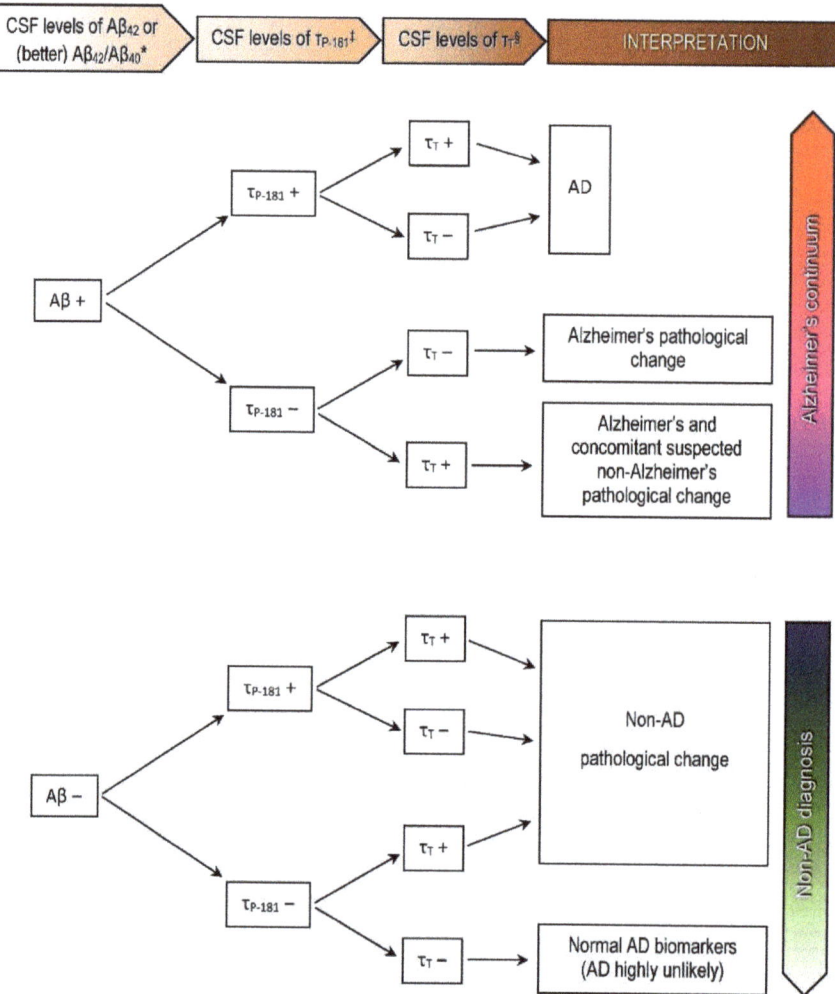

**Figure 1.** Biomarker levels in the CSF and interpretation of results for clinical purposes in our departments according to the AT(N) classification system, using the classical CSF biomarkers and structural imaging (MRI or CT) [18]. * Abnormal have decreased levels (positive result). ‡ Abnormal have increased levels (positive result). § Abnormal have increased CSF levels or atrophy in structural neuroimaging (positive result). Negative results indicate normal findings. AD: Alzheimer's disease.

## 3. Results

The demographic, clinical, neuropsychological, and CSF neurochemical data of the four patients are summarized in Table 1.

**Table 1.** Demographic, clinical, and neurochemical data of the four patients.

|  | Patient 1 | Patient 2 | Patient 3 | Patient 4 |
|---|---|---|---|---|
| Gender | Female | Female | Male | Female |
| Age (years) | 76 | 76 | 81 | 83 |
| Education (years) | 6 | 12 | 12 | 12 |
| Disease duration (years) | 4 | 3 | 4 | 3 |
| ACE-R [37] | 77/100 | 51/100 | 49/100 | 44/100 |
| MMSE [38] | 29/30 | 23/30 | 15/30 | 14/30 |
| IADL [39] | 7/8 | 8/8 | 3/8 | 2/8 |
| 5-words delayed recall [40] | 2 + 3/5 | 0 + 0/5 | 0 + 2/5 | 1 + 1/5 |
| FAB [41] | 9/18 | 10/18 | 5/18 | 3/18 |
| CLOX1 [42] | 9/15 | 12/15 | 0/15 | 4/15 |
| CLOX2 [42] | 10/15 | 12/15 | 0/15 | 6/15 |
| GDS [43] | 5/15 | 4/15 | 3/15 | 2/15 |
| CDR sum of boxes [44] | 1 | 0 | 10 | 12 |
| CDR overall [44] | 0.5 | 0 | 2 | 2 |
| Clinical diagnosis | Incipient dementia (frontal-like?) | PPA logopenic | NPH; VCI | CBS-like; VCI; NPH (?) |
| $A\beta_{42}$ (pg/mL) (normal > 500) | 492.8 ↓ | 864.5 | 262.1 ↓ | 627.9 |
| $A\beta_{40}$ (pg/mL) | 13938 | 12185 | NA | 11648 |
| $A\beta_{42}/A\beta_{40}$ (normal > 0.09) | 0.035 ↓ | 0.071 ↓ | NA | 0.054 ↓ |
| $\tau_{P\text{-}181}$ (pg/mL) (normal < 60) | 161.6 ↑ | 110.1 ↑ | 62.3 ↑ | 82.6 ↑ |
| $\tau_T$ (pg/mL) (normal < 400) | 557.7 ↑ | 490.5 ↑ | 420.1 ↑ | 427.1 ↑ |
| AT(N) profile [18] | $A^+T^+(N)^+$ | $A^+T^+(N)^+$ | $A^+T^+(N)^+$ | $A^+T^+(N)^+$ |
| Final diagnosis | AD | AD | NPH + VCI + AD | AD mixed |

ACE-R: Addenbrooke's Cognitive Examination-Revised, MMSE: Mini Mental State Examination, IADL: Instrumental Activities of Daily Living, FAB: Frontal Assessment Battery, GDS: Geriatric Depression Scale, CDR: Clinical Dementia Rating, PPA: Primary Progressive Aphasia, NPH: Normal Pressure Hydrocephalus, CBS: Corticobasal Syndrome, VCI: Vascular Cognitive Impairment, NA: not available. ↓ Decreased levels, ↑ increased levels, ? diagnostic uncertainty remains.

### 3.1. Patient 1

A seventy-six-year-old female was examined due to four years of "memory problems". She increasingly had to keep memos and frequently repeated the same questions. According to the results of the neuropsychological testing, she had incipient dementia, with a profile more compatible with a frontal or frontal-subcortical syndrome (decreased attention and concentration and executive function) rather than the typical hippocampal amnestic syndrome (Table 1). Neuroimaging showed frontal–frontoparietal atrophy and asymmetric hippocampal atrophy (Figure 2a). Biomarker assessment showed decreased $A\beta_{42}$ and $A\beta_{42}/A\beta_{40}$ ratio and increased both $\tau_{P\text{-}181}$ and $\tau_T$, compatible with AD.

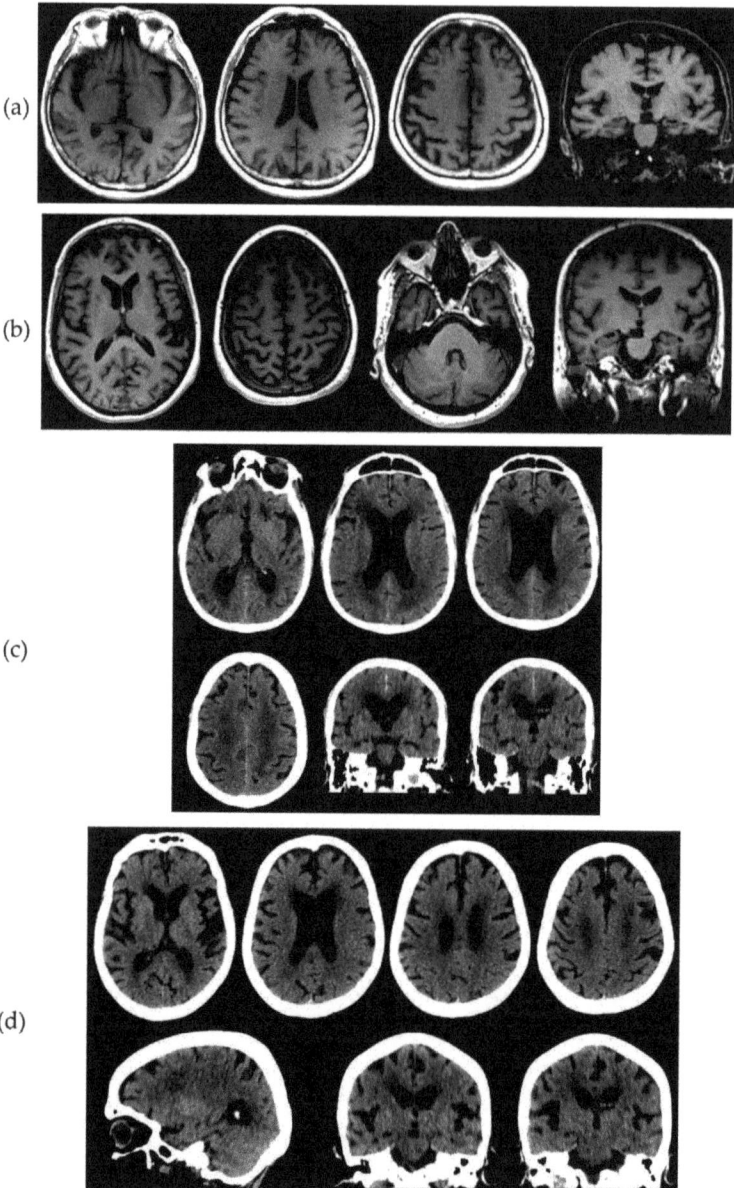

**Figure 2.** (**a**) T1 Magnetic Resonance Imaging (MRI) sequences of patient 1. Frontal (mainly), frontoparietal, perisylvian, and left hippocampal (grade 3) atrophy is observed. (**b**) T1 MRI sequences of patient 2. Atrophy in the left posterior perisylvian and parietal area is observed with preservation of the hippocampus. (**c**) Computerized tomography (CT) scan of patient 3. Some degree of frontal and parietal atrophy is seen. The white matter shows decreased density consistent with subcortical small vessel disease, in addition to periventricular caps. The parietal convexity is tight, the callosal angle is 84.4° and the Evans index has been calculated to 0.36. (**d**) CT scan of patient 4. Frontal (mainly) and parietal asymmetric atrophy are observed. Although the parietal convexity is not tight, the callosal angle is 88.4° and the Evans index has been calculated to 0.38. Decreased density of the white matter at centrum semiovale is noted, consistent with small vessel disease, with additional periventricular caps.

## 3.2. Patient 2

This seventy-six-year-old female suffered gradually progressive difficulty in speech for three years. Upon examination, she had a perfect understanding of language, but during spontaneous speech she made many pauses in an effort to "recall" the appropriate word. Upon naming testing, anomic (word-finding) difficulty was obvious, with object knowledge and single-word comprehension completely spared. Phonological errors were frequent and sentence repetition was severely affected. The motor and grammatical aspects of speech were normal. No difficulty in other cognitive domains was reported and decreased scores in neuropsychological testing were attributed mainly to the language (aphasic) disorder. She had no other significant difficulty in activities of daily living except in communication due to the aphasic disorder, which was compatible with Primary Progressive Aphasia (PPA) of the logopenic-type [49]. Atrophy was predominant in the left perisylvian and parietal areas (Figure 2b). Biomarker analysis revealed normal $A\beta_{42}$ with reduced $A\beta_{42}/A\beta_{40}$ ratio, together with increased $\tau_{P-181}$ and $\tau_T$, compatible with AD.

## 3.3. Patient 3

An eighty-one-year-old male developed a gradually progressive cognitive decline during the last four years. He had apathy, social withdrawal difficulty in performing complex tasks, mental "slowness", and reduced attention. The previous year, progressive gait difficulty was noticed, with slow and short steps, sometimes a "magnetic" gait, and occasional falls with one fracture. The previous month, urinary urgency and sometimes incontinence was added into the clinical picture. Neuropsychological testing revealed moderate-stage dementia showing a mixed profile, including significant frontal, amnestic, and visuoconstructive components. Neuroimaging revealed an increased Evans index, acute callosal angle, tight convexity and periventricular caps, suggestive of normal pressure hydrocephalus [46], but cerebral small vessel disease was also evident (Figure 2c). Consistently with the suspicion of normal pressure hydrocephalus, a spinal taping test (removal of 40 mL of CSF) resulted in a significant improvement of gait and cognition. However, CSF biomarkers analysis revealed decreased $A\beta_{42}$ and increased $\tau_{P-181}$ and $\tau_T$, compatible with the additional presence of AD.

## 3.4. Patient 4

This eighty-three-year-old female developed gradually progressive gait difficulty with slow and short steps, postural instability, and frequent falls during the last three years and was unresponsive to L-dopa treatment. In addition, apathy, mental "slowness" and reduced attention were reported. In the previous year, urinary incontinence was noted. Upon clinical examination, she was practically bed-ridden, with asymmetric parkinsonism, including limb bradykinesia and rigidity more evident in the left limbs, while pyramidal signs were additionally present, more evident in the left limbs. Frequent myoclonic jerks were observed in the upper limbs, especially the left. Cortical sensory loss and sensory neglect were present in the right limbs. Primitive reflexes (especially grasping) were also present. Neuropsychological testing revealed moderate-stage dementia showing a mixed profile, including significant frontal, amnestic and visuoconstructive components, while significant upper limb apraxia was present. The patient met clinical criteria for corticobasal syndrome [50]. Despite some degree of asymmetrical atrophy, neuroimaging revealed an increased Evans index, acute callosal angle, and periventricular caps, suggestive of normal pressure hydrocephalus [46], while some degree of cerebral small vessel disease was also evident (Figure 2d). The spinal taping test (removal of 40 mL of CSF) resulted in a significant improvement of cognition, but there was no change in gait. Analysis of CSF biomarkers showed reduced $A\beta_{42}/A\beta_{40}$ ratio, together with increased $\tau_{P-181}$ and $\tau_T$, compatible with the presence of AD.

## 4. Discussion

In the present study, we present four cognitively impaired patients with clinical presentations creating diagnostic uncertainty. The first patient was at the transition from MCI to mild dementia and, while she complained of memory problems, the total delayed recall (including memory cues) was normal, which is considered not compatible with the hippocampal amnestic disorder (typically expected in AD), but more compatible with a frontal–subcortical-type of memory decline. Despite a senile onset of disease and a presumably higher probability for AD, this is estimated to be no more than ~70% in such cases with early-stage disease and non-typical presentation [21,22], with other pathologies entering in the differential diagnosis. In the second patient, the clinical profile was compatible with PPA of the logopenic-type, which is due to AD in approximately 50–80% of patients [10,51]. However, it should be not considered synonymous with AD [49], since, in ~25%, it is caused by one of the frontotemporal pathologies [51].

Thus, in both patients 1 and 2, there was still a significant chance (at the level of 25–30%) that a non-AD pathology may be the cause of the cognitive decline. Since both patients had MMSE > 20, making them eligible for aducanumab treatment, it is necessary to increase the diagnostic certainty from 70–75% to as high as possible, in order to initiate such a specific, expensive, and with potentially serious complications, treatment. In both patients, the CSF biomarker results, according to the AT(N) classification system [18], were compatible with the presence of AD.

In patients 3 and 4, the case was quite different since they were mixed cases of dementia. Patient 3 had typical clinical and imaging characteristics of normal pressure hydrocephalus and the positive taping test was consistent with this notion. Normal-pressure hydrocephalus may occur alone, but in three-quarters of cases, AD and/or cerebrovascular disease (usual of the small vessel-type) may be additionally present [52]. In the additional presence of AD, a shunting operation may offer some degree of gait improvement, which may positively affect the quality of life [53]; however, cognitive improvement may be modest [53] and the overall improvement is traditionally thought to be moderate at best and short-lived [54]. Thus, the possible co-occurrence of AD should be known prior to the selection of optimal treatment (or treatment combinations). In patient 3, the whole picture was compatible with NPH and concomitant small vessel disease, both of which may contribute to the clinical picture. However, CSF biomarkers revealed a third significant component in this patient's dementia, that of AD.

Patient 4 was the most intriguing. She had a mixed movement and cognitive disorder, with a clinical picture typical of corticobasal *syndrome*, while neuroimaging revealed a normal pressure hydrocephalus-like picture and some degree of small vessel disease. A taping test resulted in the improvement of cognition only, but not of gait, probably because the corticobasal component of the motor disability was already severe enough to oppose any improvement. The corticobasal *syndrome* is not a disease, but a clinical picture that can be due to many neurodegenerative diseases, the most common being corticobasal *degeneration* which belongs to the 4-repeat tauopathies [50]. However, it can be caused by AD, Lewy body pathology, progressive supranuclear palsy, and even Creutzfeldt–Jakob disease [12], with AD accounting for a significant percentage of cases with corticobasal *syndrome* [55]. CSF biomarker analysis in patient 4 revealed that AD was indeed the underlying cause. Normal-pressure hydrocephalus was probably present as well (hence the cognitive improvement following the taping test), however, it was superimposed on AD.

Classical CSF biomarkers are useful in identifying the AD biochemical fingerprint in typical and atypical AD cases [27,28]. Their diagnostic performance has been validated in autopsy-proven cases [56]. They have been proven useful in cases with primary progressive aphasia [51], corticobasal syndrome [57], and cases of AD mixed with Lewy body pathology [58] or cerebrovascular disease [14,59]. They can identify the concomitant presence of AD in cases with normal pressure hydrocephalus [60,61], and possibly predict a worse neurosurgical prognosis [62], although recent data suggest that they may predict the opposite [16].

When incorporated in the AT(N) classification system, CSF biomarkers may be used effectively not only in research but also in clinical practice [36,63]. It should be noted that in patients 2 and 4, CSF levels of $A\beta_{42}$ were normal. However, the $A\beta_{42}/A\beta_{40}$ ratio was abnormally reduced in both, allowing the diagnosis of AD. Despite some concerns about the interchangeability between $A\beta_{42}$ and the $A\beta_{42}/A\beta_{40}$ ratio in the AT(N) system [64], the ratio shows better diagnostic accuracy compared to $A\beta_{42}$ alone [32,65], correlates better with amyloid imaging by positron emission tomography [32], and its better diagnostic performance has been confirmed in pathologically proven cases [32].

There are some limitations in classical CSF biomarker determination. Preanalytical factors, including CSF sampling and storage, may affect test results and internationally accepted guidelines have been formulated for this reason [47]. International quality control programs and projects have been organized, in order to identify and control for confounding factors, improve the methodologies used, optimize analytical performance, and harmonize the levels of biomarkers [66–68]. However, there is still a significant intra- and inter-laboratory variability [67,69] and each laboratory should have its own cut-off values [28]. Discordant biomarker results have been observed in different reference laboratories, especially for $A\beta_{42}$ [70]. Diagnostically gray zones also exist and, when added to the possible measurement error, they may lead to a variability of ±25% [70]. Normal levels of all three CSF classical biomarkers may be observed in normal aging, but also in psychiatric disorders which may present with cognitive complaints, sometimes entering in the differential diagnosis of frontotemporal dementia. Furthermore, the classical CSF biomarkers cannot identify additional neurodegenerative pathologies, which are not rare in older patients with AD [71]. Finally, determination of CSF biomarkers requires a lumbar puncture which is a cause of concern and anxiety in many patients and caregivers, and it cannot be easily repeated for frequent follow-up.

Other molecules are under intense investigation in an effort to optimize the differential diagnostic value of the classic biomarkers and identify possible additional neurodegenerative pathologies. They include markers of neuroinflammation such as the triggering receptor expressed on myeloid cells 2 (TREM2), progranulin, and chitinase-3-like protein-1 (YKL-40), markers of synaptic dysfunction such as neurogranin, and markers of neuronal injury such as neurofilament light (NfL) and visinin-like protein 1 (VILIP-1), while miRNAs could also be helpful [72–77]. Oligomeric forms of $A\beta_{42}$ [78], α-synuclein [79], and TAR DNA-Binding Protein 43 (TDP43) [80] are emerging biomarkers, but work must still be carried out to achieve adequate diagnostic performance. Especially for α-synuclein, which has been traditionally considered as a marker of synuclein pathology, results are conflicting [79], partially due to the effect of preanalytical and analytical factors, including differences in a-synuclein species detected by different methods [81]. Recent evidence suggests that α-, and also β- and γ-synuclein, may be effective markers of AD rather than synucleinopathy [82]. Both α- and β-synuclein may be early markers of AD, even in non-demented elder subjects [83,84], while the ratio of total tau/α-synuclein may serve as a marker of tau phosphorylation, even allowing patients with the $A^-T^+(N^+)$ profile to re-enter the AD diagnostic group [85]. Blood-based classical [86,87] and exosomal [88] biomarkers may prove helpful, especially for frequent monitoring of the biochemical effects of anti-amyloid antibodies. The AT(N) system is flexible and may expand to an ATX(N) form, incorporating such new or evolving biomarkers of AD-related or additional non-AD pathologies [89].

## 5. Conclusions

Biomarkers are not stand-alone tools and should always be interpreted along with clinical, neuropsychological, and imaging data. Keeping this in mind, analysis of classical CSF biomarkers, especially when incorporated in a classification/diagnostic system such as the AT(N), may offer a significant diagnostic tool [90,91], with both added [92] and prognostic [36] value, allowing the correct identification of AD during life, especially in cases with atypical or mixed presentations [93]. This is always important for correct therapeutic decisions, and it is of paramount importance currently, due to the recent approval of aducanumab as a disease-modifying treatment. Whether atypical cases are going to have the same benefit (from classical or newer treatments) as the typical ones, remains to be elucidated.

**Author Contributions:** Conceptualization, I.T. (Ioanna Tsantzali), F.B., E.K. and G.P.P.; methodology, I.T. (Ioanna Tsantzali), F.B., E.S., G.T., E.K. and G.P.P.; formal analysis, I.T. (Ioanna Tsantzali), F.B., E.S., A.M., M.G.P., A.F., I.T. (Ioannis Tollos), S.G.P., A.B., K.I.V., G.T., E.K. and G.P.P.; investigation, I.T. (Ioanna Tsantzali), F.B., E.S., A.M., M.G.P., A.F., I.T. (Ioannis Tollos), S.G.P., A.B., K.I.V., G.T., E.K. and G.P.P.; data curation, I.T. (Ioanna Tsantzali), F.B., E.S. and G.P.P.; writing—original draft preparation, I.T. (Ioanna Tsantzali), F.B., and G.P.P.; writing—review and editing, A.M., M.G.P., A.F., I.T. (Ioannis Tollos), S.G.P., A.B., K.I.V., G.T. and E.K.; visualization, G.T., E.K. and G.P.P.; supervision, K.I.V., G.T., E.K. and G.P.P.; project administration, G.T., E.K. and G.P.P. All authors have read and agreed to the published version of the manuscript.

**Funding:** E.K. has received research funding from ELPEN Pharmaceutical Co. Inc. and NUTRICIA.

**Institutional Review Board Statement:** The study had the approval of the Bioethics Committee and the Scientific Board of "Attikon" Hospital (approval numbers 157/16-03-2021 and A13/07-04-2021, respectively). It was performed according to the 1964 Declaration of Helsinki.

**Informed Consent Statement:** Informed consent was obtained from all subjects involved in the study and/or next of kin caregivers (depending on the severity of cognitive impairment).

**Data Availability Statement:** The data presented in this study are available upon request from the corresponding author. The data are not publicly available due to privacy restrictions.

**Acknowledgments:** We would like to thank the patients and their caregivers for their participation. We would also like to thank the laboratory technician Olga Petropoulou for her valuable assistance in sample handling and biomarker measurements.

**Conflicts of Interest:** G.P.P. receives fees from Biogen International as a consultant of the advisory board. All other authors: none. The funders had no role in the design of the study; in the collection, analyses, or interpretation of data; in the writing of the manuscript, or in the decision to publish the results.

## References

1. Hyman, B.T.; Phelps, C.H.; Beach, T.G.; Bigio, E.H.; Cairns, N.J.; Carrillo, M.C.; Dickson, D.W.; Duyckaerts, C.; Frosch, M.P.; Masliah, E.; et al. National Institute on Aging-Alzheimer's Association guidelines for the neuropathologic assessment of Alzheimer's disease. *Alzheimers Dement.* **2012**, *8*, 1–13. [CrossRef]
2. Jellinger, K.A.; Bancher, C. Neuropathology of Alzheimer's disease: A critical update. *J. Neural. Transm. Suppl.* **1998**, *54*, 77–95.
3. Braak, H.; Braak, E. Neuropathological staging of Alzheimer-related changes. *Acta Neuropathol.* **1991**, *82*, 239–259. [CrossRef]
4. Sperling, R.A.; Aisen, P.S.; Beckett, L.A.; Bennett, D.A.; Craft, S.; Fagan, A.M.; Iwatsubo, T.; Jack, C.R., Jr.; Kaye, J.; Montine, T.J.; et al. Toward defining the preclinical stages of Alzheimer's disease: Recommendations from the National Institute on Aging-Alzheimer's Association workgroups on diagnostic guidelines for Alzheimer's disease. *Alzheimers Dement.* **2011**, *7*, 280–292. [CrossRef]
5. Dubois, B.; Feldman, H.H.; Jacova, C.; Hampel, H.; Molinuevo, J.L.; Blennow, K.; DeKosky, S.T.; Gauthier, S.; Selkoe, D.; Bateman, R.; et al. Advancing research diagnostic criteria for Alzheimer's disease: The IWG-2 criteria. *Lancet Neurol.* **2014**, *13*, 614–629. [CrossRef]
6. Albert, M.S.; DeKosky, S.T.; Dickson, D.; Dubois, B.; Feldman, H.H.; Fox, N.C.; Gamst, A.; Holtzman, D.M.; Jagust, W.J.; Petersen, R.C.; et al. The diagnosis of mild cognitive impairment due to Alzheimer's disease: Recommendations from the National Institute on Aging-Alzheimer's Association workgroups on diagnostic guidelines for Alzheimer's disease. *Alzheimers Dement.* **2011**, *7*, 270–279. [CrossRef]
7. McKhann, G.M.; Knopman, D.S.; Chertkow, H.; Hyman, B.T.; Jack, C.R., Jr.; Kawas, C.H.; Klunk, W.E.; Koroshetz, W.J.; Manly, J.J.; Mayeux, R.; et al. The diagnosis of dementia due to Alzheimer's disease: Recommendations from the National Institute on Aging-Alzheimer's Association workgroups on diagnostic guidelines for Alzheimer's disease. *Alzheimers Dement.* **2011**, *7*, 263–269. [CrossRef]
8. Wagner, M.; Wolf, S.; Reischies, F.M.; Daerr, M.; Wolfsgruber, S.; Jessen, F.; Popp, J.; Maier, W.; Hüll, M.; Frölich, L.; et al. Biomarker validation of a cued recall memory deficit in prodromal Alzheimer disease. *Neurology* **2012**, *78*, 379–386. [CrossRef] [PubMed]

9. Mendez, M.F. Early-onset Alzheimer disease. *Neurol. Clin.* **2017**, *35*, 263–281. [CrossRef] [PubMed]
10. Grossman, M. Primary progressive aphasia: Clinicopathological correlations. *Nat. Rev. Neurol.* **2010**, *6*, 88–97. [CrossRef] [PubMed]
11. Mendez, M.F.; Joshi, A.; Tassniyom, K.; Teng, E.; Shapira, J.S. Clinicopathologic differences among patients with behavioral variant frontotemporal dementia. *Neurology* **2013**, *80*, 561–568. [CrossRef] [PubMed]
12. Boeve, B.F.; Josephs, K.A.; Drubach, D.A. Current and future management of the corticobasal syndrome and corticobasal degeneration. *Handb. Clin. Neurol.* **2008**, *89*, 533–548.
13. Crutch, S.J.; Lehmann, M.; Schott, J.M.; Rabinovici, G.D.; Rossor, M.N.; Fox, N.C. Posterior cortical atrophy. *Lancet Neurol.* **2012**, *11*, 170–178. [CrossRef]
14. Wallin, A.; Nordlund, A.; Jonsson, M.; Blennow, K.; Zetterberg, H.; Öhrfelt, A.; Stålhammar, J.; Eckerström, M.; Carlsson, M.; Olsson, E.; et al. Alzheimer's disease–subcortical vascular disease spectrum in a hospital-based setting: Overview of results from the Gothenburg MCI and dementia studies. *J. Cereb. Blood Flow Metab.* **2016**, *36*, 95–113. [CrossRef] [PubMed]
15. Peavy, G.M.; Edland, S.D.; Toole, B.M.; Hansen, L.A.; Galasko, D.R.; Mayo, A.M. Phenotypic differences based on staging of Alzheimer's neuropathology in autopsy-confirmed dementia with Lewy bodies. *Parkinsonism Relat. Disord.* **2016**, *31*, 72–78. [CrossRef]
16. Müller-Schmitz, K.; Krasavina-Loka, N.; Yardimci, T.; Lipka, T.; Kolman, A.G.J.; Robbers, S.; Menge, T.; Kujovic, M.; Seitz, R.J. Normal Pressure Hydrocephalus Associated with Alzheimer's Disease. *Ann. Neurol.* **2020**, *88*, 703–711. [CrossRef]
17. Graff-Radford, J.; Yong, K.X.X.; Apostolova, L.G.; Bouwman, F.H.; Carrillo, M.; Dickerson, B.C.; Rabinovici, G.D.; Schott, J.M.; Jones, D.T.; Murray, M.E. New insights into atypical Alzheimer's disease in the era of biomarkers. *Lancet Neurol.* **2021**, *20*, 222–234. [CrossRef]
18. Jack, C.R., Jr.; Bennett, D.A.; Blennow, K.; Carrillo, M.C.; Dunn, B.; Haeberlein, S.B.; Holtzman, D.M.; Jagust, W.; Jessen, F.; Karlawish, J.; et al. NIA-AA Research Framework: Toward a biological definition of Alzheimer's disease. *Alzheimers Dement.* **2018**, *14*, 535–562. [CrossRef]
19. McKhann, G.; Drachman, D.; Folstein, M.; Katzman, R.; Price, D.; Stadlan, E.M. Clinical diagnosis of Alzheimer's disease: Report of the NINCDS-ADRDA Work Group under the auspices of Department of Health and Human Services Task Force on Alzheimer's Disease. *Neurology* **1984**, *34*, 939–944. [CrossRef]
20. Lopez, O.L.; Becker, J.T.; Klunk, W.; Saxton, J.; Hamilton, R.L.; Kaufer, D.I.; Sweet, R.A.; Cidis Meltzer, C.; Wisniewski, S.; Kamboh, M.I.; et al. Research evaluation and diagnosis of probable Alzheimer's disease over the last two decades: I. *Neurology* **2000**, *55*, 1854–1862. [CrossRef]
21. Mendez, M.; Mastri, A.R.; Sung, J.H.; Frey, W.H. Clinically diagnosed Alzheimer's disease: Neuropathologic findings in 650 cases. *Alzheimer Dis. Assoc. Disord.* **1992**, *6*, 35–43. [CrossRef]
22. Nelson, P.T.; Head, E.; Schmitt, F.A.; Davis, P.R.; Neltner, J.H.; Jicha, G.A.; Abner, E.L.; Smith, C.D.; Van Eldik, L.J.; Kryscio, R.J.; et al. Alzheimer's disease is not "brain aging": Neuropathological, genetic, and epidemiological human studies. *Acta Neuropathol.* **2011**, *121*, 571–587. [CrossRef]
23. Galasko, D.; Hansen, L.A.; Katzman, R.; Wiederholt, W.; Masliah, E.; Terry, R.; Hill, L.R.; Lessin, P.; Thal, L.J. Clinical-neuropathological correlations in Alzheimer's disease and related dementias. *Arch. Neurol.* **1994**, *51*, 888–895. [CrossRef] [PubMed]
24. Johnell, K.; Religa, D.; Eriksdotter, M. Differences in drug therapy between dementia disorders in the Swedish dementia registry: A nationwide study of over 7000 patients. *Dement. Geriatr. Cogn. Disord.* **2013**, *35*, 239–248. [CrossRef] [PubMed]
25. Thomas, A.J.; Mahin-Babaei, F.; Saidi, M.; Lett, D.; Taylor, J.P.; Walker, L.; Attems, J. Improving the identification of dementia with Lewy bodies in the context of an Alzheimer's-type dementia. *Alzheimers Res. Ther.* **2018**, *10*, 27. [CrossRef] [PubMed]
26. Tagliavini, F.; Tiraboschi, P.; Federico, A. Alzheimer's disease: The controversial approval of Aducanumab. *Neurol. Sci.* **2021**, *42*, 3069–3070. [CrossRef]
27. McGrowder, D.A.; Miller, F.; Vaz, K.; Nwokocha, C.; Wilson-Clarke, C.; Anderson-Cross, M.; Brown, J.; Anderson-Jackson, L.; Williams, L.; Latore, L.; et al. Cerebrospinal Fluid Biomarkers of Alzheimer's Disease: Current Evidence and Future Perspectives. *Brain Sci.* **2021**, *11*, 215. [CrossRef]
28. Lewczuk, P.; Riederer, P.; O'Bryant, S.E.; Verbeek, M.M.; Dubois, B.; Visser, P.J.; Jellinger, K.A.; Engelborghs, S.; Ramirez, A.; Parnetti, L.; et al. Cerebrospinal fluid and blood biomarkers for neurodegenerative dementias: An update of the Consensus of the Task Force on Biological Markers in Psychiatry of the World Federation of Societies of Biological Psychiatry. *World J. Biol. Psychiatry* **2018**, *19*, 244–328. [CrossRef]
29. Sjögren, M.; Minthon, L.; Davidsson, P.; Granérus, A.K.; Clarberg, A.; Vanderstichele, H.; Vanmechelen, E.; Wallin, A.; Blennow, K. CSF levels of tau, beta-amyloid(1-42) and GAP-43 in frontotemporal dementia, other types of dementia and normal aging. *J. Neural Transm.* **2000**, *107*, 563–579.
30. Vanderstichele, H.; De Vreese, K.; Blennow, K.; Andreasen, N.; Sindic, C.; Ivanoiu, A.; Hampel, H.; Bürger, K.; Parnetti, L.; Lanari, A.; et al. Analytical performance and clinical utility of the INNOTEST PHOSPHO-TAU181P assay for discrimination between Alzheimer's disease and dementia with Lewy bodies. *Clin. Chem. Lab. Med.* **2006**, *44*, 1472–1480. [CrossRef]
31. Blennow, K.; Wallin, A.; Agren, H.; Spenger, C.; Siegfried, J.; Vanmechelen, E. Tau protein in cerebrospinal fluid: A biochemical marker for axonal degeneration in Alzheimer disease? *Mol. Chem. Neuropathol.* **1995**, *26*, 231–245. [CrossRef]

32. Niemantsverdriet, E.; Ottoy, J.; Somers, C.; De Roeck, E.; Struyfs, H.; Soetewey, F.; Verhaeghe, J.; Van den Bossche, T.; Van Mossevelde, S.; Goeman, J.; et al. The Cerebrospinal Fluid Aβ1-42/Aβ1-40 Ratio Improves Concordance with Amyloid-PET for Diagnosing Alzheimer's Disease in a Clinical Setting. *J. Alzheimers Dis.* **2017**, *60*, 561–576. [CrossRef]
33. Simonsen, A.H.; Herukka, S.K.; Andreasen, N.; Baldeiras, I.; Bjerke, M.; Blennow, K.; Engelborghs, S.; Frisoni, G.B.; Gabryelewicz, T.; Galluzzi, S.; et al. Recommendations for CSF AD biomarkers in the diagnostic evaluation of dementia. *Alzheimers Dement.* **2017**, *13*, 274–284. [CrossRef]
34. Seeburger, J.L.; Holder, D.J.; Combrinck, M.; Joachim, C.; Laterza, O.; Tanen, M.; Dallob, A.; Chappell, D.; Snyder, K.; Flynn, M.; et al. Cerebrospinal fluid biomarkers distinguish postmortem-confirmed Alzheimer's disease from other dementias and healthy controls in the OPTIMA cohort. *J. Alzheimers Dis.* **2015**, *44*, 525–539. [CrossRef]
35. Jack, C.R., Jr.; Bennett, D.A.; Blennow, K.; Carrillo, M.C.; Feldman, H.H.; Frisoni, G.B.; Hampel, H.; Jagust, W.J.; Johnson, K.A.; Knopman, D.S.; et al. A/T/N: An unbiased descriptive classification scheme for Alzheimer disease biomarkers. *Neurology* **2016**, *87*, 539–547. [CrossRef]
36. Delmotte, K.; Schaeverbeke, J.; Poesen, K.; Vandenberghe, R. Prognostic value of amyloid/tau/neurodegeneration (ATN) classification based on diagnostic cerebrospinal fluid samples for Alzheimer's disease. *Alzheimers Res. Ther.* **2021**, *13*, 84. [CrossRef]
37. Konstantinopoulou, E.; Kosmidis, M.H.; Ioannidis, P.; Kiosseoglou, G.; Karacostas, D.; Taskos, N. Adaptation of Addenbrooke's Cognitive Examination-Revised for the Greek population. *Eur. J. Neurol.* **2011**, *18*, 442–447. [CrossRef] [PubMed]
38. Fountoulakis, K.N.; Tsolaki, M.; Chantzi, H.; Kazis, A. Mini Mental State Examination (MMSE): A validation study in Greece. *Am. J. Alzheimers Dis. Other Demen.* **2000**, *15*, 342–345. [CrossRef]
39. Theotoka, I.; Kapaki, E.; Vagenas, V.; Ilias, I.; Paraskevas, G.P.; Liappas, I. Preliminary report of a validation study of Instrumental Activities of Daily Living in a Greek sample. *Percept. Mot. Skills* **2007**, *104*, 958–960. [CrossRef] [PubMed]
40. Dubois, B.; Touchon, J.; Portet, F.; Ousset, P.J.; Vellas, B.; Michel, B. "The 5 words": A simple and sensitive test for the diagnosis of Alzheimer's disease. *Presse. Med.* **2002**, *31*, 1696–1699.
41. Dubois, B.; Slachevsky, A.; Litvan, I.; Pillon, B. The FAB: A Frontal Assessment Battery at bedside. *Neurology* **2000**, *55*, 1621–1626. [CrossRef]
42. Royall, D.R.; Cordes, J.A.; Polk, M. CLOX: An executive clock drawing task. *J. Neurol. Neurosurg. Psychiatry* **1998**, *64*, 588–594. [CrossRef] [PubMed]
43. Sheikh, J.I.; Yesavage, J.A. Geriatric Depression Scale (GDS): Recent evidence and development of a shorter version. *Clin. Gerontol.* **1986**, *5*, 165–173.
44. Morris, J.C. The Clinical Dementia Rating (CDR): Current version and scoring rules. *Neurology* **1993**, *43*, 2412–2414. [CrossRef]
45. Scheltens, P.; Leys, D.; Barkhof, F.; Huglo, D.; Weinstein, H.C.; Vermersch, P.; Kuiper, M.; Steinling, M.; Wolters, E.C.; Valk, J. Atrophy of medial temporal lobes on MRI in "probable" Alzheimer's disease and normal ageing: Diagnostic value and neuropsychological correlates. *J. Neurol. Neurosurg. Psychiatry* **1992**, *55*, 967–972. [CrossRef] [PubMed]
46. Kockum, K.; Lilja-Lund, O.; Larsson, E.M.; Rosell, M.; Söderström, L.; Virhammar, J.; Laurell, K. The idiopathic normal-pressure hydrocephalus Radscale: A radiological scale for structured evaluation. *Eur. J. Neurol.* **2018**, *25*, 569–576. [CrossRef] [PubMed]
47. Del Campo, M.; Mollenhauer, B.; Bertolotto, A.; Engelborghs, S.; Hampel, H.; Simonsen, A.H.; Kapaki, E.; Kruse, N.; Le Bastard, N.; Lehmann, S.; et al. Recommendations to standardize preanalytical confounding factors in Alzheimer's and Parkinson's disease cerebrospinal fluid biomarkers: An update. *Biomark. Med.* **2012**, *6*, 419–430. [CrossRef]
48. Constantinides, V.C.; Paraskevas, G.P.; Boufidou, F.; Bourbouli, M.; Stefanis, L.; Kapaki, E. Cerebrospinal fluid biomarker profiling in corticobasal degeneration: Application of the AT(N) and other classification systems. *Parkinsonism Relat. Disord.* **2021**, *82*, 44–49. [CrossRef] [PubMed]
49. Gorno-Tempini, M.L.; Hillis, A.E.; Weintraub, S.; Kertesz, A.; Mendez, M.; Cappa, S.F.; Ogar, J.M.; Rohrer, J.D.; Black, S.; Boeve, B.F.; et al. Classification of primary progressive aphasia and its variants. *Neurology* **2011**, *76*, 1006–1014. [CrossRef] [PubMed]
50. Armstrong, M.J.; Litvan, I.; Lang, A.E.; Bak, T.H.; Bhatia, K.P.; Borroni, B.; Boxer, A.L.; Dickson, D.W.; Grossman, M.; Hallett, M.; et al. Criteria for the diagnosis of corticobasal degeneration. *Neurology* **2013**, *80*, 496–503. [CrossRef] [PubMed]
51. Paraskevas, G.P.; Kasselimis, D.; Kourtidou, E.; Constantinides, V.; Bougea, A.; Potagas, C.; Evdokimidis, I.; Kapaki, E. Cerebrospinal Fluid Biomarkers as a Diagnostic Tool of the Underlying Pathology of Primary Progressive Aphasia. *J. Alzheimers Dis.* **2017**, *55*, 1453–31461. [CrossRef] [PubMed]
52. Bech-Azeddine, R.; Hogh, P.; Juhler, M.; Gjerris, F.; Waldemar, G. Idiopathic normal-pressure hydrocephalus: Clinical comorbidity correlated with cerebral biopsy findings and outcome of cerebrospinal fluid shunting. *J. Neurol. Neurosurg. Psychiatry* **2007**, *78*, 157–161. [CrossRef]
53. Golomb, J.; Wisoff, J.; Miller, D.C.; Boksay, I.; Kluger, A.; Weiner, H.; Salton, J.; Graves, W. Alzheimer's disease comorbidity in normal pressure hydrocephalus: Prevalence and shunt response. *J. Neurol. Neurosurg. Psychiatry* **2000**, *68*, 778–781. [CrossRef]
54. Hamilton, R.; Patel, S.; Lee, E.B.; Jackson, E.M.; Lopinto, J.; Arnold, S.E.; Clark, C.M.; Basil, A.; Shaw, L.M.; Xie, S.X.; et al. Lack of shunt response in suspected idiopathic normal pressure hydrocephalus with Alzheimer disease pathology. *Ann. Neurol.* **2010**, *68*, 535–540. [CrossRef] [PubMed]
55. Schoonenboom, N.S.; Reesink, F.E.; Verwey, N.A.; Kester, M.I.; Teunissen, C.E.; van de Ven, P.M.; Pijnenburg, Y.A.; Blankenstein, M.A.; Rozemuller, A.J.; Scheltens, P.; et al. Cerebrospinal fluid markers for differential dementia diagnosis in a large memory clinic cohort. *Neurology* **2012**, *78*, 47–354. [CrossRef] [PubMed]

56. Engelborghs, S.; De Vreese, K.; Van de Casteele, T.; Vanderstichele, H.; Van Everbroeck, B.; Cras, P.; Martin, J.J.; Vanmechelen, E.; De Deyn, P.P. Diagnostic performance of a CSF-biomarker panel in autopsy-confirmed dementia. *Neurobiol. Aging* **2008**, *29*, 1143–1159. [CrossRef]
57. Benvenutto, A.; Guedj, E.; Felician, O.; Eusebio, A.; Azulay, J.P.; Ceccaldi, M.; Koric, L. Clinical Phenotypes in Corticobasal Syndrome with or without Amyloidosis Biomarkers. *J. Alzheimers Dis.* **2020**, *74*, 331–343. [CrossRef] [PubMed]
58. Winkel, I.; Ermann, N.; Żelwetro, A.; Sambor, B.; Mroczko, B.; Kornhuber, J.; Paradowski, B.; Lewczuk, P. Cerebrospinal fluid α synuclein concentrations in patients with positive AD biomarkers and extrapyramidal symptoms. *J. Neural Transm.* **2021**, *128*, 817–825. [CrossRef] [PubMed]
59. Wallin, A.; Kapaki, E.; Boban, M.; Engelborghs, S.; Hermann, D.M.; Huisa, B.; Jonsson, M.; Kramberger, M.G.; Lossi, L.; Malojcic, B.; et al. Biochemical markers in vascular cognitive impairment associated with subcortical small vessel disease—A consensus report. *BMC Neurol.* **2017**, *17*, 102. [CrossRef] [PubMed]
60. Bommarito, G.; Van De Ville, D.; Frisoni, G.B.; Garibotto, V.; Ribaldi, F.; Stampacchia, S.; Assal, F.; Allali, G.; Griffa, A. Alzheimer's Disease Biomarkers in Idiopathic Normal Pressure Hydrocephalus: Linking Functional Connectivity and Clinical Outcome. *J. Alzheimers Dis.* **2021**. [CrossRef] [PubMed]
61. Stiffel, M.; Bergeron, D.; Amari, K.M.; Poulin, É.; Roberge, X.; Meilleur-Durand, S.; Sellami, L.; Molin, P.; Nadeau, Y.; Fortin, M.P.; et al. Use of Alzheimer's Disease Cerebrospinal Fluid Biomarkers in A Tertiary Care Memory Clinic. *Can. J. Neurol. Sci.* **2021**, 1–7. [CrossRef] [PubMed]
62. Patel, S.; Lee, E.B.; Xie, S.X.; Law, A.; Jackson, E.M.; Arnold, S.E.; Clark, C.M.; Shaw, L.M.; Grady, M.S.; Trojanowski, J.Q.; et al. Phosphorylated tau/amyloid beta 1–42 ratio in ventricular cerebrospinal fluid reflects outcome in idiopathic normal pressure hydrocephalus. *Fluids Barriers C.N.S.* **2012**, *9*, 7. [CrossRef]
63. Contador, J.; Pérez-Millán, A.; Tort-Merino, A.; Balasa, M.; Falgàs, N.; Olives, J.; Castellví, M.; Borrego-Écija, S.; Bosch, B.; Fernández-Villullas, G.; et al. Longitudinal brain atrophy and CSF biomarkers in early-onset Alzheimer's disease. *Neuroimage Clin.* **2021**, *32*, 102804. [CrossRef] [PubMed]
64. Gouilly, D.; Tisserand, C.; Nogueira, L.; Saint-Lary, L.; Rousseau, V.; Benaiteau, M.; Rafiq, M.; Carlier, J.; Milongo-Rigal, E.; Pagès, J.C.; et al. Taking the A Train? Limited Consistency of Aβ42 and the Aβ42/40 Ratio in the AT(N) Classification. *J. Alzheimers Dis.* **2021**. [CrossRef] [PubMed]
65. Lewczuk, P.; Lelental, N.; Spitzer, P.; Maler, J.M.; Kornhuber, J. Amyloid-β 42/40 CSF concentration ratio in the diagnostics of Alzheimer's disease: Validation of two novel assays. *J. Alzheimers Dis.* **2015**, *43*, 183–191. [CrossRef]
66. Mattsson, N.; Andreasson, U.; Persson, S.; Arai, H.; Batish, S.D.; Bernardini, S.; Bocchio-Chiavetto, L.; Blankenstein, M.A.; Carrillo, M.C.; Chalbot, S.; et al. The Alzheimer's Association external quality control program for cerebrospinal fluid biomarkers. *Alzheimers Dement.* **2011**, *7*, 386–395. [CrossRef]
67. Mattsson, N.; Andreasson, U.; Persson, S.; Carrillo, M.C.; Collins, S.; Chalbot, S.; Cutler, N.; Dufour-Rainfray, D.; Fagan, A.M.; Heegaard, N.H.; et al. CSF biomarker variability in the Alzheimer's Association quality control program. *Alzheimers Dement.* **2013**, *9*, 251–261. [CrossRef] [PubMed]
68. EU Joint Programme—Neurodegenerative Disease Research. Biomarkers for Alzheimer's Disease and Parkinson's Disease (BIOMARKAPD). Available online: https://www.neurodegenerationresearch.eu/fileadmin/Project_Fact_Sheets/PDFs/Biomarkers/BIOMARKAPD_Fact_Sheet_Template.pdf (accessed on 11 September 2021).
69. Niemantsverdriet, E.; Goossens, J.; Struyfs, H.; Martin, J.J.; Goeman, J.; De Deyn, P.P.; Vanderstichele, H.; Engelborghs, S. Diagnostic Impact of Cerebrospinal Fluid Biomarker (Pre-)Analytical Variability in Alzheimer's Disease. *J. Alzheimers Dis.* **2016**, *51*, 97–106. [CrossRef] [PubMed]
70. Vogelgsang, J.; Vukovich, R.; Wedekind, D.; Wiltfang, J. Higher Level of Mismatch in APOEε4 Carriers for Amyloid-Beta Peptide Alzheimer's Disease Biomarkers in Cerebrospinal Fluid. *ASN Neuro.* **2019**, *11*, 1759091419845524. [CrossRef]
71. Toledo, J.B.; Brettschneider, J.; Grossman, M.; Arnold, S.E.; Hu, W.T.; Xie, S.X.; Lee, V.M.; Shaw, L.M.; Trojanowski, J.Q. CSF biomarkers cutoffs: The importance of coincident neuropathological diseases. *Acta Neuropathol.* **2012**, *124*, 23–35. [CrossRef]
72. Piccio, L.; Deming, Y.; Del-Águila, J.L.; Ghezzi, L.; Holtzman, D.M.; Fagan, A.M.; Fenoglio, C.; Galimberti, D.; Borroni, B.; Cruchaga, C. Cerebrospinal fluid soluble TREM2 is higher in Alzheimer disease and associated with mutation status. *Acta Neuropathol.* **2016**, *131*, 925–933. [CrossRef]
73. Kester, M.I.; Teunissen, C.E.; Sutphen, C.L.; Herries, E.M.; Ladenson, J.H.; Xiong, C.; Scheltens, P.; Van Der Flier, W.M.; Morris, J.C.; Holtzman, D.M.; et al. Cerebrospinal fluid VILIP-1 and YKL-40, candidate biomarkers to diagnose, predict and monitor Alzheimer's disease in a memory clinic cohort. *Alzheimer Res.* **2015**, *7*, 1–9. [CrossRef]
74. Suárez-Calvet, M.; Capell, A.; Caballero, M.; Ángel, A.; Morenas-Rodríguez, E.; Fellerer, K.; Franzmeier, N.; Kleinberger, G.; Eren, E.; Deming, Y.; et al. CSF progranulin increases in the course of Alzheimer's disease and is associated with sTREM 2, neurodegeneration and cognitive decline. *EMBO Mol. Med.* **2018**, *10*, e9712. [CrossRef]
75. Wellington, H.; Paterson, R.W.; Portelius, E.; Törnqvist, U.; Magdalinou, N.; Fox, N.C.; Blennow, K.; Schott, J.M.; Zetterberg, H. Increased CSF neurogranin concentration is specific to Alzheimer disease. *Neurology* **2016**, *86*, 829–835. [CrossRef] [PubMed]
76. Yuan, A.; Rao, M.V.; Nixon, R.A. Neurofilaments and Neurofilament Proteins in Health and Disease. *Cold Spring Harb. Perspect. Biol.* **2017**, *9*, a018309. [CrossRef]

77. McKeever, P.M.; Schneider, R.; Taghdiri, F.; Weichert, A.; Multani, N.; Brown, R.A.; Boxer, A.L.; Karydas, A.; Miller, B.; Robertson, J.; et al. MicroRNA Expression Levels Are Altered in the Cerebrospinal Fluid of Patients with Young-Onset Alzheimer's Disease. *Mol. Neurobiol.* **2018**, *55*, 8826–8841. [CrossRef]
78. Phan, L.M.; Cho, S. A Multi-Chamber Paper-Based Platform for the Detection of Amyloid β Oligomers 42 via Copper-Enhanced Gold Immunoblotting. *Biomolecules* **2021**, *11*, 948. [CrossRef] [PubMed]
79. Mollenhauer, B.; El-Agnaf, O.M.; Marcus, K.; Trenkwalder, C.; Schlossmacher, M.G. Quantification of α-synuclein in cerebrospinal fluid as a biomarker candidate: Review of the literature and considerations for future studies. *Biomark. Med.* **2010**, *4*, 683–699. [CrossRef] [PubMed]
80. Junttila, A.; Kuvaja, M.; Hartikainen, P.; Siloaho, M.; Helisalmi, S.; Moilanen, V.; Kiviharju, A.; Jansson, L.; Tienari, P.J.; Remes, A.M.; et al. Cerebrospinal fluid TDP-43 in frontotemporal lobar degeneration and amyotrophic lateral sclerosis patients with and without the C9ORF72 hexanucleotide expansion. *Dement. Geriatr. Cogn. Dis. Extra* **2016**, *6*, 142–149. [CrossRef]
81. Chalatsa, I.; Melachroinou, K.; Emmanouilidou, E.; Vekrellis, K. Assesment of cerebrospinal fluid α-synuclein as a potential biomarker in Parkinson's disease and synucleinopathies. *Neuroimmunol. Neuroinflammation* **2020**, *7*, 132–140.
82. Oeckl, P.; Metzger, F.; Nagl, M.; von Arnim, C.A.; Halbgebauer, S.; Steinacker, P.; Ludolph, A.C.; Otto, M. Alpha-, Beta-, and Gamma-synuclein Quantification in Cerebrospinal Fluid by Multiple Reaction Monitoring Reveals Increased Concentrations in Alzheimer's and Creutzfeldt-Jakob Disease but No Alteration in Synucleinopathies. *Mol. Cell Proteom.* **2016**, *15*, 3126–3138. [CrossRef]
83. Li, J.Q.; Bi, Y.L.; Shen, X.N.; Wang, H.F.; Xu, W.; Tan, C.C.; Dong, Q.; Wang, Y.J.; Tan, L.; Yu, J.T.; et al. Cerebrospinal fluid α-synuclein predicts neurodegeneration and clinical progression in non-demented elders. *Transl. Neurodegener.* **2020**, *9*, 41. [CrossRef] [PubMed]
84. Halbgebauer, S.; Oeckl, P.; Steinacker, P.; Yilmazer-Hanke, D.; Anderl-Straub, S.; von Arnim, C.; Froelich, L.; Gomes, L.A.; Hausner, L.; Huss, A.; et al. Beta-synuclein in cerebrospinal fluid as an early diagnostic marker of Alzheimer's disease. *J. Neurol. Neurosurg. Psychiatry.* **2020**. [CrossRef]
85. Shim, K.H.; Kang, M.J.; Suh, J.W.; Pyun, J.M.; Ryoo, N.; Park, Y.H.; Youn, Y.C.; Jang, J.W.; Jeong, J.H.; Park, K.W.; et al. CSF total tau/α-synuclein ratio improved the diagnostic performance for Alzheimer's disease as an indicator of tau phosphorylation. *Alzheimers Res. Ther.* **2020**, *12*, 83. [CrossRef]
86. Alcolea, D.; Delaby, C.; Muñoz, L.; Torres, S.; Estellés, T.; Zhu, N.; Barroeta, I.; Carmona-Iragui, M.; Illán-Gala, I.; Santos-Santos, M.Á.; et al. Use of plasma biomarkers for AT(N) classification of neurodegenerative dementias. *J. Neurol. Neurosurg. Psychiatry.* **2021**. [CrossRef]
87. Ashton, N.J.; Leuzy, A.; Karikari, T.K.; Mattsson-Carlgren, N.; Dodich, A.; Boccardi, M.; Corre, J.; Drzezga, A.; Nordberg, A.; Ossenkoppele, R.; et al. The validation status of blood biomarkers of amyloid and phospho-tau assessed with the 5-phase development framework for AD biomarkers. *Eur. J. Nucl. Med. Mol. Imaging* **2021**, *48*, 2140–2156. [CrossRef]
88. Kim, K.Y.; Shin, K.Y.; Chang, K.A. Brain-Derived Exosomal Proteins as Effective Biomarkers for Alzheimer's Disease: A Systematic Review and Meta-Analysis. *Biomolecules* **2021**, *11*, 980. [CrossRef] [PubMed]
89. Hampel, H.; Cummings, J.; Blennow, K.; Gao, P.; Jack, C.R., Jr.; Vergallo, A. Developing the ATX(N) classification for use across the Alzheimer disease continuum. *Nat. Rev. Neurol.* **2021**, *17*, 580–589. [CrossRef] [PubMed]
90. Blennow, K.; Zetterberg, H. The past and the future of Alzheimer's disease fluid biomarkers. *J. Alzheimers Dis.* **2018**, *62*, 1125–1140. [CrossRef]
91. Molinuevo, J.L.; Ayton, S.; Batrla, R.; Bednar, M.M.; Bittner, T.; Cummings, J.; Fagan, A.M.; Hampel, H.; Mielke, M.M.; Mikulskis, A.; et al. Current state of Alzheimer's fluid biomarkers. *Acta Neuropathol.* **2018**, *136*, 821–853. [CrossRef]
92. Álvarez, I.; Diez-Fairen, M.; Aguilar, M.; González, J.M.; Ysamat, M.; Tartari, J.P.; Carcel, M.; Alonso, A.; Brix, B.; Arendt, P.; et al. Added value of cerebrospinal fluid multimarker analysis in diagnosis and progression of dementia. *Eur. J. Neurol.* **2021**, *28*, 1142–1152. [CrossRef] [PubMed]
93. Ossenkoppele, R.; Mattsson, N.; Teunissen, C.E.; Barkhof, F.; Pijnenburg, Y.; Scheltens, P.; van der Flier, W.M.; Rabinovici, G.D. Cerebrospinal fluid biomarkers and cerebral atrophy in distinct clinical variants of probable Alzheimer's disease. *Neurobiol. Aging* **2015**, *36*, 2340–2347. [CrossRef] [PubMed]

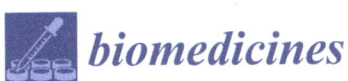 

*Review*

# Shared Molecular Mechanisms among Alzheimer's Disease, Neurovascular Unit Dysfunction and Vascular Risk Factors: A Narrative Review

Lorenzo Falsetti [1,*], Giovanna Viticchi [2], Vincenzo Zaccone [1], Emanuele Guerrieri [3], Gianluca Moroncini [4], Simona Luzzi [2] and Mauro Silvestrini [2]

1. Internal and Subintensive Medicine Department, Azienda Ospedaliero-Universitaria "Ospedali Riuniti" di Ancona, 60100 Ancona, Italy; vincenzo.zaccone@ospedaliriuniti.marche.it
2. Neurologic Clinic, Marche Polytechnic University, 60126 Ancona, Italy; giovanna.viticchi@ospedaliriuniti.marche.it (G.V.); s.luzzi@univpm.it (S.L.); m.silvestrini@univpm.it (M.S.)
3. Emergency Medicine Residency Program, Università Politecnica delle Marche, 60121 Ancona, Italy; e.guerrieri93@gmail.com
4. Clinica Medica, Marche Polytechnic University, 60124 Ancona, Italy; g.moroncini@univpm.it
* Correspondence: lorenzo.falsetti@ospedaliriuniti.marche.it; Tel.: +39-071-596-5269

**Abstract:** Alzheimer's disease (AD) is the most common type of dementia, affecting 24 million individuals. Clinical and epidemiological studies have found several links between vascular risk factors (VRF), neurovascular unit dysfunction (NVUd), blood-brain barrier breakdown (BBBb) and AD onset and progression in adulthood, suggesting a pathogenetic continuum between AD and vascular dementia. Shared pathways between AD, VRF, and NVUd/BBB have also been found at the molecular level, underlining the strength of this association. The present paper reviewed the literature describing commonly shared molecular pathways between adult-onset AD, VRF, and NVUd/BBBb. Current evidence suggests that VRF and NVUd/BBBb are involved in AD neurovascular and neurodegenerative pathology and share several molecular pathways. This is strongly supportive of the hypothesis that the presence of VRF can at least facilitate AD onset and progression through several mechanisms, including NVUd/BBBb. Moreover, vascular disease and several comorbidities may have a cumulative effect on VRF and worsen the clinical manifestations of AD. Early detection and correction of VRF and vascular disease by improving NVUd/BBBd could be a potential target to reduce the overall incidence and delay cognitive impairment in AD.

**Keywords:** Alzheimer's disease; vascular risk factors; hypertension; type 2 diabetes mellitus; dyslipidemia; cigarette smoking

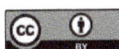

## 1. Introduction

Alzheimer's disease (AD) is the most common neurodegenerative dementia, affecting two-thirds of individuals with cognitive decline worldwide [1]. Its main pathological features are represented by neuroinflammation, extracellular amyloid-β (Aβ) peptide deposition, intracellular neurofibrillary tangles, tau protein degeneration, and neural loss with progressive deterioration of cognitive function [2–4]. Considering a doubling in 20 years, the prevalence of AD will reach 130 million people in 2050, with the greatest increase expected in the poorest countries [5]. Due to its high prevalence, several studies are focusing on reliable serum biomarkers to accurately diagnose AD [3,4].

The neuropathology of AD is characterised by structural and physiological changes that may involve different brain areas. This variability contributes to a certain heterogeneity in the final clinical manifestations in AD patients, each of whom may exhibit a variable association of different neuropsychological deficits. In fact, while the classic cognitive profile of AD is mainly characterised by episodic memory deficits due to the impairment of the temporal lobe, several recent studies have shown that in relation to the different brain areas predominantly involved, different clinical pictures may be present. For example, alterations in the medial prefrontal cortex are associated with impaired retrieval and extinction memories, whereas impairment of emotional and executive processing, similarly to the psychiatric population, reflects a probable impairment of the lateral orbitofrontal cortex or the inferior frontal gyrus [6–8]. It is worth underlining that multiple pathways are implicated in the onset and progression of neurodegeneration and specific functions, such as emotional control, are often impaired in dementia. Indeed, impairment of the prefrontal cortex causes in AD patients an impairment in emotion processing that impacts on action and motor control [7].

The AD pathophysiology is considered largely heterogeneous and characterized by both neurodegeneration—characterized by aberrant, misfolded and aggregated Aβ [9] and hyperphosphorylated tau proteins [10]—and vascular disease, with a common involvement of large [11–14] and small brain vessels. Other neurotoxic elements could also play a relevant role: oxidative stress with reactive oxygen species overproduction, mitochondrial dysfunction or metal accumulation have been extensively studied in the last years [15].

Recently a great attention was put on the interaction between neuronal (neurons and glia) and vascular tissues (endothelial cells, pericytes, and adventitial cells) that are functionally organized in the neurovascular unit (NVU). The NVU is responsible for so-called neurovascular coupling, an organized vascular response to specific neuronal stimuli aimed at modifying regional cerebral blood flow and neuronal metabolic activity [16]. The blood-brain barrier (BBB) is a part of the NVU that controls the transfer of molecules and pathogens to and from brain tissue by adopting a specific transport system in brain endothelial cells [17]. The BBB transports brain metabolic waste products from the brain interstitial fluid to the bloodstream. Thus, BBB represents the most important site of metabolic homeostasis in the central nervous system [17]. Neurovascular coupling is typically deranged in several pathological conditions such as hypertension [18], acute ischemic stroke [19] and AD [20], suggesting a potential role of NVU dysfunction (NVUd) in the progression of cognitive impairment. Of note, neurovascular coupling is strongly influenced by VRF [21–26] and atherosclerotic vascular pathology [14,27], as synthesized in Figure 1.

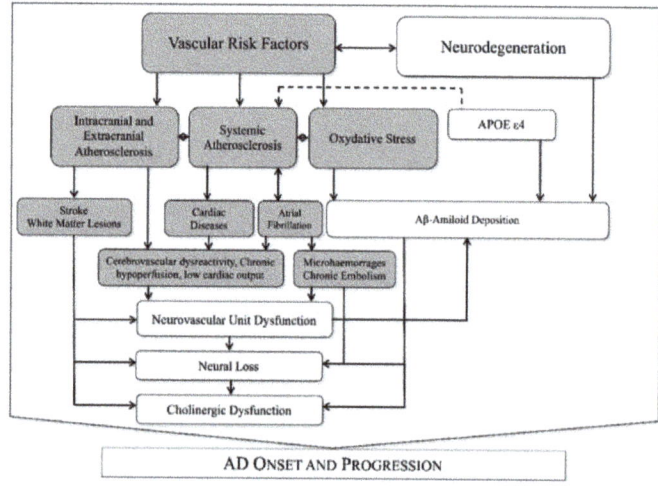

**Figure 1.** Known interactions between vascular and neurodegenerative factors in AD.

Postmortem studies emphasize an important role of vascular pathology in a large percentage of AD subjects. As first observed in the Nun study [6], the presence of neuropathologic findings of vascular lesions in AD subjects was associated with a history of worse cognitive performances. In addition, other studies have confirmed the presence of atherosclerosis of large and small vessels in AD [12]. These alterations, which could affect NVU activities, may be expressed by pathologic adaptations of cerebrovascular responsiveness to hypercapnia [26,28]. A dysfunction of the BBB has been associated with oxidative stress [29], advanced glycation end products (AGEs) and their receptor (RAGE) [30,31] and increased production of proinflammatory cytokines [32]. A blood-brain barrier breakdown (BBBb) could also contribute to AD onset and progression.

This review focuses on the main and most common vascular risk factors that can be easily detected, monitored, and addressed in common clinical practice, their impact on AD neurovascular and neurodegenerative pathology and the potential links between VRF and AD at a molecular level.

## 2. Research Strategy

The review team identified first the MeSH major terms to explore the association between AD, VRF, NVUd and BBB breakdown and performed the literature search in PubMed/Medline and Web of Science for case reports, reviews, and original research articles from 1 January 1991, to 1 December 2021. We used MeSH major terms and considered: "Alzheimer's disease" [MeSH], "Adult-onset diabetes mellitus" [MeSH], "Hypertension" [MeSH], "Dyslipidemia" [MeSH], "Cigarette smoking" [MeSH], "Neurovascular coupling" [MeSH], "Blood brain barrier" [MeSH] and "Neurovascular abnormalities" [MeSH] alone or in combination. The review team favored the inclusion of articles from the last 10 years to give up-to-date information, although they did not exclude older highly referenced reports. The reference lists of articles identified by this search strategy were also reviewed, and the working group selected relevant references. We chose to consider this time frame and all types of articles to obtain a comprehensive overview of this topic.

## 3. Discussion of the Results of the Research Strategy

According to the pre-specified research strategy, the review team selected 156 unique papers regarding the clinical, epidemiological and molecular relationships between AD, NVUd, BBBb, type 2 diabetes mellitus (T2DM), hypertension, smoking and dyslipidemia.

### 3.1. Type 2 Diabetes Mellitus

3.1.1. The Clinical and Epidemiological Link between AD and T2DM

Both AD and T2DM prevalence are progressively increasing, especially among elderly patients [1,33]. Among adults, 1 in 11 suffers from diabetes mellitus and 90% of cases are T2DM, which is a chronic, multi-organ disease characterised by a high burden of co-morbidities and a low quality of life [34]. While aging itself is the strongest risk factor for both AD [35] and T2DM [36], emerging epidemiological data suggest that T2DM and other VRFs may contribute to the pathogenesis of AD directly, in association, or as cofactors [37–39]. AD and T2DM are epidemiologically associated as AD patients appear more vulnerable to T2DM [40], and individuals with T2DM show an increased risk of dementia, including AD [41].

The Rotterdam Study confirmed that the presence of T2DM increases the risk of AD [42], and that this association is stronger in patients with a long history of T2DM. This epidemiological relationship has been confirmed in other cohorts [43]. However, despite epidemiological studies suggesting T2DM as a potential risk factor for AD, the demonstration of a complete overlap between the two diseases is lacking. Some authors have associated this effect to different insulin resistance in target organs. Cerebral hyperglycemia [44] in the absence of clinically evident T2DM has been positively associated with accelerated cognitive impairment, even adjusting for other risk factors, including age and macrovascular disease. In addition, patients with AD often exhibit both insulin resistance and insulin insufficiency even when not affected by T2DM. These observations have led to the current concept of AD as a special form of T2DM, defined by several authors as "type 3 diabetes mellitus" (T3DM) [45–47]. T3DM refers to insulin/insulin-like growth factor (IGF) deficiency and insulin/IGF resistance in brain tissue [46].

### 3.1.2. The Role of Insulin Signalling

Insulin/IGF and their receptors are widely expressed in the cortex, hippocampus, and hypothalamus of the human brain. Several investigations support the hypothesis that cognitive impairment in AD might be, at least in part, mediated by insulin resistance and deficiency of the insulin/IGF cascade in the brain [48–50]. These mechanisms activate multiple intracellular signalling pathways ensuing in intrinsic tyrosine kinases (iTK) activation starting with ligand binding to cell surface receptors, followed by iTK autophosphorylation and activation [51,52]. iTK phosphorylate IRS molecules [53–55], which transmit signals downstream by activating the extracellular/mitogen-activated signal-related kinase (ERK/MAPK) and PI3K pathways and inhibit glycogen synthase kinase 3beta (GSK3). PI3K/AKT/mTOR cascade activation leads to synaptic formation, increased neuronal cell survival [56], regional vasodilation, and regulation of cerebrovascular reactivity in the neurovascular unit [57].

Postmortem studies pointed out that, in brain samples from AD patients, insulin and insulin receptor expression were severely impaired and their levels were inversely proportional to the extent of neurodegeneration [45,58] along with impairment of insulin receptor binding capacity and reduced expression of insulin, IGF-1, IGF2 mRNA and their receptors, with a reduction in the cytosolic level of PI3K p85a and p110a subunits [59]. This was consensual with a tau protein reduction, regulated by insulin/IGF-1.

Decreased choline acetyltransferase (ChAT) expression, typically described in AD, is associated with reduced ChAT colocalization with the insulin/IGF-1 receptor, confirming that neuronal expression of tau and ChAT is regulated by insulin/IGF-1 in the human brain [46,47]. Reduced insulin and poor insulin receptor sensitivity contribute to decreased acetylcholine (ACh), further elucidating a possible biochemical link between diabetes and AD [58]. Thus, insulin resistance and deficiency in the brain could explain, at least in part, the alterations observed in AD, such as cytoskeletal collapse, retraction of neurites, synaptic disconnection, loss of neuronal plasticity, and deficiencies in ACh production. Moreover, T2DM is known to be one of the most important factors for accelerated atherosclerosis [60], and these observations suggest that cerebral vessel atherosclerosis could be another potential link between the two diseases, as confirmed by clinical studies [14].

### 3.1.3. Shared Molecular Mechanisms between AD and T2DM

Primary biological responses to insulin/IGF include increase in cell growth, survival, energy metabolism and cholinergic gene expression, and inhibition of oxidative stress and of apoptosis. These signalling pathways are activated in different cell types and tissues capable of expressing insulin/IGF receptor. Thus they are virtually universal [55,61–63]. Several authors enlightened different abnormalities in IRS-1 phosphorylation (IRS-1p) in AD brains [64]. IRS-1p on tyrosine residues is needed for insulin-stimulated responses, whereas IRS-1p on serine residues was associated to an insulin reduced response, which was consistent with insulin resistance [65].

This pathway modulates the expression of Aβ precursor protein (APP), kinesin, Abelson helper integration site-1 (AHI-1), huntingtin-associated protein-1 (HAP-1), and tau, which are all involved in the neuropathology of AD. Furthermore, neuronal and oligodendroglial cell survival and function are fully linked to the integrity of the insulin/IGF-1 pathway [46,47,49]. Impairment of these metabolic pathways leads to deficits in energy metabolism resulting in increased oxidative stress, mitochondrial dysfunction, activation of proinflammatory cytokines and APP expression. Consequently, reduced expression of neuronal and oligodendroglial specific genes and increased expression of astrocytic and microglial inflammatory genes in AD have been attributed to progressive brain insulin/IGF deficiency and resistance.

Microglial and astrocytic APP mRNA levels are increased in the early stages of neurodegeneration in AD [66]. Microglia activation promotes APP gene expression, cleavage and accumulation. Impairment of insulin/IGF signalling leads to oxidative stress and mitochondrial dysfunction that induces APP gene expression and cleavage, thus resulting in neurotoxicity due to APP-A accumulation. Tau gene expression and tau protein phosphorylation are specifically mediated by this signalling cascade [67,68].

### 3.1.4. The Role of AGE/RAGE System in AD

Glycosylation is a non-reversible and non-enzymatic reaction that occurs between proteins and glucose and eventually leads to the production of AGEs [69], which is especially observed in subjects affected by complicated T2DM [70]. The presence of AGEs marginally affects cell survival, but can significantly alter neuronal metabolism and thus brain function in several neurodegenerative disorders, such as AD [71,72]. In addition, AGEs can directly induce oxidative stress and promote the release of proinflammatory cytokines, thereby worsening cognitive dysfunction in AD [73]. AGEs and RAGEs colocalize with Aβ, senile plaques, and neurofibrillary tangles. Specifically, the interaction between RAGE and Aβ activates neuroinflammatory signalling pathways, causes the release of reactive oxygen species, and ultimately induces neuronal and mitochondrial dysfunction [31].

However, one large study observed a lack of longitudinal association between AGE-RAGE system dysfunction and dementia, suggesting a potential short-term association or reverse causality [74], thus supporting the need for further studies to explore this association.

### *3.2. Hypertension*
### 3.2.1. The Clinical and Epidemiological Link between AD and Hypertension

Aging is an important risk factor for hypertension, representing one of the epidemiological links between AD and VRF. However, the clinical association between hypertension and AD seems weaker than that with T2DM. Some studies have described this potential association [75–77] while others failed to demonstrate any link [78,79]. Papers underlining this epidemiological link have longer follow-up times [75–77]. The Rotterdam study pointed out that hypertension preceded the onset of AD by nine years [75], while in the Honolulu-Asia Aging Study, a temporal relationship of 20–26 years was observed [77].

On the other hand, some studies have shown that low blood pressure is also associated with incident dementia, and that blood pressure drops in the preclinical stages of AD, during AD, and consistently with advanced cognitive impairment [80]. Recently, a U-shaped relationship between hypertension and cognition has been confirmed, especially among the elderly [81]. Several authors have suggested that this effect might be mediated by neurodegeneration of brain structures involved in the central regulation of blood pressure (hypothalamus, amygdala, insular cortex, medial prefrontal cortex, locus coeruleus, parabrachial nucleus, pons and medulla oblongata). This hypothesis is supported by studies underlining a direct positive relationship between neuron number in pons or medulla and blood pressure in AD [82]. Further, brain atrophy has been correlated with lower blood pressure in elderly patients, regardless of dementia [83]. In addition, lower blood pressure can result in greater neuronal damage by worsening regional cerebral blood flow regulation by generating local hypoperfusion [84].

Thus, middle-aged hypertension acts as a risk factor for AD before its onset, whereas low blood pressure in the elderly should be interpreted as a consequence of neural loss, especially in advanced AD. Hypertension is known to induce cerebral vascular changes and vascular dementia. Animal models have shown that high blood pressure can also lead to AD-like neuropathology [85–87], with accumulation and deposition of Aβ.

### 3.2.2. Shared Molecular Mechanisms between AD and Hypertension

While the "classical" amyloid hypothesis suggested a cytotoxic accumulation of Aβ in the brain tissue of AD patients due to its overproduction [88], more recent evidence has shown that Aβ accumulation might be more related to an altered clearance of this molecule from the BBB due to NVU dysfunction [89].

One of the pathways linking hypertension to AD is RAGE, which modulates Aβ clearance in the BBB. Its expression is critically increased in endothelial cells and at the level of the AD brain neurovascular unit [90]. Furthermore, in experimental models, its expression is upregulated in cerebral vessels of the cortex and hippocampus after exposure to a hypertensive condition [86]. RAGE acts as a scavenger receptor for Aβ. In the BBB it mediates the passage of Aβ from the blood to the brain. It also stimulates Aβ production [91] and induces tau hyperphosphorylation [92] by activating the GSK-3 cascade. The angiotensin-II type 1 receptor suggests another link between AD and hypertension. In hypertensive subjects, activation of this receptor increased RAGE mRNA expression, suggesting a link between activation of the renin-angiotensin axis and AD progression [93]. RAGE also responds to AGEs, which are elevated in AD, especially in patients with T2DM, and this represents another possible link between VRF and AD.

The other molecular mechanism linking AD to hypertension is low-density lipoprotein receptor-related protein-1 (LRP-1). Most cell types in the neurovascular unit express LRP-1, which is able to maintain the BBB integrity and transport Aβ from the brain to the blood vessels, in a direction opposite to that by RAGE. LRP-1 acts primarily by releasing Aβ from the brain, but its soluble form (sLRP-1) can bind Aβ and remove it from the circulation, reducing its bioavailability. Interestingly, the expression of LRP-1 in endothelial cells of the neurovascular unit is reduced with aging and its activity is mediated by ApoE [94]. In murine models of hypertension, RAGE expression is increased, whereas LRP-1 expression is unchanged, suggesting increased Aβ influx that is not adequately counteracted by increased efflux [95]. Furthermore, the presence of oxidative stress, as commonly observed in association with the presence of VRF, decreases sLRP-1 activity and increases serum levels of Aβ, which negatively correlates with cognition [96].

Finally, hypertensive patients often show increased serum levels of several markers of endothelial damage, such as soluble intercellular adhesion molecule-1 (sICAM-1), soluble vascular cell adhesion molecule-1 (sVCAM-1), and endothelin-1 (ET-1), which might be implicated in the dysregulation of cerebrovascular reactivity in AD and other neurodegenerative diseases by promoting vasoconstriction [97–99].

*3.3. Dyslipidaemia*

3.3.1. The Clinical and Epidemiological Link between AD and Dyslipidaemia

Dyslipidaemias are a heterogeneous group of diseases defined as disorders of lipid metabolism that lead, alone or in association with other VRFs, to cerebral and systemic atherosclerosis. The current management of dyslipidaemias is closely dependent on the presence and extent of other VRFs, and current guidelines suggest treatment according to the patient's overall cardiovascular risk, as assessed by formal scores [100]. The systematic assessment and proper management of cardiovascular risk is leading to a progressive reduction in the incidence of atherosclerosis. However, this disease remains one of the leading causes of mortality and morbidity worldwide [100]. The link between dyslipidaemia and AD has been described at several levels. Epidemiological evidence suggests an association between high serum cholesterol levels and AD, with a potential role for lipids in modulating AD expression. Total cholesterol serum levels appear to be independently associated with increased AD prevalence, with a potential modulation of the effect by ApoE genotype [101]. Similar to hypertension, increased serum total cholesterol in middle age also appears to be strongly associated with the risk of AD, with a 3-fold increase in the likelihood of development, independent of ApoE genotype [102]. High levels of LDL cholesterol (LDL-C) correlate with lower global cognition in the absence of clinical dementia [103], and with more rapid cognitive decline in individuals who will develop AD [104]. Some authors underlined a paradoxically protective effect of increased serum cholesterol levels from dementia in late life [105], underlining the detrimental role of dyslipidaemia in younger subjects [106]. In addition, intracranial and extracranial atherosclerosis, one of the major consequences of inadequately treated dyslipidaemia, is significantly associated with the risk of AD onset and progression [14,107].

3.3.2. Shared Molecular Mechanisms between AD and Dyslipidaemia

Increased serum cholesterol levels are presumed to induce neuronal apoptosis, oxidative stress, and tau hyperphosphorylation [108]. Brain lipid composition appears to be directly involved in APP processing and Aβ production: increased endosomal cholesterol levels appear to unbalance APP processing, thereby promoting the amyloid-genic pathway [109,110]. A cholesterol-rich membrane might also alter the activity of membrane secretases, thus inducing Aβ production [111]. Furthermore, dyslipidemia is thought to be associated with BBB disruption, which is commonly observed in AD [112]. Animal models, particularly low-density lipoprotein receptor (LDL-R) knock-out mice, confirm these observations: dyslipidemia increases the severity of cognitive dysfunction, especially learning and memory, and Aβ-associated neurotoxicity [113].

Recent studies have emphasized a genetic overlap between AD, C-reactive protein, and plasma lipids [114]. Genome-wide association studies emphasize a strong association between dyslipidemia and AD in several genes. ApoE genotype has been confirmed central to this interaction [115]. ApoE is the most abundant apolipoprotein in the human brain whose role is to transport lipids and facilitate brain homeostasis by removing debris from the interstitial fluid of the brain by interacting with endothelial cells, the basement membrane and glia [116]. In AD, APOE promotes Aβ clearance. The efficiency of Aβ clearance through the BBB depends on the activity of transport proteins such as APOE and APOJ, and receptors such as LRP-1 and RAGE. In particular, it has been observed that APOE ε2 and APOE ε3 genotypes bind with high affinity with LRP-1, whereas APOE ε4 binds with LDL-R [117]. The lack of interaction between APOE ε4 and LRP-1 has been associated with reduced cyclophilin A (CypA) inhibition leading to a proinflammatory state and BBB breakdown [118]. This effect appears to be mediated in pericytes by an NFB-dependent matrix metalloproteinase 9 (MMP-9), which disrupts endothelial tight junctions [117,119]. In addition, CypA has been associated with systemic atherosclerosis [117].

Other single nucleotide polymorphisms of genes implicated in lipid metabolism, such as CLU and ABCA7, have been associated with AD, underscoring a strong link between lipid homeostasis and cognitive function [120]. Of note, several genes implicated in the modulation of inflammation, such as CR1, HLA-DRB5 and TREM, have also been identified as associated with AD [120].

*3.4. Cigarette Smoking*

3.4.1. The Clinical and Epidemiological Link between AD and Cigarette Smoking

Some cross-sectional studies, supported by the tobacco industry, reported a lower AD prevalence among smokers [121]. However, when analysing incident cases and controlling for tobacco industry affiliation [122], it was observed that smoking consistently increased the risk for AD and cognitive decline [123]. This increased risk was found in both APOE ε4 allele carriers [124] and non-carriers [125]. Particularly, mid-life smoking was associated to an increased AD risk [126]. Smoking habit shows its detrimental effects in cognition at different levels. Compared to non-smokers, middle-aged, active smokers showed poorer neurocognitive performances in executive domains (processing speed, learning and memory). Such cognitive dysfunctions were associated with a reduced volume and thickness in hippocampal, cortical, and subcortical areas, reduced neuronal and BBB integrity and neurobiological alterations like those found in early-stage AD, with a dose-dependent effect. Elderly, active-smoking subjects showed worse executive functions, processing speed, learning and memory, a greater cortical atrophy and lower grey matter density in specific brain areas when compared to non-smokers. Former smokers showed intermediate abnormalities between smokers and non-smokers. Patients with chronic obstructive pulmonary disease (COPD), which is commonly caused by smoking, often show worse cognitive performances [127] that seem to be partially preserved by long-term oxygen therapy [128]. A midlife COPD diagnosis is associated to an increased risk of a later-life cognitive deterioration [129]. However, COPD and lung function impairment seem to affect only marginally incident AD [130].

### 3.4.2. Shared Molecular Mechanisms between AD and Cigarette Smoking

The only potential neuroprotective effect of smoking on the brain relies on the finding that nicotine showed neuroprotective activity against glutamate toxicity via α4 and α7 subunits, which can inhibit the neuronal apoptosis process similarly to therapeutic acetylcholinesterase inhibitors [131]. Cigarette smoking, however, has been associated to a downregulation of nicotinic acetylcholine receptors (nAChrs) subunit α7 expression on astrocytes [132] with a reduction of the neuroprotection offered. Furthermore, nicotine strongly affects brain endothelial function, since brain endothelium expresses several nicotinic receptor subunits (α3, α5, α7, β2 and β3) [133]. Nicotine increases BBB permeability by reducing tight junctions expression [134]. The detrimental effects of nicotine on tight junctions' permeability are worsened by oxidative stress and hypoxia. Moreover, nicotine downregulates NOTCH-4 expression in brain endothelial cells: a reduced NOTCH-4 expression is also associated to BBB breakdown [133]. Chronic cigarette smoking has been associated to an increased Aβ deposition and amyloid burden, tau phosphorylation, neuroinflammation with microglial activation, and plaque formation in a dose-dependent manner [135]. On the other side, it has been demonstrated that different central nervous system cells express nicotinic subunits (α3, α4, α5, α6, α7, β2, β4) in the context of nAChrs with a wide variability of expression within different areas of the brain.

Smoking attitude increases oxidative stress by unbalancing the production of reactive oxygen/nitrogen species and their reduction by natural antioxidants [136,137]. Notably, oxidative damage acts on nucleic acids, proteins and lipid membranes of NVU cells [136,137]. Oxidative stress induces cytokine-mediated activation of inflammation in the NVU, thus inducing neuronal cell death and BBBb.

There is a narrow link between neurodegenerative diseases, as AD, and chronic lung pathologies, as COPD [138]. Chronic brain hypoxia, which is commonly observed in advanced COPD and worsened by the occurrence of significant carotid atherosclerosis, seems to worsen cognition by increasing Aβ deposition and tau hyperphosphorylation [139,140]. Moreover, chronic hypoxia acts on VMSCs by downregulating LRP-1 [140], favouring a hypercontractile, non Aβ-clearing phenotype [141]. Moreover, chronic hypoxia has other detrimental effects on cognition: it activates microglia inducing a proinflammatory state that downregulates Aβ receptors and induces a BBB breakdown [140].

### 3.5. Association between VRF and NVU Dysfunction in AD

Neurovascular imbalance is sufficient to initiate neuronal damage and induce accumulation of Aβ. VRF aggregation leads to atherosclerosis, and both factors can induce NVU dysfunction and BBB disruption. These two alterations are associated with increased entry and defective clearance of neurotoxic compounds into brain tissues and reduced energy metabolites and oxygen delivery to activated areas of the brain resulting in neuronal damage. Furthermore, by regulating small vessel blood flow, neurovascular coupling aims to reduce local thrombosis by balancing pro-thrombotic and anti-thrombotic pathways. Its alteration is associated with increased vascular damage. Different combinations of VRF have been associated with cognitive impairment [26,39], especially in the presence of altered cerebrovascular reactivity [142]. Large vessels atherosclerosis is the most prominent effect of a long-term VRF combination, has been associated with an imbalance in cerebrovascular reactivity and more rapid cognitive deterioration [27,143].

At the cellular level, vascular muscle smooth cells (VMSCs) in AD exhibit a "hypercontractile phenotype," which appears to be critically involved in the dysregulation of local cerebral blood flow by inducing chronic hypoxia and hypoperfusion that facilitates neural loss [141]. In addition, AD-VMSCs exhibit impaired capacity to clear Aβ, facilitating cerebral amyloid angiopathy, which in turn leads to impaired cerebral hemodynamic adaptability [144].

BBB disruption appears to be associated with increased production and reduced clearance of Aβ, which promotes the accumulation of amyloidogenic molecules, typically present in advanced AD. BBB dysfunction is favoured by genetic traits, such as APOE ε4. APOE ε4 carriers show accelerated pericyte degeneration due to activation of the

CypA MMP-9 pathway, which is associated with BBB dysfunction with tight junctions and alteration of core proteins [145]. In addition, APOE ε4 carriers often show impaired cerebrovascular reactivity that could affect cerebral perfusion [38,146,147].

## 4. Conclusions

This narrative review aimed to focus on the major vascular risk factors that may contribute to AD genesis and progression (as shown in Figure 2). The reviewed literature highlights correlations between VRF, NVU dysfunction, BBB breakdown and AD onset and progression. Older and emerging data suggest data suggest the urgent need for increased attention on VRF detection, monitoring, and correction in all the ageing populations in order to reduce the burden of cognitive deterioration. In addition, these observations suggest—especially in elderly patients—that a global assessment should be carried out, considering 'classical' VRF and their aggregation [26]. Moreover, special attention should be paid to various pathological conditions, which are particularly frequent in elderly people such as extracranial and intracranial atherosclerosis [107,148], atrial fibrillation [38,149], chronic lung [129] and kidney [150] disease that could have a detrimental effect on cognition. The strongest link between AD and VRF can be observed in the presence of NVUd and BBB breakdown. In these conditions most of the molecular alterations have been observed. However, although several authors underlined this correlation, less is known on neurovascular unit and blood-brain barrier function after intensive correction of VRF, especially at a molecular level. The current treatment strategy for AD progression has currently focused mainly on correcting neurodegenerative aspects, by also using Aβ-directed monoclonal antibodies [151]. In prospective, especially among elderly, multicomorbid patients with AD, a comprehensive, multi-target approach could be comprehensive not only of an early and intensive VRF correction, but also a of a personalized management of comorbidities in later life to reduce the risk of AD onset and to contain the progression of cognitive impairment also at a vascular level.

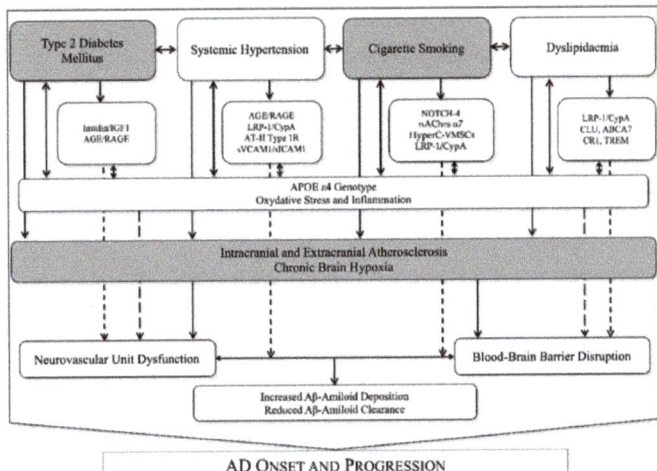

**Figure 2.** Shared molecular mechanisms linking vascular risk factors, vascular pathology, APOE genotype, neurovascular unit dysfunction, blood-brain barrier dysfunction and Alzheimer's disease onset and progression. Legend: AGE: advanced glycation end products; AT-II: angiotensin receptor 2; CypA: cyclophilin A; HyperC-VMSCs: hyper-contractile phenotype vascular muscular smoot cells; LRP-1: low-density lipoprotein receptor-related protein-1; nAChrs: nicotinic acetylcholine receptors subunit α7; IGF1: insulin growth factor; RAGE: advanced glycation end products receptor; sICAM1: soluble intercellular adhesion molecule-1; sVCAM1: soluble vascular cell adhesion molecule 1.

## 5. Future Directions

Midlife VRF correction by drugs [152] or physical activity [153,154] has been associated to a reduction of incident dementia, especially AD, and cognitive deterioration in later life. Antihypertensive drugs have already been shown to reduce both the risk and progression of cognitive decline [155]. Oral antidiabetics and insulin seem able to reduce cognitive impairment in AD [156]. Statin use is not associated with an increased risk of cognitive impairment, and some small observational studies seem to associate this treatment with a potentially favourable role in the setting of AD [157]. Long-term oxygen therapy, also, seems to improve cognition hypoxemic patients affected by AD [128]. Recently, 5-phosphodiesterase inhibitors, such as sildenafil, have been shown to improve neurovascular and neurometabolic function in AD [158,159], and are currently under investigation as repurposed drugs for AD treatment by improving NVU function [160]. Analyses of small groups of subjects show that the correction of extracranial carotid stenosis could be associated to an improvement of NVU dysfunction and a reduction of cognitive decline [161]. However, all these observations are largely based on retrospective or non-randomized prospective cohort studies. Larger, robust and long-term trials are required to assess the role of neurometabolic and neurovascular treatment to prevent AD onset and progression. At the present time, in conjunction with the evaluation of the possible benefits of the most modern therapies as Aβ directed treatment or brain stimulation techniques, it could be useful to pay attention to the potential role of carotid surgery or drugs that improve neurovascular and neurometabolic balance [162–164].

**Author Contributions:** Conceptualization: L.F., G.V., S.L. and M.S.; methodology: L.F. and G.V.; validation: L.F., G.V., V.Z., E.G., S.L., M.S.; investigation, L.F., G.V., V.Z., E.G.; writing- original draft preparation: L.F., G.V., V.Z., E.G., G.M., S.L., M.S.; writing—review and editing: L.F., G.V., V.Z., E.G.; supervision: G.M., S.L., M.S. All authors have read and agreed to the published version of the manuscript.

**Funding:** This research received no external funding.

**Institutional Review Board Statement:** Not applicable.

**Informed Consent Statement:** Not applicable.

**Data Availability Statement:** Not applicable.

**Conflicts of Interest:** The authors declare no conflict of interest.

## References

1. Nichols, E.; Szoeke, C.E.I.; Vollset, S.E.; Abbasi, N.; Abd-Allah, F.; Abdela, J.; Aichour, M.T.E.; Akinyemi, R.O.; Alahdab, F.; Asgedom, S.W.; et al. Global, regional, and national burden of Alzheimer's disease and other dementias, 1990–2016: A systematic analysis for the Global Burden of Disease Study 2016. *Lancet Neurol.* **2019**, *18*, 88–106. [CrossRef]
2. Fan, L.; Mao, C.; Hu, X.; Zhang, S.; Yang, Z.; Hu, Z.; Sun, H.; Fan, Y.; Dong, Y.; Yang, J.; et al. New Insights Into the Pathogenesis of Alzheimer's Disease. *Front. Neurol.* **2020**, *10*, 1312. [CrossRef]
3. Török, N.; Tanaka, M.; Vécsei, L. Searching for Peripheral Biomarkers in Neurodegenerative Diseases: The Tryptophan-Kynurenine Metabolic Pathway. *Int. J. Mol. Sci.* **2020**, *21*, 9338. [CrossRef] [PubMed]
4. Tanaka, M.; Toldi, J.; Vécsei, L. Exploring the Etiological Links behind Neurodegenerative Diseases: Inflammatory Cytokines and Bioactive Kynurenines. *Int. J. Mol. Sci.* **2020**, *21*, 2431. [CrossRef]
5. Alzheimer's Association. 2021 Alzheimer's disease facts and figures. *Alzheimers Dement.* **2021**, *17*, 327–406. [CrossRef] [PubMed]
6. Battaglia, S.; Garofalo, S.; di Pellegrino, G. Context-dependent extinction of threat memories: Influences of healthy aging. *Sci. Rep.* **2018**, *8*, 12592. [CrossRef] [PubMed]
7. Battaglia, S.; Serio, G.; Scarpazza, C.; D'Ausilio, A.; Borgomaneri, S. Frozen in (e)motion: How reactive motor inhibition is influenced by the emotional content of stimuli in healthy and psychiatric populations. *Behav. Res. Ther.* **2021**, *146*, 103963. [CrossRef] [PubMed]
8. Battaglia, S.; Harrison, B.J.; Fullana, M.A. Does the human ventromedial prefrontal cortex support fear learning, fear extinction or both? A commentary on subregional contributions. *Mol. Psychiatry* **2021**. [CrossRef]
9. van der Kant, R.; Goldstein, L.S.B.; Ossenkoppele, R. Amyloid-β-independent regulators of tau pathology in Alzheimer disease. *Nat. Rev. Neurosci.* **2020**, *21*, 21–35. [CrossRef]

10. Iqbal, K.; Alonso, A.d.C.; Chen, S.; Chohan, M.O.; El-Akkad, E.; Gong, C.-X.; Khatoon, S.; Li, B.; Liu, F.; Rahman, A.; et al. Tau pathology in Alzheimer disease and other tauopathies. *Biochim. Biophys. Acta Mol. Basis Dis.* **2005**, *1739*, 198–210. [CrossRef]
11. Snowdon, D.A.; Greiner, L.H.; Mortimer, J.A.; Riley, K.P.; Greiner, P.A.; Markesbery, W.R. Brain infarction and the clinical expression of Alzheimer disease. The Nun Study. *JAMA* **1997**, *277*, 813–817. [CrossRef] [PubMed]
12. Arvanitakis, Z.; Capuano, A.W.; Leurgans, S.E.; Bennett, D.A.; Schneider, J.A. Relation of cerebral vessel disease to Alzheimer's disease dementia and cognitive function in elderly people: A cross-sectional study. *Lancet Neurol.* **2016**, *15*, 934–943. [CrossRef]
13. Yarchoan, M.; Xie, S.X.; Kling, M.A.; Toledo, J.B.; Wolk, D.A.; Lee, E.B.; Van Deerlin, V.; Lee, V.M.-Y.; Trojanowski, J.Q.; Arnold, S.E. Cerebrovascular atherosclerosis correlates with Alzheimer pathology in neurodegenerative dementias. *Brain* **2012**, *135*, 3749–3756. [CrossRef] [PubMed]
14. Silvestrini, M.; Viticchi, G.; Falsetti, L.; Balucani, C.; Vernieri, F.; Cerqua, R.; Luzzi, S.; Bartolini, M.; Provinciali, L. The role of carotid atherosclerosis in Alzheimer's disease progression. *J. Alzheimers Dis.* **2011**, *25*, 719–726. [CrossRef] [PubMed]
15. Ibrahim, M.; Gabr, M. Multitarget therapeutic strategies for Alzheimer's disease. *Neural Regen. Res.* **2019**, *14*, 437–440. [CrossRef]
16. Girouard, H.; Iadecola, C. Neurovascular coupling in the normal brain and in hypertension, stroke, and Alzheimer disease. *J. Appl. Physiol.* **2006**, *100*, 328–335. [CrossRef]
17. Zhao, Z.; Nelson, A.R.; Betsholtz, C.; Zlokovic, B.V. Establishment and Dysfunction of the Blood-Brain Barrier. *Cell* **2015**, *163*, 1064–1078. [CrossRef]
18. Presa, J.L.; Saravia, F.; Bagi, Z.; Filosa, J.A. Vasculo-Neuronal Coupling and Neurovascular Coupling at the Neurovascular Unit: Impact of Hypertension. *Front. Physiol.* **2020**, *11*, 584135. [CrossRef]
19. Silvestrini, M.; Vernieri, F.; Pasqualetti, P.; Matteis, M.; Passarelli, F.; Troisi, E.; Caltagirone, C. Impaired Cerebral Vasoreactivity and Risk of Stroke in Patients With Asymptomatic Carotid Artery Stenosis. *JAMA* **2000**, *283*, 2122–2127. [CrossRef]
20. Viticchi, G.; Falsetti, L.; Vernieri, F.; Altamura, C.; Altavilla, R.; Luzzi, S.; Bartolini, M.; Provinciali, L.; Silvestrini, M. Apolipoprotein E genotype and cerebrovascular alterations can influence conversion to dementia in patients with mild cognitive impairment. *J. Alzheimers Dis.* **2014**, *41*, 401–410. [CrossRef]
21. Mogi, M.; Horiuchi, M. Neurovascular Coupling in Cognitive Impairment Associated With Diabetes Mellitus. *Circ. J.* **2011**, *75*, 1042–1048. [CrossRef]
22. Boms, N.; Yonai, Y.; Molnar, S.; Rosengarten, B.; Bornstein, N.M.; Csiba, L.; Olah, L. Effect of Smoking Cessation on Visually Evoked Cerebral Blood Flow Response in Healthy Volunteers. *J. Vasc. Res.* **2010**, *47*, 214–220. [CrossRef] [PubMed]
23. Jennings, J.R.; Muldoon, M.F.; Ryan, C.; Price, J.C.; Greer, P.; Sutton-Tyrrell, K.; van der Veen, F.M.; Meltzer, C.C. Reduced cerebral blood flow response and compensation among patients with untreated hypertension. *Neurology* **2005**, *64*, 1358–1365. [CrossRef] [PubMed]
24. Czuba, E.; Steliga, A.; Lietzau, G.; Kowiański, P. Cholesterol as a modifying agent of the neurovascular unit structure and function under physiological and pathological conditions. *Metab. Brain Dis.* **2017**, *32*, 935–948. [CrossRef] [PubMed]
25. Hu, B.; Yan, L.-F.; Sun, Q.; Yu, Y.; Zhang, J.; Dai, Y.-J.; Yang, Y.; Hu, Y.-C.; Nan, H.-Y.; Zhang, X.; et al. Disturbed neurovascular coupling in type 2 diabetes mellitus patients: Evidence from a comprehensive fMRI analysis. *NeuroImage Clin.* **2019**, *22*, 101802. [CrossRef]
26. Viticchi, G.; Falsetti, L.; Buratti, L.; Luzzi, S.; Bartolini, M.; Acciarri, M.C.; Provinciali, L.; Silvestrini, M. Metabolic syndrome and cerebrovascular impairment in Alzheimer's disease. *Int. J. Geriatr. Psychiatry* **2015**, *30*, 1164–1170. [CrossRef] [PubMed]
27. Buratti, L.; Balucani, C.; Viticchi, G.; Falsetti, L.; Altamura, C.; Avitabile, E.; Provinciali, L.; Vernieri, F.; Silvestrini, M. Cognitive deterioration in bilateral asymptomatic severe carotid stenosis. *Stroke* **2014**, *45*, 2072–2077. [CrossRef]
28. Buratti, L.; Viticchi, G.; Falsetti, L.; Balucani, C.; Altamura, C.; Petrelli, C.; Provinciali, L.; Vernieri, F.; Silvestrini, M. Thresholds of impaired cerebral hemodynamics that predict short-term cognitive decline in asymptomatic carotid stenosis. *J. Cereb. Blood Flow Metab.* **2016**, *36*, 1804–1812. [CrossRef]
29. Huang, W.-J.; Zhang, X.; Chen, W.-W. Role of oxidative stress in Alzheimer's disease. *Biomed. Rep.* **2016**, *4*, 519–522. [CrossRef]
30. Sasaki, N.; Fukatsu, R.; Tsuzuki, K.; Hayashi, Y.; Yoshida, T.; Fujii, N.; Koike, T.; Wakayama, I.; Yanagihara, R.; Garruto, R.; et al. Advanced Glycation End Products in Alzheimer's Disease and Other Neurodegenerative Diseases. *Am. J. Pathol.* **1998**, *153*, 1149–1155. [CrossRef]
31. Kong, Y.; Wang, F.; Wang, J.; Liu, C.; Zhou, Y.; Xu, Z.; Zhang, C.; Sun, B.; Guan, Y. Pathological Mechanisms Linking Diabetes Mellitus and Alzheimer's Disease: The Receptor for Advanced Glycation End Products (RAGE). *Front. Aging Neurosci.* **2020**, *12*, 217. [CrossRef] [PubMed]
32. Swardfager, W.; Lanctôt, K.; Rothenburg, L.; Wong, A.; Cappell, J.; Herrmann, N. A Meta-Analysis of Cytokines in Alzheimer's Disease. *Biol. Psychiatry* **2010**, *68*, 930–941. [CrossRef] [PubMed]
33. Khan, M.A.B.; Hashim, M.J.; King, J.K.; Govender, R.D.; Mustafa, H.; Al Kaabi, J. Epidemiology of Type 2 Diabetes—Global Burden of Disease and Forecasted Trends. *J. Epidemiol. Glob. Health* **2020**, *10*, 107–111. [CrossRef] [PubMed]
34. Zheng, Y.; Ley, S.H.; Hu, F.B. Global aetiology and epidemiology of type 2 diabetes mellitus and its complications. *Nat. Rev. Endocrinol.* **2018**, *14*, 88–98. [CrossRef] [PubMed]
35. Guerreiro, R.; Bras, J. The age factor in Alzheimer's disease. *Genome Med.* **2015**, *7*, 106. [CrossRef]
36. Fazeli, P.K.; Lee, H.; Steinhauser, M.L. Aging Is a Powerful Risk Factor for Type 2 Diabetes Mellitus Independent of Body Mass Index. *Gerontology* **2020**, *66*, 209–210. [CrossRef]

37. Qiu, C.; De Ronchi, D.; Fratiglioni, L. The epidemiology of the dementias: An update. *Curr. Opin. Psychiatry* **2007**, *20*, 380–385. [CrossRef]
38. Falsetti, L.; Viticchi, G.; Buratti, L.; Grigioni, F.; Capucci, A.; Silvestrini, M. Interactions between Atrial Fibrillation, Cardiovascular Risk Factors, and ApoE Genotype in Promoting Cognitive Decline in Patients with Alzheimer's Disease: A Prospective Cohort Study. *J. Alzheimers Dis.* **2018**, *62*, 713–725. [CrossRef]
39. Viticchi, G.; Falsetti, L.; Buratti, L.; Boria, C.; Luzzi, S.; Bartolini, M.; Provinciali, L.; Silvestrini, M. Framingham risk score can predict cognitive decline progression in Alzheimer's disease. *Neurobiol. Aging* **2015**, *36*, 2940–2945. [CrossRef]
40. Janson, J.; Laedtke, T.; Parisi, J.E.; O'Brien, P.; Petersen, R.C.; Butler, P.C. Increased Risk of Type 2 Diabetes in Alzheimer Disease. *Diabetes* **2004**, *53*, 474–481. [CrossRef]
41. Biessels, G.J.; Staekenborg, S.; Brunner, E.; Brayne, C.; Scheltens, P. Risk of dementia in diabetes mellitus: A systematic review. *Lancet Neurol.* **2006**, *5*, 64–74. [CrossRef]
42. Hofman, A.; Ott, A.; Breteler, M.M.; Bots, M.L.; Slooter, A.J.; van Harskamp, F.; van Duijn, C.N.; Van Broeckhoven, C.; Grobbee, D.E. Atherosclerosis, apolipoprotein E, and prevalence of dementia and Alzheimer's disease in the Rotterdam Study. *Lancet* **1997**, *349*, 151–154. [CrossRef]
43. Kloppenborg, R.P.; van den Berg, E.; Kappelle, L.J.; Biessels, G.J. Diabetes and other vascular risk factors for dementia: Which factor matters most? A systematic review. *Eur. J. Pharmacol.* **2008**, *585*, 97–108. [CrossRef] [PubMed]
44. Crane, P.K.; Walker, R.; Hubbard, R.A.; Li, G.; Nathan, D.M.; Zheng, H.; Haneuse, S.; Craft, S.; Montine, T.J.; Kahn, S.E.; et al. Glucose Levels and Risk of Dementia. *N. Engl. J. Med.* **2013**, *369*, 540–548. [CrossRef]
45. Steen, E.; Terry, B.M.; Rivera, E.J.; Cannon, J.L.; Neely, T.R.; Tavares, R.; Xu, X.J.; Wands, J.R.; de la Monte, S.M. Impaired insulin and insulin-like growth factor expression and signaling mechanisms in Alzheimer's disease—Is this type 3 diabetes? *J. Alzheimers Dis.* **2005**, *7*, 63–80. [CrossRef]
46. de la Monte, S.M.; Wands, J.R. Alzheimer's Disease is Type 3 Diabetes—Evidence Reviewed. *J. Diabetes Sci. Technol.* **2008**, *2*, 1101–1113. [CrossRef]
47. de la Monte, S.M.; Tong, M.; Lester-Coll, N.; Plater, M., Jr.; Wands, J.R. Therapeutic rescue of neurodegeneration in experimental type 3 diabetes: Relevance to Alzheimer's disease. *J. Alzheimers Dis.* **2006**, *10*, 89–109. [CrossRef]
48. de la Monte, S.M. Brain Insulin Resistance and Deficiency as Therapeutic Targets in Alzheimers Disease. *Curr. Alzheimer Res.* **2012**, *9*, 35–66. [CrossRef]
49. Lester-Coll, N.; Rivera, E.J.; Soscia, S.J.; Doiron, K.; Wands, J.R.; de la Monte, S.M. Intracerebral streptozotocin model of type 3 diabetes: Relevance to sporadic Alzheimer's disease. *J. Alzheimers Dis.* **2006**, *9*, 13–33. [CrossRef]
50. de la Monte, S.M.; Ganju, N.; Banerjee, K.; Brown, N.V.; Luong, T.; Wands, J.R. Partial rescue of ethanol-induced neuronal apoptosis by growth factor activation of phosphoinositol-3-kinase. *Alcohol. Clin. Exp. Res.* **2000**, *24*, 716–726. [CrossRef]
51. Myers, M.G.; Sun, X.J.; White, M.F. The IRS-1 signaling system. *Trends Biochem. Sci.* **1994**, *19*, 289–293. [CrossRef]
52. Ullrich, A.; Bell, J.R.; Chen, E.Y.; Herrera, R.; Petruzzelli, L.M.; Dull, T.J.; Gray, A.; Coussens, L.; Liao, Y.-C.; Tsubokawa, M.; et al. Human insulin receptor and its relationship to the tyrosine kinase family of oncogenes. *Nature* **1985**, *313*, 756–761. [CrossRef] [PubMed]
53. Sun, X.J.; Rothenberg, P.; Kahn, C.R.; Backer, J.M.; Araki, E.; Wilden, P.A.; Cahill, D.A.; Goldstein, B.J.; White, M.F. Structure of the insulin receptor substrate IRS-1 defines a unique signal transduction protein. *Nature* **1991**, *352*, 73–77. [CrossRef] [PubMed]
54. White, M.F.; Maron, R.; Kahn, C.R. Insulin rapidly stimulates tyrosine phosphorylation of a Mr-185,000 protein in intact cells. *Nature* **1985**, *318*, 183–186. [CrossRef] [PubMed]
55. Sun, X.J.; Crimmins, D.L.; Myers, M.G.; Miralpeix, M.; White, M.F. Pleiotropic insulin signals are engaged by multisite phosphorylation of IRS-1. *Mol. Cell. Biol.* **1993**, *13*, 7418–7428. [CrossRef] [PubMed]
56. Matsuda, S.; Nakagawa, Y.; Tsuji, A.; Kitagishi, Y.; Nakanishi, A.; Murai, T. Implications of PI3K/AKT/PTEN Signaling on Superoxide Dismutases Expression and in the Pathogenesis of Alzheimer's Disease. *Diseases* **2018**, *6*, 28. [CrossRef]
57. Chang, C.-Z.; Wu, S.-C.; Chang, C.-M.; Lin, C.-L.; Kwan, A.-L. Arctigenin, a Potent Ingredient of *Arctium lappa* L., Induces Endothelial Nitric Oxide Synthase and Attenuates Subarachnoid Hemorrhage-Induced Vasospasm through PI3K/Akt Pathway in a Rat Model. *BioMed Res. Int.* **2015**, *2015*, 490209. [CrossRef]
58. Rivera, E.J.; Goldin, A.; Fulmer, N.; Tavares, R.; Wands, J.R.; de la Monte, S.M. Insulin and insulin-like growth factor expression and function deteriorate with progression of Alzheimer's disease: Link to brain reductions in acetylcholine. *J. Alzheimers Dis.* **2005**, *8*, 247–268. [CrossRef]
59. Moloney, A.M.; Griffin, R.J.; Timmons, S.; O'Connor, R.; Ravid, R.; O'Neill, C. Defects in IGF-1 receptor, insulin receptor and IRS-1/2 in Alzheimer's disease indicate possible resistance to IGF-1 and insulin signalling. *Neurobiol. Aging* **2010**, *31*, 224–243. [CrossRef]
60. Basta, G.; Schmidt, A.M.; De Caterina, R. Advanced glycation end products and vascular inflammation: Implications for accelerated atherosclerosis in diabetes. *Cardiovasc. Res.* **2004**, *63*, 582–592. [CrossRef]
61. Burgering, B.M.T.; Coffer, P.J. Protein kinase B (c-Akt) in phosphatidylinositol-3-OH kinase signal transduction. *Nature* **1995**, *376*, 599–602. [CrossRef]
62. Delcommenne, M.; Tan, C.; Gray, V.; Rue, L.; Woodgett, J.; Dedhar, S. Phosphoinositide-3-OH kinase-dependent regulation of glycogen synthase kinase 3 and protein kinase B/AKT by the integrin-linked kinase. *Proc. Natl. Acad. Sci. USA* **1998**, *95*, 11211–11216. [CrossRef] [PubMed]

63. Kulik, G.; Klippel, A.; Weber, M.J. Antiapoptotic signalling by the insulin-like growth factor I receptor, phosphatidylinositol 3-kinase, and Akt. *Mol. Cell. Biol.* **1997**, *17*, 1595–1606. [CrossRef] [PubMed]
64. Talbot, K.; Wang, H.-Y.; Kazi, H.; Han, L.-Y.; Bakshi, K.P.; Stucky, A.; Fuino, R.L.; Kawaguchi, K.R.; Samoyedny, A.J.; Wilson, R.S.; et al. Demonstrated brain insulin resistance in Alzheimer's disease patients is associated with IGF-1 resistance, IRS-1 dysregulation, and cognitive decline. *J. Clin. Investig.* **2012**, *122*, 1316–1338. [CrossRef]
65. Hirosumi, J.; Tuncman, G.; Chang, L.; Görgün, C.Z.; Uysal, K.T.; Maeda, K.; Karin, M.; Hotamisligil, G.S. A central role for JNK in obesity and insulin resistance. *Nature* **2002**, *420*, 333–336. [CrossRef]
66. de la Monte, S.M.; Wands, J.R. Molecular indices of oxidative stress and mitochondrial dysfunction occur early and often progress with severity of Alzheimer's disease. *J. Alzheimers Dis.* **2006**, *9*, 167–181. [CrossRef]
67. Schubert, M.; Brazil, D.P.; Burks, D.J.; Kushner, J.A.; Ye, J.; Flint, C.L.; Farhang-Fallah, J.; Dikkes, P.; Warot, X.M.; Rio, C.; et al. Insulin Receptor Substrate-2 Deficiency Impairs Brain Growth and Promotes Tau Phosphorylation. *J. Neurosci.* **2003**, *23*, 7084–7092. [CrossRef] [PubMed]
68. Schubert, M.; Gautam, D.; Surjo, D.; Ueki, K.; Baudler, S.; Schubert, D.; Kondo, T.; Alber, J.; Galldiks, N.; Küstermann, E.; et al. Role for neuronal insulin resistance in neurodegenerative diseases. *Proc. Natl. Acad. Sci. USA* **2004**, *101*, 3100–3105. [CrossRef]
69. Bunn, H.; Higgins, P. Reaction of monosaccharides with proteins: Possible evolutionary significance. *Science* **1981**, *213*, 222–224. [CrossRef]
70. Simó, R.; Ciudin, A.; Simó-Servat, O.; Hernández, C. Cognitive impairment and dementia: A new emerging complication of type 2 diabetes—The diabetologist's perspective. *Acta Diabetol.* **2017**, *54*, 417–424. [CrossRef]
71. Miranda, H.V.; Outeiro, T.F. The sour side of neurodegenerative disorders: The effects of protein glycation. *J. Pathol.* **2010**, *221*, 13–25. [CrossRef] [PubMed]
72. Salahuddin, P.; Rabbani, G.; Khan, R. The role of advanced glycation end products in various types of neurodegenerative disease: A therapeutic approach. *Cell. Mol. Biol. Lett.* **2014**, *19*, 407–437. [CrossRef] [PubMed]
73. Yan, S.D.; Chen, X.; Fu, J.; Chen, M.; Zhu, H.; Roher, A.; Slattery, T.; Zhao, L.; Nagashima, M.; Morser, J.; et al. RAGE and amyloid-β peptide neurotoxicity in Alzheimer's disease. *Nature* **1996**, *382*, 685–691. [CrossRef] [PubMed]
74. Chen, J.; Mooldijk, S.S.; Licher, S.; Waqas, K.; Ikram, M.K.; Uitterlinden, A.G.; Zillikens, M.C.; Ikram, M.A. Assessment of Advanced Glycation End Products and Receptors and the Risk of Dementia. *JAMA Netw. Open* **2021**, *4*, e2033012. [CrossRef] [PubMed]
75. Portegies, M.L.P.; Mirza, S.S.; Verlinden, V.J.A.; Hofman, A.; Koudstaal, P.J.; Swanson, S.A.; Ikram, M.A. Mid- to Late-Life Trajectories of Blood Pressure and the Risk of Stroke. *Hypertension* **2016**, *67*, 1126–1132. [CrossRef]
76. Kivipelto, M.; Helkala, E.-L.; Laakso, M.; Hänninen, T.; Hallikainen, M.; Alhainen, K.; Soininen, H.; Tuomilehto, J.; Nissinen, A. Midlife vascular risk factors and Alzheimer's disease in later life: Longitudinal, population based study. *BMJ* **2001**, *322*, 1447–1451. [CrossRef]
77. Launer, L.J.; Ross, G.W.; Petrovitch, H.; Masaki, K.; Foley, D.; White, L.R.; Havlik, R.J. Midlife blood pressure and dementia: The Honolulu–Asia aging study☆. *Neurobiol. Aging* **2000**, *21*, 49–55. [CrossRef]
78. Posner, H.B.; Tang, M.-X.; Luchsinger, J.; Lantigua, R.; Stern, Y.; Mayeux, R. The relationship of hypertension in the elderly to AD, vascular dementia, and cognitive function. *Neurology* **2002**, *58*, 1175–1181. [CrossRef]
79. Yoshitake, T.; Kiyohara, Y.; Kato, I.; Ohmura, T.; Iwamoto, H.; Nakayama, K.; Ohmori, S.; Nomiyama, K.; Kawano, H.; Ueda, K.; et al. Incidence and risk factors of vascular dementia and Alzheimer's disease in a defined elderly Japanese population: The Hisayama Study. *Neurology* **1995**, *45*, 1161–1168. [CrossRef]
80. Skoog, I.; Nilsson, L.; Persson, G.; Lernfelt, B.; Landahl, S.; Palmertz, B.; Andreasson, L.-A.; Odén, A.; Svanborg, A. 15-year longitudinal study of blood pressure and dementia. *Lancet* **1996**, *347*, 1141–1145. [CrossRef]
81. van Dalen, J.W.; Brayne, C.; Crane, P.K.; Fratiglioni, L.; Larson, E.B.; Lobo, A.; Lobo, E.; Marcum, Z.A.; van Charante, E.P.M.; Qiu, C.; et al. Association of Systolic Blood Pressure With Dementia Risk and the Role of Age, U-Shaped Associations, and Mortality. *JAMA Intern. Med.* **2021**. [CrossRef] [PubMed]
82. Burke, W.J.; Coronado, P.G.; Schmitt, C.A.; Gillespie, K.M.; Chung, H.D. Blood pressure regulation in alzheimer's disease. *J. Auton. Nerv. Syst.* **1994**, *48*, 65–71. [CrossRef]
83. Skoog, I.; Andreasson, L.-A.; Landahl, S.; Lernfelt, B. A Population-Based Study on Blood Pressure and Brain Atrophy in 85-Year-Olds. *Hypertension* **1998**, *32*, 404–409. [CrossRef] [PubMed]
84. de la Torre, J.C. Cerebral Hypoperfusion, Capillary Degeneration, and Development of Alzheimer Disease. *Alzheimer Dis. Assoc. Disord.* **2000**, *14*, S72–S81. [CrossRef]
85. Carnevale, D.; Lembo, G. 'Alzheimer-like' pathology in a murine model of arterial hypertension. *Biochem. Soc. Trans.* **2011**, *39*, 939–944. [CrossRef]
86. Carnevale, D.; Mascio, G.; D'Andrea, I.; Fardella, V.; Bell, R.D.; Branchi, I.; Pallante, F.; Zlokovic, B.; Yan, S.S.; Lembo, G. Hypertension Induces Brain β-Amyloid Accumulation, Cognitive Impairment, and Memory Deterioration Through Activation of Receptor for Advanced Glycation End Products in Brain Vasculature. *Hypertension* **2012**, *60*, 188–197. [CrossRef]
87. Carnevale, D.; Mascio, G.; Ajmone-Cat, M.A.; D'Andrea, I.; Cifelli, G.; Madonna, M.; Cocozza, G.; Frati, A.; Carullo, P.; Carnevale, L.; et al. Role of neuroinflammation in hypertension-induced brain amyloid pathology. *Neurobiol. Aging* **2012**, *33*, 205.e19–205.e29. [CrossRef]
88. Hardy, J.; Higgins, G. Alzheimer's disease: The amyloid cascade hypothesis. *Science* **1992**, *256*, 184–185. [CrossRef]

89. Zlokovic, B.V. Cerebrovascular transport of Alzheimer's amyloid β and apolipoproteins J and E: Possible anti-amyloidogenic role of the blood-brain barrier. *Life Sci.* **1996**, *59*, 1483–1497. [CrossRef]
90. Deane, R.; Du Yan, S.; Submamaryan, R.K.; LaRue, B.; Jovanovic, S.; Hogg, E.; Welch, D.; Manness, L.; Lin, C.; Yu, J.; et al. RAGE mediates amyloid-β peptide transport across the blood-brain barrier and accumulation in brain. *Nat. Med.* **2003**, *9*, 907–913. [CrossRef]
91. Chen, C.; Li, X.-H.; Tu, Y.; Sun, H.-T.; Liang, H.-Q.; Cheng, S.-X.; Zhang, S. Aβ-AGE aggravates cognitive deficit in rats via RAGE pathway. *Neuroscience* **2014**, *257*, 1–10. [CrossRef] [PubMed]
92. Li, X.-H.; Lv, B.-L.; Xie, J.-Z.; Liu, J.; Zhou, X.-W.; Wang, J.-Z. AGEs induce Alzheimer-like tau pathology and memory deficit via RAGE-mediated GSK-3 activation. *Neurobiol. Aging* **2012**, *33*, 1400–1410. [CrossRef] [PubMed]
93. Nakamura, K.; Yamagishi, S.; Nakamura, Y.; Takenaka, K.; Matsui, T.; Jinnouchi, Y.; Imaizumi, T. Telmisartan inhibits expression of a receptor for advanced glycation end products (RAGE) in angiotensin-II-exposed endothelial cells and decreases serum levels of soluble RAGE in patients with essential hypertension. *Microvasc. Res.* **2005**, *70*, 137–141. [CrossRef] [PubMed]
94. Shibata, M.; Yamada, S.; Kumar, S.R.; Calero, M.; Bading, J.; Frangione, B.; Holtzman, D.M.; Miller, C.A.; Strickland, D.K.; Ghiso, J.; et al. Clearance of Alzheimer's amyloid-β1-40 peptide from brain by LDL receptor–related protein-1 at the blood-brain barrier. *J. Clin. Investig.* **2000**, *106*, 1489–1499. [CrossRef]
95. Shih, Y.-H.; Wu, S.-Y.; Yu, M.; Huang, S.-H.; Lee, C.-W.; Jiang, M.-J.; Lin, P.-Y.; Yang, T.-T.; Kuo, Y.-M. Hypertension Accelerates Alzheimer's Disease-Related Pathologies in Pigs and 3xTg Mice. *Front. Aging Neurosci.* **2018**, *10*, 73. [CrossRef]
96. Sagare, A.P.; Deane, R.; Zetterberg, H.; Wallin, A.; Blennow, K.; Zlokovic, B.V. Impaired Lipoprotein Receptor-Mediated Peripheral Binding of Plasma Amyloid-β is an Early Biomarker for Mild Cognitive Impairment Preceding Alzheimer's Disease. *J. Alzheimers Dis.* **2011**, *24*, 25–34. [CrossRef]
97. Uiterwijk, R.; Huijts, M.; Staals, J.; Rouhl, R.P.W.; De Leeuw, P.W.; Kroon, A.A.; Van Oostenbrugge, R.J. Endothelial Activation Is Associated With Cognitive Performance in Patients With Hypertension. *Am. J. Hypertens.* **2016**, *29*, 464–469. [CrossRef]
98. Rosei, E.A.; Rizzoni, D.; Muiesan, M.L.; Sleiman, I.; Salvetti, M.; Monteduro, C.; Porteri, E. Effects of candesartan cilexetil and enalapril on inflammatory markers of atherosclerosis in hypertensive patients with non-insulin-dependent diabetes mellitus. *J. Hypertens.* **2005**, *23*, 435–444. [CrossRef]
99. Akter, S.; Jesmin, S.; Iwashima, Y.; Hideaki, S.; Rahman, M.A.; Islam, M.M.; Moroi, M.; Shimojo, N.; Yamaguchi, N.; Miyauchi, T.; et al. Higher circulatory level of endothelin-1 in hypertensive subjects screened through a cross-sectional study of rural Bangladeshi women. *Hypertens. Res.* **2015**, *38*, 208–212. [CrossRef]
100. Visseren, F.L.J.; Mach, F.; Smulders, Y.M.; Carballo, D.; Koskinas, K.C.; Bäck, M.; Benetos, A.; Biffi, A.; Boavida, J.-M.; Capodanno, D.; et al. 2021 ESC Guidelines on cardiovascular disease prevention in clinical practice. *Eur. Heart J.* **2021**, *42*, 3227–3337. [CrossRef]
101. Notkola, I.-L.; Sulkava, R.; Pekkanen, J.; Erkinjuntti, T.; Ehnholm, C.; Kivinen, P.; Tuomilehto, J.; Nissinen, A. Serum Total Cholesterol, Apolipoprotein E {FC12}e4 Allele, and Alzheimer's Disease. *Neuroepidemiology* **1998**, *17*, 14–20. [CrossRef]
102. Kivipelto, M.; Helkala, E.-L.; Laakso, M.P.; Hänninen, T.; Hallikainen, M.; Alhainen, K.; Iivonen, S.; Mannermaa, A.; Tuomilehto, J.; Nissinen, A.; et al. Apolipoprotein E ε4 Allele, Elevated Midlife Total Cholesterol Level, and High Midlife Systolic Blood Pressure Are Independent Risk Factors for Late-Life Alzheimer Disease. *Ann. Intern. Med.* **2002**, *137*, 149–155. [CrossRef] [PubMed]
103. Yaffe, K.; Barrett-Connor, E.; Lin, F.; Grady, D. Serum Lipoprotein Levels, Statin Use, and Cognitive Function in Older Women. *Arch. Neurol.* **2002**, *59*, 378–384. [CrossRef] [PubMed]
104. Helzner, E.P.; Luchsinger, J.A.; Scarmeas, N.; Cosentino, S.; Brickman, A.M.; Glymour, M.M.; Stern, Y. Contribution of Vascular Risk Factors to the Progression in Alzheimer Disease. *Arch. Neurol.* **2009**, *66*, 343–348. [CrossRef]
105. Mielke, M.M.; Zandi, P.P.; Sjogren, M.; Gustafson, D.; Ostling, S.; Steen, B.; Skoog, I. High total cholesterol levels in late life associated with a reduced risk of dementia. *Neurology* **2005**, *64*, 1689–1695. [CrossRef] [PubMed]
106. Whitmer, R.A.; Sidney, S.; Selby, J.; Johnston, S.C.; Yaffe, K. Midlife cardiovascular risk factors and risk of dementia in late life. *Neurology* **2005**, *64*, 277–281. [CrossRef] [PubMed]
107. Roher, A.E.; Esh, C.; Kokjohn, T.A.; Kalback, W.; Luehrs, D.C.; Seward, J.D.; Sue, L.I.; Beach, T.G. Circle of Willis Atherosclerosis Is a Risk Factor for Sporadic Alzheimer's Disease. *Arterioscler. Thromb. Vasc. Biol.* **2003**, *23*, 2055–2062. [CrossRef] [PubMed]
108. McLaurin, J.; Darabie, A.A.; Morrison, M.R. Cholesterol, a Modulator of Membrane-Associated Aβ-Fibrillogenesis. *Ann. N. Y. Acad. Sci.* **2002**, *977*, 376–383. [CrossRef]
109. Sun, F.; Chen, L.; Wei, P.; Chai, M.; Ding, X.; Xu, L.; Luo, S.-Z. Dimerization and Structural Stability of Amyloid Precursor Proteins Affected by the Membrane Microenvironments. *J. Chem. Inf. Model.* **2017**, *57*, 1375–1387. [CrossRef]
110. Brown, A.M.; Bevan, D.R. Influence of sequence and lipid type on membrane perturbation by human and rat amyloid β-peptide (1–42). *Arch. Biochem. Biophys.* **2017**, *614*, 1–13. [CrossRef]
111. Abad-Rodriguez, J.; Ledesma, M.D.; Craessaerts, K.; Perga, S.; Medina, M.; Delacourte, A.; Dingwall, C.; De Strooper, B.; Dotti, C.G. Neuronal membrane cholesterol loss enhances amyloid peptide generation. *J. Cell Biol.* **2004**, *167*, 953–960. [CrossRef] [PubMed]
112. Bowman, G.L.; Kaye, J.A.; Quinn, J.F. Dyslipidemia and Blood-Brain Barrier Integrity in Alzheimer's Disease. *Curr. Gerontol. Geriatr. Res.* **2012**, *2012*, 184042. [CrossRef] [PubMed]

113. de Oliveira, J.; Moreira, E.L.G.; dos Santos, D.B.; Piermartiri, T.C.; Dutra, R.C.; Pinton, S.; Tasca, C.I.; Farina, M.; Prediger, R.D.S.; de Bem, A.F. Increased Susceptibility to Amyloid-β-Induced Neurotoxicity in Mice Lacking the Low-Density Lipoprotein Receptor. *J. Alzheimers Dis.* 2014, *41*, 43–60. [CrossRef] [PubMed]
114. Desikan, R.S.; Schork, A.J.; Wang, Y.; Thompson, W.K.; Dehghan, A.; Ridker, P.M.; Chasman, D.I.; McEvoy, L.K.; Holland, D.; Chen, C.-H.; et al. Polygenic Overlap Between C-Reactive Protein, Plasma Lipids, and Alzheimer Disease. *Circulation* 2015, *131*, 2061–2069. [CrossRef] [PubMed]
115. Coon, K.D.; Myers, A.J.; Craig, D.W.; Webster, J.A.; Pearson, J.V.; Lince, D.H.; Zismann, V.L.; Beach, T.G.; Leung, D.; Bryden, L.; et al. A High-Density Whole-Genome Association Study Reveals That APOE Is the Major Susceptibility Gene for Sporadic Late-Onset Alzheimer's Disease. *J. Clin. Psychiatry* 2007, *68*, 613–618. [CrossRef]
116. Flowers, S.A.; Rebeck, G.W. APOE in the normal brain. *Neurobiol. Dis.* 2020, *136*, 104724. [CrossRef]
117. Bell, R.D. The Imbalance of Vascular Molecules in Alzheimer's Disease. *J. Alzheimers Dis.* 2012, *32*, 699–709. [CrossRef]
118. Nikolakopoulou, A.M.; Wang, Y.; Ma, Q.; Sagare, A.P.; Montagne, A.; Huuskonen, M.T.; Rege, S.V.; Kisler, K.; Dai, Z.; Körbelin, J.; et al. Endothelial LRP1 protects against neurodegeneration by blocking cyclophilin A. *J. Exp. Med.* 2021, *218*, e20202207. [CrossRef]
119. Nigro, P.; Satoh, K.; O'Dell, M.R.; Soe, N.N.; Cui, Z.; Mohan, A.; Abe, J.; Alexis, J.D.; Sparks, J.D.; Berk, B.C. Cyclophilin A is an inflammatory mediator that promotes atherosclerosis in apolipoprotein E-deficient mice. *J. Exp. Med.* 2011, *208*, 53–66. [CrossRef]
120. Karch, C.M.; Cruchaga, C.; Goate, A.M. Alzheimer's disease genetics: From the bench to the clinic. *Neuron* 2014, *83*, 11–26. [CrossRef]
121. Fratiglioni, L.; Wang, H.-X. Smoking and Parkinson's and Alzheimer's disease: Review of the epidemiological studies. *Behav. Brain Res.* 2000, *113*, 117–120. [CrossRef]
122. Anstey, K.J.; von Sanden, C.; Salim, A.; O'Kearney, R. Smoking as a Risk Factor for Dementia and Cognitive Decline: A Meta-Analysis of Prospective Studies. *Am. J. Epidemiol.* 2007, *166*, 367–378. [CrossRef] [PubMed]
123. Cataldo, J.K.; Prochaska, J.J.; Glantz, S.A. Cigarette Smoking is a Risk Factor for Alzheimer's Disease: An Analysis Controlling for Tobacco Industry Affiliation. *J. Alzheimers Dis.* 2010, *19*, 465–480. [CrossRef] [PubMed]
124. Rusanen, M.; Rovio, S.; Ngandu, T.; Nissinen, A.; Tuomilehto, J.; Soininen, H.; Kivipelto, M. Midlife Smoking, Apolipoprotein E and Risk of Dementia and Alzheimer's Disease: A Population-Based Cardiovascular Risk Factors, Aging and Dementia Study. *Dement. Geriatr. Cogn. Disord.* 2010, *30*, 277–284. [CrossRef]
125. Merchant, C.; Tang, M.-X.; Albert, S.; Manly, J.; Stern, Y.; Mayeux, R. The influence of smoking on the risk of Alzheimer's disease. *Neurology* 1999, *52*, 1408. [CrossRef]
126. Rusanen, M.; Kivipelto, M.; Quesenberry, C.P.; Zhou, J.; Whitmer, R.A. Heavy Smoking in Midlife and Long-term Risk of Alzheimer Disease and Vascular Dementia. *Arch. Intern. Med.* 2011, *171*, 333–339. [CrossRef]
127. Incalzi, R.A.; Gemma, A.; Marra, C.; Muzzolon, R.; Capparella, O.; Carbonin, P. Chronic obstructive pulmonary disease: An original model of cognitive decline. *Am. Rev. Respir. Dis.* 1993, *148*, 418–424. [CrossRef]
128. Dal Negro, R.W.; Bonadiman, L.; Bricolo, F.P.; Tognella, S.; Turco, P. Cognitive dysfunction in severe chronic obstructive pulmonary disease (COPD) with or without Long-Term Oxygen Therapy (LTOT). *Multidiscip. Respir. Med.* 2015, *10*, 17. [CrossRef]
129. Rusanen, M.; Ngandu, T.; Laatikainen, T.; Tuomilehto, J.; Soininen, H.; Kivipelto, M. Chronic obstructive pulmonary disease and asthma and the risk of mild cognitive impairment and dementia: A population based CAIDE study. *Curr. Alzheimer Res.* 2013, *10*, 549–555. [CrossRef]
130. Lutsey, P.L.; Chen, N.; Mirabelli, M.C.; Lakshminarayan, K.; Knopman, D.S.; Vossel, K.A.; Gottesman, R.F.; Mosley, T.H.; Alonso, A. Impaired Lung Function, Lung Disease, and Risk of Incident Dementia. *Am. J. Respir. Crit. Care Med.* 2019, *199*, 1385–1396. [CrossRef]
131. Akaike, A.; Takada-Takatori, Y.; Kume, T.; Izumi, Y. Mechanisms of Neuroprotective Effects of Nicotine and Acetylcholinesterase Inhibitors: Role of α4 and α7 Receptors in Neuroprotection. *J. Mol. Neurosci.* 2010, *40*, 211–216. [CrossRef] [PubMed]
132. Teaktong, T.; Graham, A.J.; Johnson, M.; Court, J.A.; Perry, E.K. Selective changes in nicotinic acetylcholine receptor subtypes related to tobacco smoking: An immunohistochemical study. *Neuropathol. Appl. Neurobiol.* 2004, *30*, 243–254. [CrossRef] [PubMed]
133. Egleton, R.D.; Abbruscato, T. Drug Abuse and the Neurovascular Unit. *Adv. Pharmacol.* 2014, *71*, 451–480. [PubMed]
134. Abbruscato, T.J.; Lopez, S.P.; Mark, K.S.; Hawkins, B.T.; Davis, T.P. Nicotine and Cotinine Modulate Cerebral Microvascular Permeability and Protein Expression of ZO-1 through Nicotinic Acetylcholine Receptors Expressed on Brain Endothelial Cells. *J. Pharm. Sci.* 2002, *91*, 2525–2538. [CrossRef] [PubMed]
135. Moreno-Gonzalez, I.; Estrada, L.D.; Sanchez-Mejias, E.; Soto, C. Smoking exacerbates amyloid pathology in a mouse model of Alzheimer's disease. *Nat. Commun.* 2013, *4*, 1495. [CrossRef] [PubMed]
136. Wang, X.; Michaelis, E.K. Selective neuronal vulnerability to oxidative stress in the brain. *Front. Aging Neurosci.* 2010, *2*, 12. [CrossRef]
137. Durazzo, T.C.; Mattsson, N.; Weiner, M.W. Alzheimer's Disease Neuroimaging Initiative. Smoking and increased Alzheimer's disease risk: A review of potential mechanisms. *Alzheimers Dement.* 2014, *10*, S122–S145. [CrossRef]
138. Falsetti, L.; Viticchi, G.; Zaccone, V.; Tarquinio, N.; Nobili, L.; Nitti, C.; Salvi, A.; Moroncini, G.; Silvestrini, M. Chronic respiratory diseases and neurodegenerative disorders: A primer for the practicing clinician. *Med. Princ. Pract.* 2021, *30*, 501–507. [CrossRef]
139. Zhang, F.; Niu, L.; Li, S.; Le, W. Pathological impacts of chronic hypoxia on alzheimer's disease. *ACS Chem. Neurosci.* 2019, *10*, 902–909. [CrossRef]

140. Zhang, X.; Le, W. Pathological role of hypoxia in Alzheimer's disease. *Exp. Neurol.* **2010**, *223*, 299–303. [CrossRef]
141. Chow, N.; Bell, R.D.; Deane, R.; Streb, J.W.; Chen, J.; Brooks, A.; Van Nostrand, W.; Miano, J.M.; Zlokovic, B.V. Serum response factor and myocardin mediate arterial hypercontractility and cerebral blood flow dysregulation in Alzheimer's phenotype. *Proc. Natl. Acad. Sci. USA* **2007**, *104*, 823–828. [CrossRef] [PubMed]
142. Viticchi, G.; Falsetti, L.; Vernieri, F.; Altamura, C.; Bartolini, M.; Luzzi, S.; Provinciali, L.; Silvestrini, M. Vascular predictors of cognitive decline in patients with mild cognitive impairment. *Neurobiol. Aging* **2012**, *33*, 1127.e1–1127.e9. [CrossRef] [PubMed]
143. Balucani, C.; Viticchi, G.; Falsetti, L.; Silvestrini, M. Cerebral hemodynamics and cognitive performance in bilateral asymptomatic carotid stenosis. *Neurology* **2012**, *79*, 1788–1795. [CrossRef] [PubMed]
144. Nelson, A.R.; Sweeney, M.D.; Sagare, A.P.; Zlokovic, B.V. Neurovascular dysfunction and neurodegeneration in dementia and Alzheimer's disease. *Biochim. Biophys. Acta—Mol. Basis Dis.* **2016**, *1862*, 887–900. [CrossRef]
145. Halliday, M.R.; Pomara, N.; Sagare, A.P.; Mack, W.J.; Frangione, B.; Zlokovic, B.V. Relationship Between Cyclophilin A Levels and Matrix Metalloproteinase 9 Activity in Cerebrospinal Fluid of Cognitively Normal Apolipoprotein E4 Carriers and Blood-Brain Barrier Breakdown. *JAMA Neurol.* **2013**, *70*, 1198–1200. [CrossRef]
146. Viticchi, G.; Falsetti, L.; Buratti, L.; Sajeva, G.; Luzzi, S.; Bartolini, M.; Provinciali, L.; Silvestrini, M. Framingham Risk Score and the Risk of Progression from Mild Cognitive Impairment to Dementia. *J Alzheimers Dis.* **2017**, *59*, 67–75. [CrossRef]
147. Suri, S.; Mackay, C.E.; Kelly, M.E.; Germuska, M.; Tunbridge, E.M.; Frisoni, G.B.; Matthews, P.M.; Ebmeier, K.P.; Bulte, D.P.; Filippini, N. Reduced cerebrovascular reactivity in young adults carrying the APOE ε4 allele. *Alzheimers Dement.* **2015**, *11*, 648–657. [CrossRef]
148. Buratti, L.; Balestrini, S.; Altamura, C.; Viticchi, G.; Falsetti, L.; Luzzi, S.; Provinciali, L.; Vernieri, F.; Silvestrini, M. Markers for the risk of progression from mild cognitive impairment to Alzheimer's disease. *J. Alzheimers Dis.* **2015**, *45*, 883–890. [CrossRef]
149. Viticchi, G.; Falsetti, L.; Burattini, M.; Zaccone, V.; Buratti, L.; Bartolini, M.; Moroncini, G.; Silvestrini, M. Atrial Fibrillation on Patients with Vascular Dementia: A Fundamental Target for Correct Management. *Brain Sci.* **2020**, *10*, 420. [CrossRef]
150. Stanciu, G.D.; Ababei, D.C.; Bild, V.; Bild, W.; Paduraru, L.; Gutu, M.M.; Tamba, B.-I. Renal Contributions in the Pathophysiology and Neuropathological Substrates Shared by Chronic Kidney Disease and Alzheimer's Disease. *Brain Sci.* **2020**, *10*, 563. [CrossRef]
151. Ferrero, J.; Williams, L.; Stella, H.; Leitermann, K.; Mikulskis, A.; O'Gorman, J.; Sevigny, J. First-in-human, double-blind, placebo-controlled, single-dose escalation study of aducanumab (BIIB037) in mild-to-moderate Alzheimer's disease. *Alzheimers Dement. Transl. Res. Clin. Interv.* **2016**, *2*, 169–176. [CrossRef] [PubMed]
152. Tariq, S.; Barber, P.A. Dementia risk and prevention by targeting modifiable vascular risk factors. *J. Neurochem.* **2018**, *144*, 565–581. [CrossRef] [PubMed]
153. Stephen, R.; Hongisto, K.; Solomon, A.; Lönnroos, E. Physical Activity and Alzheimer's Disease: A Systematic Review. *J. Gerontol. Ser. A Biol. Sci. Med. Sci.* **2017**, *72*, 733–739. [CrossRef] [PubMed]
154. Jeon, S.Y.; Byun, M.S.; Yi, D.; Lee, J.-H.; Ko, K.; Sohn, B.K.; Lee, J.-Y.; Ryu, S.-H.; Lee, D.W.; Shin, S.A.; et al. Midlife Lifestyle Activities Moderate APOE ε4 Effect on in vivo Alzheimer's Disease Pathologies. *Front. Aging Neurosci.* **2020**, *12*, 42. [CrossRef]
155. Nagai, M.; Hoshide, S.; Kario, K. Hypertension and Dementia. *Am. J. Hypertens.* **2010**, *23*, 116–124. [CrossRef]
156. Alkasabera, A.; Onyali, C.B.; Anim-Koranteng, C.; Shah, H.E.; Ethirajulu, A.; Bhawnani, N.; Mostafa, J.A. The Effect of Type-2 Diabetes on Cognitive Status and the Role of Anti-diabetes Medications. *Cureus* **2021**, *13*, e19176. [CrossRef]
157. Olmastroni, E.; Molari, G.; De Beni, N.; Colpani, O.; Galimberti, F.; Gazzotti, M.; Zambon, A.; Catapano, A.L.; Casula, M. Statin use and risk of dementia or Alzheimer's disease: A systematic review and meta-analysis of observational studies. *Eur. J. Prev. Cardiol.* **2021**. [CrossRef]
158. Sheng, M.; Lu, H.; Liu, P.; Li, Y.; Ravi, H.; Peng, S.-L.; Diaz-Arrastia, R.; Devous, M.D.; Womack, K.B. Sildenafil Improves Vascular and Metabolic Function in Patients with Alzheimer's Disease. *J. Alzheimers Dis.* **2017**, *60*, 1351–1364. [CrossRef]
159. Sanders, O. Sildenafil for the Treatment of Alzheimer's Disease: A Systematic Review. *J. Alzheimers Dis. Rep.* **2020**, *4*, 91–106. [CrossRef]
160. Zuccarello, E.; Acquarone, E.; Calcagno, E.; Argyrousi, E.K.; Deng, S.-X.; Landry, D.W.; Arancio, O.; Fiorito, J. Development of novel phosphodiesterase 5 inhibitors for the therapy of Alzheimer's disease. *Biochem. Pharmacol.* **2020**, *176*, 113818. [CrossRef]
161. Lattanzi, S.; Carbonari, L.; Pagliariccio, G.; Bartolini, M.; Cagnetti, C.; Viticchi, G.; Buratti, L.; Provinciali, L.; Silvestrini, M. Neurocognitive functioning and cerebrovascular reactivity after carotid endarterectomy. *Neurology* **2018**, *90*, e307–e315. [CrossRef] [PubMed]
162. Buss, S.S.; Fried, P.J.; Pascual-Leone, A. Therapeutic noninvasive brain stimulation in Alzheimer's disease and related dementias. *Curr. Opin. Neurol.* **2019**, *32*, 292–304. [CrossRef] [PubMed]
163. Borgomaneri, S.; Battaglia, S.; Avenanti, A.; di Pellegrino, G. Don't Hurt Me No More: State-dependent Transcranial Magnetic Stimulation for the treatment of specific phobia. *J. Affect. Disord.* **2021**, *286*, 78–79. [CrossRef] [PubMed]
164. Borgomaneri, S.; Battaglia, S.; Sciamanna, G.; Tortora, F.; Laricchiuta, D. Memories are not written in stone: Re-writing fear memories by means of non-invasive brain stimulation and optogenetic manipulations. *Neurosci. Biobehav. Rev.* **2021**, *127*, 334–352. [CrossRef] [PubMed]

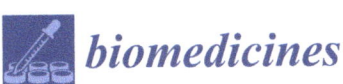 

*Opinion*

# Plasma Phospho-Tau-181 as a Diagnostic Aid in Alzheimer's Disease

Ioanna Tsantzali [†], Aikaterini Foska [†], Eleni Sideri, Evdokia Routsi, Effrosyni Tsomaka, Dimitrios K. Kitsos, Christina Zompola, Anastasios Bonakis, Sotirios Giannopoulos, Konstantinos I. Voumvourakis, Georgios Tsivgoulis and George P. Paraskevas *

2nd Department of Neurology, School of Medicine, National and Kapodistrian University of Athens, "Attikon" General University Hospital, 12462 Athens, Greece; docjo1989@gmail.com (I.T.); dkfoska@gmail.com (A.F.); elenisideri1985@gmail.com (E.S.); evd.routsi@hotmail.com (E.R.); tsomaka@gmail.com (E.T.); dkitsos@icloud.com (D.K.K.); chriszompola@yahoo.gr (C.Z.); bonakistasos@med.uoa.gr (A.B.); sgiannop@uoi.gr (S.G.); cvoumvou@otenet.gr (K.I.V.); tsivgoulisgiorg@yahoo.gr (G.T.)
* Correspondence: geoprskvs44@gmail.com; Tel.: +30-2105832466
† These authors contributed equally to this work.

**Abstract:** Cerebrospinal fluid (CSF) biomarkers remain the gold standard for fluid-biomarker-based diagnosis of Alzheimer's disease (AD) during life. Plasma biomarkers avoid lumbar puncture and allow repeated sampling. Changes of plasma phospho-tau-181 in AD are of comparable magnitude and seem to parallel the changes in CSF, may occur in preclinical or predementia stages of the disease, and may differentiate AD from other causes of dementia with adequate accuracy. Plasma phospho-tau-181 may offer a useful alternative to CSF phospho-tau determination, but work still has to be done concerning the optimal method of determination with the highest combination of sensitivity and specificity and cost-effect parameters.

**Keywords:** Alzheimer's disease; cerebrospinal fluid; plasma; biomarkers; phospho-tau

## 1. Introduction

Cerebrospinal fluid (CSF) levels of amyloid peptide β with 42 amino acids (Aβ$_{42}$), tau protein phosphorylated at a threonine residue at position 181 ($\tau_{P-181}$) and total tau protein ($\tau_T$) constitute the three established (classical) biomarkers for Alzheimer's disease (AD) [1]. They have been studied extensively during the last two decades and, with estimated sensitivities and specificities approaching or exceeding 90%, they have been incorporated in diagnostic criteria [2] and recommendations [3]. More recently, they have been considered as core features for the definition of AD as an in vivo biological process [4], regardless of the presence or absence of symptoms and their type or severity (mild cognitive impairment or dementia). They have proven to be useful as diagnostic tools for the diagnostic work-up of dementia [5–8] and some movement disorders [9,10] during life. Additional candidate CSF biomarkers, including α-synuclein [11,12] and the transactive response DNA binding protein-43 (TDP-43) [13], are being thoroughly investigated, but work still has to be done before they become established biomarkers.

Over the last few years, blood-based biomarkers for AD, especially the classical Aβ$_{42}$, $\tau_{P-181}$ and $\tau_T$, have received much attention [14,15]. It has been observed that plasma biomarkers show changes almost simultaneously with CSF biomarkers, following similar trajectories [16]. Although the range of changes for plasma Aβ$_{42}$ and $\tau_T$ is lower compared to CSF changes, it is similar for $\tau_{P-181}$ [16]. Thus, the later could serve as a surrogate biomarker for AD.

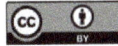

## 2. Why Plasma Biomarkers? Blood vs. CSF Sampling

Since the CSF is in close contact with extracellular/interstitial fluid, it is expected to reflect the biochemical changes occurring within the central nervous system with adequate accuracy and thus, it may be preferable to blood [17]. However, CSF sampling requires lumbar puncture (LP). It is a routine procedure in neurological wards, well-tolerated, with a very low incidence of complications, the most frequent being post-LP headache [18]. The use of atraumatic needles reduces the likelihood of headache [18] and, in dementia patients, a headache incidence of <4.5% has been repeatedly reported [19] even with the use of Quincke-type needles [20].

Despite the above, LP is a relatively (minimally) invasive procedure, rarely performed by non-neurologists, requiring hospitalization in some countries or institutions, and it is a source of concern or anxiety for some patients or relatives. Furthermore, the amount of CSF collected is not unlimited. On the other hand, blood sampling is a non-invasive, much more easy-to-perform and acceptable procedure, has no complications, requires no hospitalization, and it can be performed in outpatient wards or in the community, permitting the collection of a larger sample volume which, in turn, facilitates biochemical determination of a wider spectrum of analytes, whilst repeated venipuncture (if necessary for equivocal or conflicting results, for additional biochemical assessments or for follow-up) is far more easy and acceptable than repeated LP.

## 3. Plasma $\tau_{P-181}$ and Alzheimer's Disease

Plasma $\tau_{P-181}$ levels significantly correlate with the cerebrospinal fluid levels [16] and with the Aβ and τ protein load in the cerebral parenchyma, according to studies using Positron Emission Tomography-scan [21] (Table 1). Plasma $\tau_{P-181}$ levels are 3.5-fold increased in patients with AD as compared to controls, and this change is greater than the one of any other plasma biomarker [16,21–23]. In asymptomatic individuals and in patients with mild cognitive impairment, increased plasma $\tau_{P-181}$ levels predict future transition to Alzheimer's dementia [23], indicating that $\tau_{P-181}$ levels may become abnormal during the pre-dementia or even the presymptomatic stage of AD.

From the clinical point of view, plasma $\tau_{P-181}$ levels may show a significant diagnostic value, in order to discriminate Alzheimer's disease from other neurodegenerative disorders, with an area under the curve (AUC) reaching 0.94–0.98 [23]. This discriminative value may prove useful for the differential diagnosis of AD from frontotemporal dementia [24], with an AUC at the level of 0.88 [22]. For the discrimination from vascular dementia AUC reaches 0.92, for the discrimination from progressive supranuclear palsy and corticobasal degeneration, AUC reaches 0.88, and for the discrimination from Parkinson disease or multiple system atrophy, AUC may reach 0.82 [25]. Furthermore, plasma $\tau_{P-181}$ may identify an additional AD pathology in patients with Lewy body diseases [26]. Based on the above, the diagnostic value of plasma $\tau_{P-181}$ may approach that of CSF $\tau_{P-181}$ [25], introducing the former as a promising surrogate biomarker for AD.

Plasma levels of $\tau_{P-181}$ may also have prognostic value, since they may predict cortical brain atrophy in AD [27], AD pathology at least 8 years prior to pathologic diagnosis [28] and progression to AD dementia even in presymptomatic subjects [29–31]. Indeed, longitudinal changes in plasma levels seem to correlate with the progression of the AD neurodegenerative process [32–35]. Recently, it has been suggested that $\tau_{P-217}$ may perform better than $\tau_{P-181}$ [31,32,36].

Table 1. The major conclusions of the latest studies concerning the role of plasma $\tau_{P-181}$ in the diagnosis of Alzheimer's disease.

| Conclusions | References |
|---|---|
| Plasma $\tau_{P-181}$ levels correlate with CSF levels | [16] |
| Plasma $\tau_{P-181}$ levels are significantly higher in AD patients compared to controls | [16,21–23] |
| Plasma $\tau_{P-181}$ levels may also increase in pre-symptomatic or mildly demented patients and serve as a possible predictive biomarker | [23,28,29] |
| Plasma $\tau_{P-181}$ levels may act as a discriminative biomarker between Alzheimer's and other types of dementia | [24,25,27] |

## 4. Comparison with Other Plasma Biomarkers

### 4.1. Beta Amyloid Levels

Shin et al. [37] had observed a statistically significant decrease of $A\beta_{42}$ in the plasma of patients with Alzheimer's disease, without alteration of $A\beta_{40}$ as compared to the control group. However, the $A\beta_{42}/A\beta_{40}$ ratio made this difference even more conspicuous. Likewise, Janelidze et al. [38] observed a significant reduction of $A\beta_{42}$ and $A\beta_{42}/A\beta_{40}$ in plasma, without change of $A\beta_{40}$ levels. The findings of two other studies [39,40] were headed towards the same direction, showing statistically significant differences; however, the $A\beta_{42}/A\beta_{40}$ ratio (although greater than $A\beta_{42}$ level alone) showed a moderate capacity to separate sporadic presenile Alzheimer's disease cases from normal individuals, with an area under the Receiver Operating Characteristics curve reaching 0.76 and a sensitivity and specificity that did not exceed 70% [39], due to an adequate amount of overlapping values between Alzheimer's disease and other groups [38,40]. Nonetheless, through the use of more developed and precise detection techniques (including multiplexed, densely aligned sensor array), the $A\beta_{42}/A\beta_{40}$ ratio may have the potential to reach a more compensatory capacity to separate Alzheimer's disease from the control group with an area under the curve 0.925 and a sensitivity and specificity that accedes to 90% [41].

The plasma $A\beta_{42}/A\beta_{40}$ ratio seems to predict the amount of cerebral amyloid burden, irrespective of the presence of cognitive deterioration [40,42,43], a fact that could be useful for the early (pre-symptomatic) diagnosis of Alzheimer's disease and the incorporation of pre-symptomatic patients in research for new medications. An abnormal $A\beta_{42}/A\beta_{40}$ ratio recognizes the presence of amyloid in cerebral parenchyma with an area under the curve reaching 0.88, and increasing to 0.94 with APOE4 addition, whilst it recognizes the presence of increased cerebrospinal fluid levels of $\tau_{P-181}$ with an area under the curve reaching 0.85 [44]. In addition to these, diminished levels of $A\beta_{42}$ are associated with decreased hippocampal volume and a higher risk of Alzheimer's disease occurrence [45].

Not all studies are in agreement with the above data; Feinkohl et al. did not conclude to a statistically significant difference between $A\beta_{42}$, $A\beta_{40}$ and $A\beta_{42}/A\beta_{40}$ in the plasma of AD patients [46], while two other studies have found an increased plasma $A\beta_{42}$ level as compared to the control group [47,48]. Most of the above studies use more advanced methodologies, like highly sensitive immunoassays, mass spectrometry, Simoa (single molecule array), Luminex xMAP®, ή IMR (immunomagnetic reduction). The use of those techniques is associated to a higher cost, regarding that the low-cost technical infrastructure of Enzyme-linked Immunosorbent Assay (ELISA), which is used for the measurement of classical cerebrospinal fluid biomarkers, cannot generally be reclaimed in the measurement of plasma biomarkers.

### 4.2. Total Tau Levels and Other Biomarkers

Despite some initial indications of reduction [49], the level of $\tau_T$ is elevated in the plasma of Alzheimer's disease patients, although not significantly correlated to the cerebrospinal fluid level [50,51]. Nevertheless, an elevation of total tau protein has been observed in other disorders, including frontotemporal dementia [52], thus limiting the specificity of this biomarker, whose determination demands a Single Molecule Array (Simoa) assay.

Neurofilament light chain (NFL) level is another indicator of axonal damage that presents a significant increase in the plasma of Alzheimer's disease patients [53] and in other neurodegenerative disorders; therefore, it consists of another sensitive but not specific biomarker [15].

The plasma level of α-synuclein, which is increased in Parkinson's disease patients [54], would be considered as a suitable biomarker for the separation between Alzheimer's disease and Lewy body synucleinopathies. However, there are several restrictions that require further research to estimate the diagnostic value of this biomarker [15]; those restrictions are mainly related to the nature of the molecule under determination (monomer or oligomeric protein, total, phosphorylated) and other pre-analytical factors.

## 5. Some Preanalytical Aspects

As with CSF collection and handling, pre-analytical aspects in plasma biomarkers determination (including $\tau_{P-181}$) may be extremely important for diagnostic accuracy. It seems that K2- or K3-EDTA is the preferable anticoagulant for blood collection [55]. Centrifugation should be performed within <1 h after blood collection (preferably < 30 min), followed by aliquoting in tubes filled to >75% of their volume and storage at $-80$ °C within 1 h from sampling [56–60]. Polypropylene should be the material of collecting and storage tubes. Those techniques and preanalytical protocols have been established by numerous study groups, including the Alzheimer's Biomarkers Standardization Initiative. The conditions and temporal limits under which the blood sample is centrifuged and stored may affect the levels of tau protein and β-amyloid in the sample under test. Other anticoagulants, such as Li-heparin or Na-citrate, can dramatically reduce the levels of tau protein compared to K3-EDTA. In addition, a reduction in β-amyloid levels in a plasma sample separated after 6 hours compared to a freshly separated sample has been noted. Finally, the sequalae of freeze/thaw cycles are shown to minimally affect the levels of plasma biomarkers. It is therefore important that a sample is obtained, separated, and stored under conditions that do not affect the quality of results [56–58].

## 6. New Disease-Modifying Treatments and Plasma $\tau_{P-181}$

Among the various disease modifying treatments tested for AD, the monoclonal antibody aducanumab has been recently approved by the Food and Drug Administration in the USA (accelerated approval pathway) [60], but not by the EMA, while other monoclonal antibodies are currently under clinical trials. Although these antibodies act by removing brain parenchymal amyloid, they also lead to a decrease of CSF phospho-tau [61]. The latter may be used to monitor the biochemical treatment effect, although there is not necessarily a correlation between the efficacy of the drug and modification of the CSF biomarker levels. Plasma phospho-tau may prove a good alternative, allowing frequent biochemical follow up, more convenient to the patient compared to repeated lumbar punctures and less costly compared to repeated positron emission tomography for amyloid load. Indeed, new data from aducanumab trials indicate a significant decrease of plasma $\tau_{P-181}$ following treatment [62,63].

Furthermore, since disease-modifying treatments may be more effective at early stages of the disease, the diagnosis of AD during the preclinical stages by blood (and not CSF) sampling could open new perspectives in wide population screening.

## 7. Emerging Plasma $\tau_{P-271}$

The phosphorylation of tau proteins can emerge at multiple sites. Recent studies have shown an increased capacity of another phospho-tau protein, $\tau_{P-271}$, to discriminate patients between Alzheimer's disease and other dementias. Studies on CSF levels of $\tau_{P-271}$ have shown to accurately discriminate amyloid-PET-positive from amyloid-PET-negative patients. Those promising findings have led to studies involving the accuracy of plasma levels of $\tau_{P-271}$ in early diagnosis of AD, alone or compared to $\tau_{P-181}$. Further studies are needed to determine the possible applications of this new biomarker and its contingent superiority upon $\tau_{P-181}$ [32,36,64].

## 8. Conclusions

It seems that plasma levels of $\tau_{P-181}$ may prove helpful (and probably better than other blood-based biomarkers) in AD diagnosis, and prediction of progression. The additional combined use of other plasma biomarkers may not offer advantage over $\tau_{P-181}$ alone. Furthermore, it may prove a useful tool for frequent biochemical follow-up of patients under disease-modifying treatments. Despite the above encouraging data, plasma biomarkers including $\tau_{P-181}$ cannot be considered as established biomarkers yet. There are still questions concerning the optimal method of determination, and some recent studies raise doubts about the diagnostic help of $\tau_{P-181}$, which may be lower compared to the value of other plasma biomarkers such as the combination of $A\beta_{42}$ and neurofilament light chain (NFL). Still, much work has to be done, including extensive real-world studies, testing various combinations of plasma biomarkers and cost-effect analyses.

**Author Contributions:** Conceptualization, I.T., E.S., G.T. and G.P.P.; critical review of the literature, I.T., A.F., E.S., E.R., E.T., D.K.K., C.Z., A.B., S.G., K.I.V., G.T. and G.P.P.; original draft preparation, I.T., A.F., E.S., E.R., E.T., D.K.K., C.Z. and G.P.P.; manuscript review and editing: I.T., A.F., E.S., E.R., E.T., D.K.K., C.Z., A.B., S.G., K.I.V., G.T. and G.P.P.; supervision, A.B., S.G., K.I.V., G.T. and G.P.P. All authors have read and agreed to the published version of the manuscript.

**Funding:** This research received no external funding.

**Institutional Review Board Statement:** Not applicable.

**Informed Consent Statement:** Not applicable.

**Data Availability Statement:** Not applicable.

**Conflicts of Interest:** G.P.P. has received fees from Biogen International as a consultant of advisory board. All other authors none.

## References

1. Blennow, K.; Zetterberg, H. Biomarkers for Alzheimer's disease: Current status and prospects for the future. *J. Intern. Med.* **2018**, *284*, 643–663. [CrossRef] [PubMed]
2. Dubois, B.; Feldman, H.H.; Jacova, C.; Hampel, H.; Molinuevo, J.L.; Blennow, K.; DeKosky, S.T.; Gauthier, S.; Selkoe, D.; Bateman, R.; et al. Advancing research diagnostic criteria for Alzheimer's disease: The IWG-2 criteria. *Lancet Neurol.* **2014**, *13*, 614–629. [CrossRef]
3. Simonsen, A.H.; Herukka, S.K.; Andreasen, N.; Baldeiras, I.; Bjerke, M.; Blennow, K.; Engelborghs, S.; Frisoni, G.B.; Gabryelewicz, T.; Galluzzi, S.; et al. Recommendations for CSF AD biomarkers in the diagnostic evaluation of dementia. *Alzheimers Dement.* **2017**, *13*, 274–284. [CrossRef] [PubMed]
4. Jack, C.R., Jr.; Bennett, D.A.; Blennow, K.; Carrillo, M.C.; Dunn, B.; Haeberlein, S.B.; Holtzman, D.M.; Jagust, W.; Jessen, F.; Karlawish, J.; et al. NIA-AA Research Framework: Toward a biological definition of Alzheimer's disease. *Alzheimers Dement.* **2018**, *14*, 535–562. [CrossRef] [PubMed]
5. McGrowder, D.A.; Miller, F.; Vaz, K.; Nwokocha, C.; Wilson-Clarke, C.; Anderson-Cross, M.; Brown, J.; Anderson-Jackson, L.; Williams, L.; Latore, L.; et al. Cerebrospinal Fluid Biomarkers of Alzheimer's Disease: Current Evidence and Future Perspectives. *Brain Sci.* **2021**, *11*, 215. [CrossRef]
6. Paraskevas, G.P.; Kapaki, E. Cerebrospinal Fluid Biomarkers for Alzheimer's Disease in the Era of Disease-Modifying Treatments. *Brain Sci.* **2021**, *11*, 1258. [CrossRef]
7. Paraskevas, G.P.; Constantinides, V.C.; Pyrgelis, E.S.; Kapaki, E. Mixed Small Vessel Disease in a Patient with Dementia with Lewy Bodies. *Brain Sci.* **2019**, *9*, 159. [CrossRef]
8. Tsantzali, I.; Boufidou, F.; Sideri, E.; Mavromatos, A.; Papaioannou, M.G.; Foska, A.; Tollos, I.; Paraskevas, S.G.; Bonakis, A.; Voumvourakis, K.I.; et al. From Cerebrospinal Fluid Neurochemistry to Clinical Diagnosis of Alzheimer's Disease in the Era of Anti-Amyloid Treatments. Report of Four Patients. *Biomedicines* **2021**, *9*, 1376. [CrossRef]
9. Constantinides, V.C.; Paraskevas, G.P.; Emmanouilidou, E.; Petropoulou, O.; Bougea, A.; Vekrellis, K.; Evdokimidis, I.; Stamboulis, E.; Kapaki, E. CSF biomarkers β-amyloid, tau proteins and a-synuclein in the differential diagnosis of Parkinson-plus syndromes. *J. Neurol. Sci.* **2017**, *382*, 91–95. [CrossRef]

10. Katayama, T.; Sawada, J.; Takahashi, K.; Yahara, O. Cerebrospinal Fluid Biomarkers in Parkinson's Disease: A Critical Overview of the Literature and Meta-Analyses. *Brain Sci.* **2020**, *10*, 466. [CrossRef]
11. Kapaki, E.; Paraskevas, G.P.; Emmanouilidou, E.; Vekrellis, K. The diagnostic value of CSF α-synuclein in the differential diagnosis of dementia with Lewy bodies vs. normal subjects and patients with Alzheimer's disease. *PLoS ONE* **2013**, *8*, e81654. [CrossRef] [PubMed]
12. Constantinides, V.C.; Majbour, N.K.; Paraskevas, G.P.; Abdi, I.; Safieh-Garabedian, B.; Stefanis, L.; El-Agnaf, O.M.; Kapaki, E. Cerebrospinal Fluid α-Synuclein Species in Cognitive and Movements Disorders. *Brain Sci.* **2021**, *11*, 119. [CrossRef] [PubMed]
13. Bourbouli, M.; Rentzos, M.; Bougea, A.; Zouvelou, V.; Constantinides, V.C.; Zaganas, I.; Evdokimidis, I.; Kapaki, E.; Paraskevas, G.P. Cerebrospinal Fluid TAR DNA-Binding Protein 43 Combined with Tau Proteins as a Candidate Biomarker for Amyotrophic Lateral Sclerosis and Frontotemporal Dementia Spectrum Disorders. *Dement. Geriatr. Cogn. Disord.* **2017**, *44*, 144–152. [CrossRef] [PubMed]
14. Zetterberg, H.; Blennow, K. Blood Biomarkers: Democratizing Alzheimer's Diagnostics. *Neuron* **2020**, *106*, 881–883. [CrossRef]
15. Obrocki, P.; Khatun, A.; Ness, D.; Senkevich, K.; Hanrieder, J.; Capraro, F.; Mattsson, N.; Andreasson, U.; Portelius, E.; Ashton, N.J.; et al. Perspectives in fluid biomarkers in neurodegeneration from the 2019 biomarkers in neurodegenerative diseases course—A joint PhD student course at University College London and University of Gothenburg. *Alzheimers Res. Ther.* **2020**, *12*, 20. [CrossRef]
16. Palmqvist, S.; Insel, P.S.; Stomrud, E.; Janelidze, S.; Zetterberg, H.; Brix, B.; Eichenlaub, U.; Dage, J.L.; Chai, X.; Blennow, K.; et al. Cerebrospinal fluid and plasma biomarker trajectories with increasing amyloid deposition in Alzheimer's disease. *EMBO Mol. Med.* **2019**, *11*, e11170. [CrossRef] [PubMed]
17. Shetty, A.K.; Zanirati, G. The Interstitial System of the Brain in Health and Disease. *Aging Dis.* **2020**, *11*, 200–211.
18. Engelborghs, S.; Niemantsverdriet, E.; Struyfs, H.; Blennow, K.; Brouns, R.; Comabella, M.; Dujmovic, I.; van der Flier, W.; Frölich, L.; Galimberti, D.; et al. Consensus guidelines for lumbar puncture in patients with neurological diseases. *Alzheimers Dement.* **2017**, *8*, 111–126. [CrossRef]
19. Andreasen, N.; Minthon, L.; Davidsson, P.; Vanmechelen, E.; Vanderstichele, H.; Winblad, B.; Blennow, K. Evaluation of CSF-tau and CSF-Abeta42 as diagnostic markers for Alzheimer disease in clinical practice. *Arch. Neurol.* **2001**, *58*, 373–379. [CrossRef]
20. Kapaki, E.; Paraskevas, G.P.; Zalonis, I.; Zournas, C. CSF tau protein and beta-amyloid (1-42) in Alzheimer's disease diagnosis: Discrimination from normal ageing and other dementias in the Greek population. *Eur. J. Neurol.* **2003**, *10*, 119–128. [CrossRef]
21. Mielke, M.M.; Hagen, C.E.; Xu, J.; Chai, X.; Vemuri, P.; Lowe, V.J.; Airey, D.C.; Knopman, D.S.; Roberts, R.O.; Machulda, M.M.; et al. Plasma phospho-tau181 increases with Alzheimer's disease clinical severity and is associated with tau- and amyloid-positron emission tomography. *Alzheimers Dement.* **2018**, *14*, 989–997. [CrossRef] [PubMed]
22. Thijssen, E.H.; La Joie, R.; Wolf, A.; Strom, A.; Wang, P.; Iaccarino, L.; Bourakova, V.; Cobigo, Y.; Heuer, H.; Spina, S.; et al. Diagnostic value of plasma phosphorylated tau181 in Alzheimer's disease and frontotemporal lobar degeneration. *Nat. Med.* **2020**, *26*, 387–397. [CrossRef] [PubMed]
23. Janelidze, S.; Mattsson, N.; Palmqvist, S.; Smith, R.; Beach, T.G.; Serrano, G.E.; Chai, X.; Proctor, N.K.; Eichenlaub, U.; Zetterberg, H.; et al. Plasma P-tau181 in Alzheimer's disease: Relationship to other biomarkers, differential diagnosis, neuropathology and longitudinal progression to Alzheimer's dementia. *Nat. Med.* **2020**, *26*, 379–386. [CrossRef] [PubMed]
24. Ntymenou, S.; Tsantzali, I.; Kalamatianos, T.; Voumvourakis, K.I.; Kapaki, E.; Tsivgoulis, G.; Stranjalis, G.; Paraskevas, G.P. Blood Biomarkers in Frontotemporal Dementia: Review and Meta-Analysis. *Brain Sci.* **2021**, *11*, 244. [CrossRef] [PubMed]
25. Karikari, T.K.; Pascoal, T.A.; Ashton, N.J.; Janelidze, S.; Benedet, A.L.; Rodriguez, J.L.; Chamoun, M.; Savard, M.; Kang, M.S.; Therriault, J.; et al. Blood phosphorylated tau 181 as a biomarker for Alzheimer's disease: A diagnostic performance and prediction modelling study using data from four prospective cohorts. *Lancet Neurol.* **2020**, *19*, 422–433. [CrossRef]
26. Hall, S.; Janelidze, S.; Londos, E.; Leuzy, A.; Stomrud, E.; Dage, J.L.; Hansson, O. Plasma Phospho-Tau Identifies Alzheimer's Co-Pathology in Patients with Lewy Body Disease. *Mov. Disord.* **2021**, *36*, 767–771. [CrossRef]
27. Tissot, C.; Benedet, A.L.; Therriault, J.; Pascoal, T.A.; Lussier, F.Z.; Saha-Chaudhuri, P.; Chamoun, M.; Savard, M.; Mathotaarachchi, S.S.; Bezgin, G.; et al. Plasma pTau181 predicts cortical brain atrophy in aging and Alzheimer's disease. *Alzheimers Res. Ther.* **2021**, *13*, 69. [CrossRef]
28. Lantero Rodriguez, J.; Karikari, T.K.; Suárez-Calvet, M.; Troakes, C.; King, A.; Emersic, A.; Aarsland, D.; Hye, A.; Zetterberg, H.; Blennow, K.; et al. Plasma p-tau181 accurately predicts Alzheimer's disease pathology at least 8 years prior to post-mortem and improves the clinical characterisation of cognitive decline. *Acta Neuropathol.* **2020**, *140*, 267–278. [CrossRef]
29. O'Connor, A.; Karikari, T.K.; Poole, T.; Ashton, N.J.; Lantero Rodriguez, J.; Khatun, A.; Swift, I.; Heslegrave, A.J.; Abel, E.; Chung, E.; et al. Plasma phospho-tau181 in presymptomatic and symptomatic familial Alzheimer's disease: A longitudinal cohort study. *Mol. Psychiatry* **2021**, *26*, 5967–5976. [CrossRef]
30. Karikari, T.K.; Benedet, A.L.; Ashton, N.J.; Lantero Rodriguez, J.; Snellman, A.; Suárez-Calvet, M.; Saha-Chaudhuri, P.; Lussier, F.; Kvartsberg, H.; Rial, A.M.; et al. Diagnostic performance and prediction of clinical progression of plasma phospho-tau181 in the Alzheimer's Disease Neuroimaging Initiative. *Mol. Psychiatry* **2021**, *26*, 429–442. [CrossRef]
31. Brickman, A.M.; Manly, J.J.; Honig, L.S.; Sanchez, D.; Reyes-Dumeyer, D.; Lantigua, R.A.; Lao, P.J.; Stern, Y.; Vonsattel, J.P.; Teich, A.F.; et al. Plasma p-tau181, p-tau217, and other blood-based Alzheimer's disease biomarkers in a multi-ethnic, community study. *Alzheimers Dement.* **2021**, *17*, 1353–1364. [CrossRef] [PubMed]

32. Janelidze, S.; Berron, D.; Smith, R.; Strandberg, O.; Proctor, N.K.; Dage, J.L.; Stomrud, E.; Palmqvist, S.; Mattsson-Carlgren, N.; Hansson, O. Associations of Plasma Phospho-Tau217 Levels with Tau Positron Emission Tomography in Early Alzheimer Disease. *JAMA Neurol.* **2021**, *78*, 149–156. [CrossRef]
33. Moscoso, A.; Grothe, M.J.; Ashton, N.J.; Karikari, T.K.; Lantero Rodríguez, J.; Snellman, A.; Suárez-Calvet, M.; Blennow, K.; Zetterberg, H.; Schöll, M.; et al. Longitudinal Associations of Blood Phosphorylated Tau181 and Neurofilament Light Chain with Neurodegeneration in Alzheimer Disease. *JAMA Neurol.* **2021**, *78*, 396–406. [CrossRef]
34. Moscoso, A.; Grothe, M.J.; Ashton, N.J.; Karikari, T.K.; Rodriguez, J.L.; Snellman, A.; Suárez-Calvet, M.; Zetterberg, H.; Blennow, K.; Schöll, M.; et al. Time course of phosphorylated-tau181 in blood across the Alzheimer's disease spectrum. *Brain* **2021**, *144*, 325–339. [CrossRef] [PubMed]
35. Hansson, O.; Cullen, N.; Zetterberg, H.; Alzheimer's Disease Neuroimaging Initiative; Blennow, K.; Mattsson-Carlgren, N. Plasma phosphorylated tau181 and neurodegeneration in Alzheimer's disease. *Ann. Clin. Transl. Neurol.* **2021**, *8*, 259–265. [CrossRef]
36. Thijssen, E.H.; La Joie, R.; Strom, A.; Fonseca, C.; Iaccarino, L.; Wolf, A.; Spina, S.; Allen, I.E.; Cobigo, Y.; Heuer, H.; et al. Plasma phosphorylated tau 217 and phosphorylated tau 181 as biomarkers in Alzheimer's disease and frontotemporal lobar degeneration: A retrospective diagnostic performance study. *Lancet Neurol.* **2021**, *20*, 739–752. [CrossRef]
37. Shin, H.S.; Lee, S.K.; Kim, S.; Kim, H.J.; Chae, W.S.; Park, S.A. The Correlation Study between Plasma Aβ Proteins and Cerebrospinal Fluid Alzheimer's Disease Biomarkers. *Dement. Neurocogn. Disord.* **2016**, *15*, 122–128. [CrossRef]
38. Janelidze, S.; Stomrud, E.; Palmqvist, S.; Zetterberg, H.; van Westen, D.; Jeromin, A.; Song, L.; Hanlon, D.; Tan Hehir, C.A.; Baker, D.; et al. Plasma β-amyloid in Alzheimer's disease and vascular disease. *Sci. Rep.* **2016**, *6*, 26801. [CrossRef] [PubMed]
39. Kim, H.J.; Park, K.W.; Kim, T.E.; Im, J.Y.; Shin, H.S.; Kim, S.; Lee, D.H.; Ye, B.S.; Kim, J.H.; Kim, E.J.; et al. Elevation of the Plasma Aβ40/Aβ42 Ratio as a Diagnostic Marker of Sporadic Early-Onset Alzheimer's Disease. *J. Alzheimers Dis.* **2015**, *48*, 1043–1050. [CrossRef] [PubMed]
40. Verberk, I.M.W.; Slot, R.E.; Verfaillie, S.C.J.; Heijst, H.; Prins, N.D.; van Berckel, B.N.M.; Scheltens, P.; Teunissen, C.E.; van der Flier, W.M. Plasma Amyloid as Prescreener for the Earliest Alzheimer Pathological Changes. *Ann. Neurol.* **2018**, *84*, 648–658. [CrossRef]
41. Kim, K.; Kim, M.J.; Kim, D.W.; Kim, S.Y.; Park, S.; Park, C.B. Clinically accurate diagnosis of Alzheimer's disease via multiplexed sensing of core biomarkers in human plasma. *Nat. Commun.* **2020**, *11*, 119. [CrossRef] [PubMed]
42. Doecke, J.D.; Pérez-Grijalba, V.; Fandos, N.; Fowler, C.; Villemagne, V.L.; Masters, C.L.; Pesini, P.; Sarasa, M.; AIBL Research Group. Total Aβ$_{42}$/Aβ$_{40}$ ratio in plasma predicts amyloid-PET status, independent of clinical AD diagnosis. *Neurology* **2020**, *94*, e1580–e1591. [CrossRef]
43. Vergallo, A.; Mégret, L.; Lista, S.; Cavedo, E.; Zetterberg, H.; Blennow, K.; Vanmechelen, E.; De Vos, A.; Habert, M.O.; Potier, M.C.; et al. Alzheimer Precision Medicine Initiative (APMI). Plasma amyloid β 40/42 ratio predicts cerebral amyloidosis in cognitively normal individuals at risk for Alzheimer's disease. *Alzheimers Dement.* **2019**, *15*, 764–775. [CrossRef] [PubMed]
44. Schindler, S.E.; Bollinger, J.G.; Ovod, V.; Mawuenyega, K.G.; Li, Y.; Gordon, B.A.; Holtzman, D.M.; Morris, J.C.; Benzinger, T.L.S.; Xiong, C.; et al. High-precision plasma β-amyloid 42/40 predicts current and future brain amyloidosis. *Neurology* **2019**, *93*, e1647–e1659. [CrossRef]
45. Hilal, S.; Wolters, F.J.; Verbeek, M.M.; Vanderstichele, H.; Ikram, M.K.; Stoops, E.; Ikram, M.A.; Vernooij, M.W. Plasma amyloid-β levels, cerebral atrophy and risk of dementia: A population-based study. *Alzheimers Res. Ther.* **2018**, *10*, 63. [CrossRef]
46. Feinkohl, I.; Schipke, C.G.; Kruppa, J.; Menne, F.; Winterer, G.; Pischon, T.; Peters, O. Plasma Amyloid Concentration in Alzheimer's Disease: Performance of a High-Throughput Amyloid Assay in Distinguishing Alzheimer's Disease Cases from Controls. *J. Alzheimers Dis.* **2020**, *74*, 1285–1294. [CrossRef]
47. Teunissen, C.E.; Chiu, M.-J.; Yang, C.-C.; Yang, S.-Y.; Scheltens, P.; Zetterberg, H.; Blennow, K. Plasma amyloid-beta (Abeta42) correlates with cerebrospinal fluid Abeta42 in Alzheimer's disease. *J. Alzheimers Dis.* **2018**, *62*, 1857–1863. [CrossRef] [PubMed]
48. Fan, L.-Y.; Tzen, K.-Y.; Chen, Y.-F.; Chen, T.-F.; Lai, Y.-M.; Yen, R.-F.; Huang, Y.Y.; Shiue, C.Y.; Yang, S.Y.; Chiu, M.J. The relation between Brain amyloid deposition, cortical atrophy, and plasma biomarkers in amnesic mild cognitive impairment and Alzheimer's disease. *Front. Aging Neurosci.* **2018**, *10*, 175. [CrossRef]
49. Sparks, D.L.; Kryscio, R.J.; Sabbagh, M.N.; Ziolkowski, C.; Lin, Y.; Sparks, L.M.; Liebsack, C.; Johnson-Traver, S. Tau is reduced in AD plasma and validation of employed ELISA methods. *Am. J. Neurodegener. Dis.* **2012**, *1*, 99–106.
50. Zetterberg, H.; Wilson, D.; Andreasson, U.; Minthon, L.; Blennow, K.; Randall, J.; Hansson, O. Plasma tau levels in Alzheimer's disease. *Alzheimers Res. Ther.* **2013**, *5*, 9. [CrossRef]
51. Molinuevo, J.L.; Ayton, S.; Batrla, R.; Bednar, M.M.; Bittner, T.; Cummings, J.; Fagan, A.M.; Hampel, H.; Mielke, M.M.; Mikulskis, A.; et al. Current state of Alzheimer's fluid biomarkers. *Acta Neuropathol.* **2018**, *136*, 821–853. [CrossRef] [PubMed]
52. Foiani, M.S.; Woollacott, I.O.; Heller, C.; Bocchetta, M.; Heslegrave, A.; Dick, K.M.; Russell, L.L.; Marshall, C.R.; Mead, S.; Schott, J.M.; et al. Plasma tau is increased in frontotemporal dementia. *J. Neurol. Neurosurg. Psychiatry* **2018**, *89*, 804–807. [CrossRef] [PubMed]
53. Mattsson, N.; Andreasson, U.; Zetterberg, H.; Blennow, K. Association of Plasma Neurofilament Light with Neurodegeneration in patients with Alzheimer disease. *JAMA Neurol.* **2017**, *74*, 557–566. [CrossRef]
54. Bougea, A.; Stefanis, L.; Paraskevas, G.P.; Emmanouilidou, E.; Vekrelis, K.; Kapaki, E. Plasma alpha-synuclein levels in patients with Parkinson's disease: A systematic review and meta-analysis. *Neurol. Sci.* **2019**, *40*, 929–938. [CrossRef] [PubMed]
55. Rózga, M.; Bittner, T.; Batrla, R.; Karl, J. Preanalytical sample handling recommendations for Alzheimer's disease plasma biomarkers. *Alzheimers Dement.* **2019**, *11*, 291–300. [CrossRef] [PubMed]

56. Verberk, I.M.W.; Misdorp, E.O.; Koelewijn, J.; Ball, A.J.; Blennow, K.; Dage, J.L.; Fandos, N.; Hansson, O.; Hirtz, C.; Janelidze, S.; et al. Characterization of Pre-Analytical Sample Handling Effects on a Panel of Alzheimer's Disease-Related Blood-Based Biomarkers: Results from the Standardization of Alzheimer's Blood Biomarkers (SABB) Working Group. *Alzheimers Dement.* 2021; ahead of print. [CrossRef]
57. Vanderstichele, H.; Bibl, M.; Engelborghs, S.; Le Bastard, N.; Lewczuk, P.; Molinuevo, J.L.; Parnetti, L.; Perret-Liaudet, A.; Shaw, L.M.; Teunissen, C.; et al. Standardization of preanalytical aspects of cerebrospinal fluid biomarker testing for Alzheimer's disease diagnosis: A consensus paper from the Alzheimer's Biomarkers Standardization Initiative. *Alzheimers Dement.* 2012, *8*, 65–73. [CrossRef] [PubMed]
58. Liu, H.C.; Chiu, M.J.; Lin, C.H.; Yang, S.Y. Stability of Plasma Amyloid-β 1-40, Amyloid-β 1-42, and Total Tau Protein over Repeated Freeze/Thaw Cycles. *Dement. Geriatr. Cogn. Disord. Extra* 2020, *10*, 46–55. [CrossRef]
59. O'Bryant, S.E.; Gupta, V.; Henriksen, K.; Edwards, M.; Jeromin, A.; Lista, S.; Bazenet, C.; Soares, H.; Lovestone, S.; Hampel, H.; et al. Guidelines for the standardization of preanalytic variables for blood-based biomarker studies in Alzheimer's disease research. *Alzheimers Dement.* 2015, *11*, 549–560. [CrossRef]
60. Keshavan, A.; Heslegrave, A.; Zetterberg, H.; Schott, J.M. Stability of blood-based biomarkers of Alzheimer's disease over multiple freeze-thaw cycles. *Alzheimers Dement.* 2018, *10*, 448–451. [CrossRef]
61. Tagliavini, F.; Tiraboschi, P.; Federico, A. Alzheimer's disease: The controversial approval of Aducanumab. *Neurol. Sci.* 2021, *42*, 3069–3070. [CrossRef]
62. Tolar, M.; Abushakra, S.; Hey, J.A.; Porsteinsson, A.; Sabbagh, M. Aducanumab, gantenerumab, BAN2401, and ALZ-801-the first wave of amyloid-targeting drugs for Alzheimer's disease with potential for near term approval. *Alzheimers Res. Ther.* 2020, *12*, 95. [CrossRef] [PubMed]
63. Biogen. New Phase 3 Data Show Positive Correlation Between ADUHELM™ Treatment Effect on Biomarkers and Reduction in Clinical Decline in Alzheimer's Disease, 11 November 2021. Available online: https://investors.biogen.com/news-releases/news-release-details/new-phase-3-data-show-positive-correlation-between-aduhelmtm (accessed on 13 February 2022).
64. Palmqvist, S.; Janelidze, S.; Quiroz, Y.T.; Zetterberg, H.; Lopera, F.; Stomrud, E.; Su, Y.; Chen, Y.; Serrano, G.E.; Leuzy, A.; et al. Discriminative Accuracy of Plasma Phospho-tau217 for Alzheimer Disease vs Other Neurodegenerative Disorders. *JAMA* 2020, *324*, 772–781. [CrossRef] [PubMed]

MDPI
St. Alban-Anlage 66
4052 Basel
Switzerland
www.mdpi.com

*Biomedicines* Editorial Office
E-mail: biomedicines@mdpi.com
www.mdpi.com/journal/biomedicines

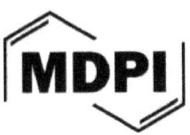

Disclaimer/Publisher's Note: The statements, opinions and data contained in all publications are solely those of the individual author(s) and contributor(s) and not of MDPI and/or the editor(s). MDPI and/or the editor(s) disclaim responsibility for any injury to people or property resulting from any ideas, methods, instructions or products referred to in the content.